AF572323

Coagulation and Lipids

Editor

Robert F. A. Zwaal, Ph.D
Department of Biochemistry
University of Limburg
Maastricht, The Netherlands

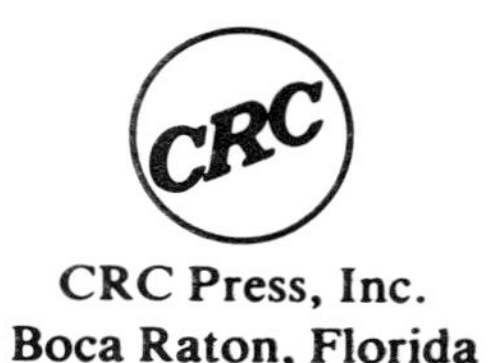

CRC Press, Inc.
Boca Raton, Florida

Library of Congress Cataloging-in-Publication Data

Coagulation and lipids.

Includes bibliographies and index.
1. Blood--Coagulation. 2. Membrane lipids.
3. Phospholipids--Physiological effect. I. Zwaal,
R. F. A. [DNLM: 1. Blood Coagulation. 2. Lipids--
blood. WH 310 C652]
QP93.5.C63 1988 612′.115 87–36818
ISBN 0–8493–6762–X

Direct all inquiries to CRC Press, Inc., 2000 Corporate Blvd., N.W., Boca Raton, Florida, 33431.

International Standard Book Number 0–8493–6762–X

Library of Congress Number 87–36818

Printed in the United States

PREFACE

The crucial role of lipids in blood coagulation has been appreciated for many years. They participate in several steps in the coagulation cascade, increasing the rate with which thrombin is formed. The medical importance of this process is obvious: excess of thrombin production may lead to arterial and venous thrombosis, whereas a short measure of thrombin formation gives rise to bleeding disorders. Although the whole of thrombotic and bleeding disorders is responsible for more than half of the causes of death in western societies, the importance is nevertheless underrated. This occurs not only among people with medical training but is equally true for biochemists if you consider the relatively small fraction that studies blood coagulation. They should not underrate this importance, if only for scientific reasons, and we hope that this volume will convince them.

The objectives of this book are to present a coherent and up-to-date volume on the various biochemical mechanisms by which lipids partake in the process of blood coagulation. Essential background information on blood coagulation, membrane lipids, and platelets is contained in three introductory chapters. The next section deals with the biophysical mechanisms involved in adsorption of coagulation factors at lipid-water interfaces, as well as with biochemical mechanisms by which lipids promote the catalytic activity of the different proteases in the coagulation cascade. This includes the function of phospholipids in the extrinsic pathway and the role of sulfolipids in the intrinsic pathway of blood coagulation. Since platelet membrane phospholipids play a significant role in two consecutive and crucial reactions in coagulation, i.e., factor X and prothrombin activation, a number of membrane phenomena involved in the exposure of procoagulant lipids during platelet activation will be dealt within the final section of this volume.

We hope that the work will not only provide useful reference to investigators in the field but will also stimulate workers in related areas such as enzyme kinetics and biological membranes.

R. F. A. Zwaal
October 1987

THE EDITOR

Robert F. A. Zwaal, Ph. D., (born 1942) is full professor of biochemistry at the Medical Faculty of the University of Limburg, Maastricht, The Netherlands. He is also a member of the faculty board in the capacity of medical research at the University of Limburg.

From 1959 to 1965, Dr. Zwaal studied chemistry, physics, and biochemistry at the University of Utrecht and received a Ph.D. in biochemistry in 1970, supervised by Prof. Laurens van Deenen, Department of Biochemistry, University of Utrecht. In 1973 and 1974, he spent 1 year as a postdoctoral fellow under Prof. Peter Zahler at the Theodor Kocher Institute, Berne, Switzerland. In 1977, he was appointed Associate Professor in the Department of Biochemistry (headed by Prof. Coen Hemker) of the University of Limburg. He became full professor of biochemistry in 1980. He is currently teaching biochemistry to medical students.

Dr. Zwaal has presented nearly 100 invited papers at international meetings including several plenary lectures and guest lectures in a variety of institutes in most European countries, as well as in North and South America and Asia. He has taken an active part in the organization of four international workshops on lipids, membranes, and blood coagulation in The Netherlands and France. At present he has published about 130 papers on lipid-protein interactions, red cell and platelet membranes, membrane phospholipid asymmetry, and blood coagulation. In addition, he is the editor of Volume 13 of *New Comprehensive Biochemistry on Blood Coagulation,* Elsevier, Amsterdam. He is a member of the Editorial Board of *Biochimica Biophysica Acta,* and a member of the Section for Biochemistry and Biophysics of the Dutch Royal Academy of Sciences.

His present research interest is focused on the role of platelet membranes and lipids in blood coagulation, and he is recipient of a 7-year program grant from the Dutch Foundation for Medical and Health Research.

CONTRIBUTORS

J. W. N. Akkerman, Ph.D.
Department of Hematology
University Hospital
Utrecht, The Netherlands

Rogier M. Bertina, Ph.D.
Biochemist
Haemostasis and Thrombosis
Research Unit
University Hospital Leiden
Leiden, The Netherlands

Edouard M. Bevers, Ph.D.
Department of Biochemistry
University of Limburg
Maastricht, The Netherlands

Victor J. Bom
Haemostasis and Thrombosis
Research Unit
University Hospital Leiden
Leiden, The Netherlands

H. Coenraad Hemker, M.D.
Professor
Department of Biochemistry
University of Limburg
Maastricht, The Netherlands

Wim Th. Hermens, Ph.D.
Department of Biophysics
University of Limburg
Maastricht, The Netherlands

Jos M. M. Kop, B.A.
Department of Biochemistry
University of Limburg
Maastricht, The Netherlands

Jos A. F. Op den Kamp, Ph.D.
Department of Biochemistry
University of Utrecht
Utrecht, The Netherlands

Ben Roelofsen, Ph.D.
Department of Biochemistry
University of Utrecht
Utrecht, The Netherlands

Jan Rosing, Ph.D.
Department of Biochemistry
University of Limburg
Maastricht, The Netherlands

Guido Tans, Ph.D.
Department of Biochemistry
University of Limburg
Maastricht, The Netherlands

Ton M. H. P. van den Besselaar, Ph.D.
Haemostasis and Thrombosis
Research Unit
University Hospital
Leiden, The Netherlands

George M. Willems, Ph.D.
Department of Biophysics
University of Limburg
Maastricht, The Netherlands

Robert F. A. Zwaal, Prof. Dr.
Department of Biochemistry
University of Limburg
Maastricht, The Netherlands

TABLE OF CONTENTS

Chapter 1

INTRODUCTION TO THE MECHANISM OF BLOOD COAGULATION

H. Coenraad Hemker

TABLE OF CONTENTS

I. INTRODUCTION

Blood coagulation, in the strict sense of the word, is the conversion of liquid blood into a jelly-like substance. The phenomenon has been observed for ages, and it has been attributed to drying or settling of the blood, cooling, loss of "vis vitalis", the contact with air, etc. Not earlier than in the second half of the last century it became clear that blood coagulation is a process akin to the curdling of milk, where an enzyme (rennin) converts a soluble protein (casein) into an insoluble one.[1] It was understood that thrombin solidifies fibrinogen, and that this process is the basic phenomenon of blood coagulation.

The term "blood coagulation" is sometimes used to encompass the whole field of hemostasis and thrombosis, including the cell biology of thrombocytes and the vessel wall, as well as the reactions in the plasma leading to the appearance and disappearance of a clot. In this chapter we will use the term in a restricted sense to indicate the reactions that lead to the formation and disappearance of the blood clotting enzyme, thrombin. Neither the formation of fibrin nor the breakdown by fibrinolysis will be treated, nor hemeostasis in the wide sense of the word. It is only in the reactions that govern the generation of thrombin that protein-lipid interactions play an important role. This, therefore, is the useful scope for this book. Limited as it may seem, it should be recognized that thrombin formation is the essential phenomenon around which all hemostasis and thrombosis pivots. This can be judged from the fact that all patients in which thrombin formation is impaired beyond a certain limit will bleed. On the other hand, thrombosis can be effectively prevented only by those drugs or treatments that impair the appearance of thrombin, to wit, heparins and vitamin K antagonists.

It is vitally important for survival of the individual that the formation of thrombin occurs promptly where necessary, but remains limited to the region where it is needed. Hemorrhage or thrombosis will be the fate of patients that produce either not enough or too much thrombin for their needs. It is therefore comprehensible that thrombin generation is a biochemical mechanism of intermediate complexity, the velocity of which is regulated by a series of positive and negative feedback mechanisms. The reaction mechanism is complex enough to create a nonlinear system,[2] i.e., a system in which all-or-none phenomena can occur, trigger thresholds can exist, etc. Also, transport phenomena by diffusion and convection play an important role in vivo. As thrombin formation occurs under different conditions of blood flow, the latter transport phenomena give rise to (patho)-physiological results that may be quite variable. They vary from hemostatic plug formation, to the genesis of red or white thrombi, or to the advent of intravascular coagulation. Yet the chemical mechanism behind these different pathophysiological reactions is one and the same.

Perhaps the most interesting property of thrombin generation from a biochemical point of view is that it is a form of heterogenous biocatalysis,[3] a series of reactions confined to the interface of a liquid phase (plasma) and a lipid phase (cell membranes) — a system that, unlike most other processes that occur at biological membranes, forms *ad hoc* at the interface at the moment that it is needed. Thrombin formation, therefore, is an interesting subject of study for the biochemist who is interested in membrane processes in the wide sense of the word, be it membrane transport, oxydative phosphorylation, membrane asymmetry, signal transduction, etc., because many essential features of biochemical two-phase systems can be more easily studied in a system that arises *ad hoc* from soluble components than in a system that is intrinsically membrane-bound.

II. LIMITED PROTEOLYSIS

Activation of proenzymes to enzymes by limited proteolysis is the key mechanism of the reaction sequence that leads to the formation of thrombin. In fact, prothrombin, the inactive precursor of thrombin, was the first proenzyme to be recognized as such.[4] Prothrombin is a 60-kdalton single-chain glycoprotein, the plasma concentration of which is 1.5 to 2 μM. One single proteolytic cleavage brings about the changes that activate proteolytic capacities. As in all other clotting factors, the active center is a serine residue. The product after one cleavage is called meizothrombin. It is a two-chain molecule because the two parts of prothrombin resulting from the cleavage remain attached via a disulfide bond. It has the capacity to split small peptides and esters such as t-gly-pro-arg-pNA the way thrombin does. Before being able to carry out the physiological functions of thrombin, however, a second cleavage is necessary. This cleavage splits the protein in half and separates the thrombin part from the large activation peptide called fragment 1,2.[5-10]

Thrombin has a series of very specific actions, notably on clotting factors V, VIII, XIII, and I (fibrinogen), on blood platelets, on protein C, and on endothelial cells.[11,12] All these actions cannot be carried out by meizothrombin. This is a good illustration of the fact that not only is an active site required for enzymatic activity, but in coagulation also secondary and tertiary binding sites are important.

The primary binding site is located in the immediate vicinity of the active serine. In all coagulation proteases it closely resembles that of chymotrypsin. As such this site is capable of splitting small esters such as tosyl arginine methyl esters. It is possible to make substrates that are more specific for a given clotting protease. For instance, t-gly-pro-arg-pNA is readily split by thrombin and not by the close relative factor X_a. This type of substrate shows a tri- or tetrapeptide structure, and it is evident that specificity must be based on secondary binding sites around the active center.[13]

Binding to more distant sites also plays a role in the reaction of blood coagulation. Meizothrombin is perfectly capable to split the same oligopeptide substrate which thrombin splits, but it is not able to activate factor VIII or to clot fibrinogen. Another example can be found in the action of the antiprotease α_2-macroglobulin. Thrombin bound to this protein is unable to split any protein, but it retains activity towards small molecular weight substrates.[14,15]

Another example of the importance of distant sites can be found in the action of staphylocoagulase.[16] This protein, secreted by certain strains of staphylococci, binds tightly to prothrombin without splitting it. The complex is capable of clotting fibrinogen and of splitting small molecular weight substrates, but it will not activate factors V, VIII, or XIII.

It is evident that the configuration of a protein, even at great distance from the active center, is very important for biological action. Sometimes this may be due to specific tertiary binding sites, sometimes to conformational changes and steric hindrance, more often to a combination of these effects. We will see later how changes of tertiary binding sites allow thrombin to switch from positive feedback reactions near the site of a wound to negative feedback reactions in intact vessels.

III. THE MAIN PATHWAY OF THROMBIN FORMATION

As will be explained in Chapter 6, the initiation of coagulation occurs by the combination between factor VII and an intracellular lipoprotein known as thromboplastin. Factor VII binds to both the lipid and the protein part of thromboplastin and in this way acquires the capability to activate factor X.

Factor X is a two-chain proenzyme circulating in the plasma in a concentration of about 200 nM. Factor VII is a one-chain proenzyme present in a concentration of about 15 nM. Factor VII has a small but nonneglectible proteolytic activity even when not activated. This activity is enhanced by its combination with thromboplastin. Thus, it can split factor X and activate it. Once activated, factor X retroactivates factor VII. This is the first feedback activation in the system. Factor X_a can activate prothrombin if procoagulant phospholipids are present (see Chapter 2). In this way the first molecules of thrombin can be formed.

Using open arrows to indicate proteolytic activation, the backbone of coagulation can thus be rendered as:

$$\mathrm{VII} \rightleftarrows \mathrm{X} \Rightarrow \mathrm{II}$$

The kinetic effect of such an enzyme cascade is evident. If the enzyme factor X_a is formed with a constant velocity, then the product, thrombin, will be formed with the velocity that increases linearly in time. The amount of thrombin will thus increase as a parabolic function of time as long as the substrate is not exhausted. For a more extensive treatment of the kinetics involved see Reference 17.

There is also a series of processes that eliminates thrombin. Antithrombins inactivate it, and diffusion and convection tend to transport it away from the site where the tissue thromboplastin is available, i.e., the wound. Therefore, if a significant concentration of thrombin is to be achieved, it is important that the thrombin formation velocity exceeds a certain threshold.

Theoretically, a three-step enzyme cascade will eventually reach this threshold velocity. If the amount of thromboplastin is small, however, the time necessary may be dangerously long. In that case a four-step cascade, in which the final product (thrombin) increases as a third-order function of time, would be more adequate.

Because factor VII can also activate factor IX, which in turn activates factor X, such a four-step cascade indeed exists in parallel with the three-step cascade.[18-21]

$$\begin{array}{c} \mathrm{VII} \rightleftarrows \mathrm{X} \Rightarrow \mathrm{II} \\ \Updownarrow \;\; \nearrow \\ \mathrm{IX} \end{array}$$

Because the activation of factor IX is slower than that of factor X, the contribution of the reinforcement loop constituted by this extra factor will be neglectable during the first moments after coagulation starts. With the progress of the reaction, importance grows because of the accumulation of factor IX_a (see Chapter 6).

Factor IX is an antihemophilic factor (AHF-B). It may be significant that hemophiliacs tend to bleed in thromboplastin-poor organs such as skin, joints, and muscle, whereas bleeding in thromboplastin-rich organs (brain and lung) occurs much more rarely.[22] The reinforcement loop was first recognized by the French investigator François Josso (1927 to 1981); for this reason we will call it the Josso loop.

It is significant to note that classical coagulation research almost always uses an "optimal" amount of tissue thromboplastin, i.e., such a high concentration that the shortest possible thromboplastin-induced clotting time is found ("quick time": 12 sec). Under these circumstances the Josso loop does not contribute significantly to the reaction velocity; hemophiliacs have a normal quick time.

Classical coagulation research also occupied itself extensively with the clotting of blood in complete absence of thromboplastin, but initiated by glass, kaolin, ellagic acid, etc. In that case the so-called "contact factors" (Factors XII and XI, prekallikrein, and high molecular weight kininogen) interact after absorption to the "foreign" surfaces, and this interaction results in the formation of factor XI_a. Factor XI_a can activate factor IX. Classical coagulation[23] therefore recognized two pathways of coagulation: the extrinsic pathway

$$\mathrm{VII} \rightleftarrows \mathrm{X} \Rightarrow \mathrm{II}$$

and the intrinsic pathway

$$\mathrm{XII} \Rightarrow \mathrm{XI} \Rightarrow \mathrm{IX} \Rightarrow \mathrm{X} \Rightarrow \mathrm{II}$$

Indeed, it is probable that blood clots via these pathways in the presence of either an excess amount of thromboplastin or in a glass tube. Foreign surfaces are, however, rare in pathophysiology, unless one subjects a patient to artificial organs and extracorporeal circulation. An excess of thromboplastin is equally rare unless massive damage to brain, lung, or placenta occurs. The most physiological of all triggers probably is a small amount of thromboplastin. That is why we prefer to propose the FVII-(FIX)-FX-FII pathway as the triangle that forms the core of our coagulation scheme. Recognition of the Josso loop explains a conceptual difficulty from the clinical observation, that is, the fact that hemophiliacs (i.e., FIX deficiency or deficiency of cofactor FVIII) have a severe bleeding syndrome, whereas deficiencies of the contact factors usually go unnoticed.

IV. COFACTORS

Before starting the description of the different stages of thrombin formation, it is necessary to discuss briefly the role of the cofactors in clotting factor activation. For a detailed description the reader is referred to Chapter 7 of this book.

As stated before, activated factor X is capable of converting prothrombin into thrombin, be it at a very slow rate and with a very low affinity to the substrate: k_{cat} is low and K_m is high. In fact, one molecule of free factor X_a can activate one molecule of prothrombin every 4 min if the enzyme is half saturated. To obtain half saturation, a prothrombin concentration of 20 μM is necessary, i.e., ten times that present in normal plasma. Under the conditions prevailing in plasma, one molecule of factor X_a would produce one or two molecules of thrombin per hour. For all practical purposes the reaction is, therefore, completely dependent upon accelerators. There are two of these, phospholipids and factor V_a. Phospholipids adsorb both the enzyme and the substrate. The effect is often described as a "concentration of the reactant at the surface".[24] It will be clear that this explanation is not satisfactory, because adsorption at a surface — so as could be achieved by $BaSO_4$ or $Al(OH)_3$ — fixes the molecules and prevents interaction. If concentration by adsorption would play a role, then it would be necessary for the reactants to maintain lateral mobility at the surface. This is not inconceivable, but recent results obtained indirectly by kinetic experiments[25,26] and more directly by the application of ellipsometric methods[27] show that this does not contribute to the phospholipid effect. In fact, it appears that upon adsorption, the binding properties of the enzyme for the substrate change so that the enzyme is more readily saturated. In order to be effective in these reactions the phospholipids should be in a liquid crystalline state, i.e., above the transition temperature.[28]

The other cofactor is a protein, factor V_a. It also adsorbs at the phospholipid surface. The effect is twofold: it increases the affinity of the enzyme (Factor X_a) for the phospholipid surface and it increases the turnover number of the enzyme. In the factor X-activating enzyme complex (tenase), factor VIII_a is the protein cofactor. In tissue thromboplastin the cofactor and the lipids are intimately linked and present as a lipoprotein complex from the wounded cells (Figure 1).

V. THE STAGES OF THROMBIN FORMATION

The formation of thrombin is a continuous process of complicated interactions. To facilitate visualization it can be thought to consist of several phases. In fact, these phases overlap and the processes belonging to the different phases occur simultaneously. Still, stages can be recognized according to the preponderant reactions. We thus distinguish:

1. Lag phase
2. Feedback phase

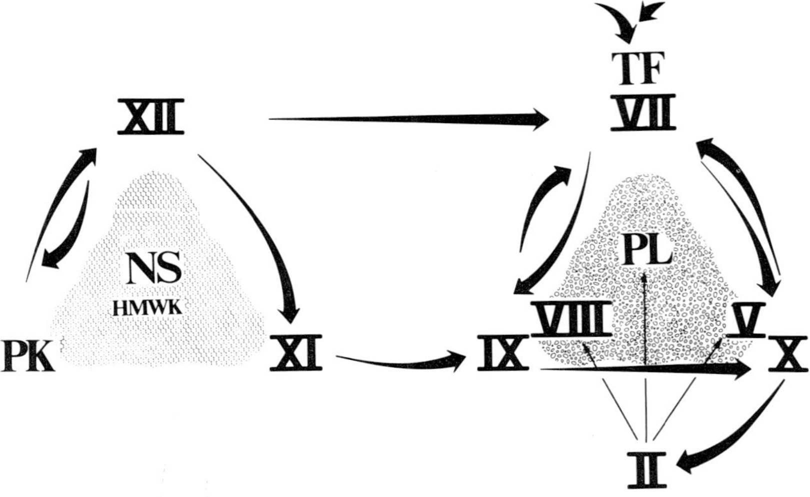

FIGURE 1. A scheme of blood coagulation. The arrows indicate activation; double arrows indicate reciprocal activation. The shaded areas indicate surfaces. NS = negatively charged (foreign) surface, PL = phospholipid procoagulant surface, and TF = tissue factor. The two small arrows above indicate a lesion that makes tissue factor available. (Copyright H. C. Hemker.)

3. Explosive phase
4. Decay phase
5. Negative feedback phase

During the *lag phase* blood coagulation is initiated by the contact of blood plasma with tissue thromboplastin and procoagulant phospholipids. The reactions occurring are those described in the previous paragraph. They allow the slow formation of minute amounts of thrombin. Recent research in our laboratory indicates that the lag phase can be appreciably prolonged by the presence of 0.05 U/mℓ of hirudin. This concentration neutralizes about 4 nmol of thrombin. This means that concentrations of thrombin that represent two promille of prothrombin present in the plasma play an essential role here.

Thrombin formation is slow in this phase because the activated form of the protein cofactors (FV_a and $FVIII_a$) is still missing. Also, there is a continuous inactivation of thrombin. This reaction is pseudo-first order with regard to the thrombin generation. Any steady *rate* of thrombin formation thus causes a proportional *level* of thrombin concentration in the plasma.

The lag phase is the phase in which the pathway

$$\text{Thromboplastin} + \text{VII} \Rightarrow (\text{IX}) \Rightarrow \text{X} \Rightarrow \text{II}$$

generates a low concentration of thrombin that enables the onset of the next phase. It is in the lag phase that the coagulation process is most vulnerable to inhibition. In the presence of heparin, for instance, the decay constant of thrombin in plasma is markedly increased. Therefore, the levels of thrombin that can be obtained at a given thrombin formation velocity are much lower. This markedly prolongs the lag phase. Low concentrations of heparin (<0.08 U/mℓ), which do not prevent the actual burst in thrombin formation in platelet-rich plasma in the explosive phase, will yet retard this burst appreciably. It is probably via this mechanism that low-dose heparin therapy exerts antithrombotic action.[29]

Once a certain (low) concentration of thrombin can be maintained in the blood for a certain time, the conditions are created to produce more thrombin by the feedback reactions that are described in the next section. The conditions for attaining these concentrations are both chemical and physical. The chemical conditions are (1) a sufficient amount of tissue thromboplastin, (2) a functioning VII ⇒ IX ⇒ X ⇒ II pathway, and probably (3) some phosphatidylserine-containing phospholipid surface. It is not clear yet whether the phospholipids that come as an intrinsic part of tissue thromboplastin would be sufficient to support the action of factor X_a on prothrombin.

The physical conditions are the possibilities to maintain a local concentration of thrombin which is not diluted by the bloodstream. As a wound usually involves large pressure gradients and hence high streaming velocities, the formation of a macroscopic fibrin clot as such is not a feature of normal hemostasis! Very probably thrombin can only build up in the microscopic surroundings of the blood platelets aggregating at the site of the wound.

The thrombin thus formed provokes the aggregation of more platelets. Electron microscopical studies[30] show that in normal blood fibrin forms in platelet aggregates as soon as they can possibly be detected. It thus appears that one of the functions of the platelet aggregate is to serve as a sponge in which the plasma is not disturbed by flow and can develop thrombin.

VI. THE FEEDBACK REACTIONS

Thrombin enhances formation of itself because it activates the clotting factors V and VIII and contributes to exposure of procoagulant phospholipid in blood platelets. It thus provides the cofactors for its own formation. Factor V, as it occurs in plasma, is a 300-kdalton protein. Thrombin splits it in three places, and two of the four resulting chains recombine via a Ca^{2+} ion to form factor V_a.[31] Factor V_a is the protein cofactor of factor X_a in prothrombin activation.

In a quite similar manner factor VIII is split by thrombin to yield factor VIII_a, the protein cofactor of factor IX_a.[32] In circulation factor VIII is bound to the von Willebrand factor, a protein that is essential for the attachment of blood platelets to subendothelial microfibrils.

It has been shown beyond doubt that the activations of both factor V and VIII are essential in a normal coagulation reaction mechanism. In vivo studies on the state of activation of factor V and VIII in the blood emerging from a capillary wound show that factor VIII activation does occur within 20 sec after the wound is made, clearly indicating that this reaction is part of the physiological hemostatic process.[33]

In this place we can be very short about the role of platelets in coagulation, as they will be extensively treated in Chapters 3, 8, and 9. We only mention that small concentrations of thrombin (0.1 to 1 n*M*) already provoke the release reaction, which causes factor V to be shed out in the surrounding medium. The platelets in platelet-rich plasma will in this way increase the ambient concentration of factor V from ~25 to ~30 μ*M*. This seems a rather insignificant contribution.[33] In a platelet aggregate, however, the ratio of platelets to plasma is much higher then in platelet-rich plasma. We can only guess the local concentrations in these situations. It seems by no means far-fetched, however, to assume that the factor V from the platelets helps to raise the factor V concentration in the plasma immediately surrounding the platelets to levels that are comparable to the factor X concentration, i.e., around 200 n*M*. In the presence of thrombin and collagen, washed platelets show the flip-flop reaction and in this way provide procoagulant phospholipids (see Chapters 8 and 9).

VII. THE THROMBIN EXPLOSION

Once sufficient procoagulant phospholipids, factors V_a and VIII_a are present, the rate of thrombin production increases two or more orders of magnitude and the thrombin concentrations reach the level of 200 to 800 n*M*, depending upon the conditions. In stagnant blood, clotting will be the inevitable result. Fibrinogen is converted into fibrin that spontaneously polymerizes and forms a network in which erythrocytes and leukocytes are caught.

In physiology this phenomenon is seen after hemostasis as such occurred, in the cavity of a wound and in the vessels shut off by the hemostatic plug. In pathology it is observed there where thrombus formation occurs under conditions of low flow, i.e., in venous thrombosis. The fact that thrombin makes blood clot and that clotting is hardly seen in normal hemostasis and arterial thrombosis has led to an almost uncorrectable conceptual mistake about blood clotting, hemostasis, and thrombosis. All too often primary hemostasis and arterial thrombosis are seen as functions of the blood platelets, whereas blood clotting and venous thrombosis are thought to be the phenomena that are dependent upon the coagulation phenomenon. This idea is as attractive as it is simple, and is as false as it is attractive. All existing evidence points at the importance of the activating cross-reactions between thrombin formation and platelet response.

VIII. THE DECAY PHASE

Several antiproteases exist in plasma. These proteins combine irreversibly with a protease molecule so as to render it incapable of splitting other proteins. They have a certain specificity in that they react more readily with one protease than with another. This specificity is not absolute, and the majority of proteases, when brought into contact with plasma, will react with two or more antiproteases to an extent which is dependent upon the concentration and the affinity constants.

The situation with clotting factors is relatively simple. As long as they are confined at the surface of phospholipids, they are protected from the action of antiproteases. Thus, during blood coagulation, thrombin, being the only activated factor that is readily liberated in solution, is the only one to be inactivated to a significant extent. The most important among the antithrombins is antithrombin (AT) III that accounts for about 70% of the antithrombin capacity of plasma. The next important is α_2-macroglobulin, that captures about 20%; 10% is inactivated by other antiproteases, the most important of which is probably α_1-antithrombin. In a recent study we found that in defibrinated whole plasma, thrombin in good approximation disappears in an apparent first-order reaction with a reaction constant of 1.25 min^{-1}, that can be decomposed in 0.80 for AT III, 0.29 for α_2-macroglobulin, and 0.16 for the others.[34]

These results are obtained on pooled normal plasma, but in individual plasmas the figures may be different. The most important change that can be brought about in the decay pattern is by heparin. In normal plasma 0.05 U/mℓ will increase the decay constant due to antithrombin from 0.80 to 3.00 min^{-1}. These figures hold for thrombin generated in the plasma but in absence of fibrinogen and platelets. Exogenous thrombin disappears about twice as fast[29] as endogenous thrombin does. This unexpected observation is probably explained by the fact that newly generated thrombin partly remains bound at the surface of the phospholipids, probably attached to its activation peptides. Again, even in the presence of heparin, the other clotting factors remain largely immune to plasma antiproteases as long as they are bound to phospholipid and a protein cofactor.

The inhibition of thrombin by α_2-macroglobulin is of a special kind, in that this antiprotease, unlike the others, does not capture proteolytic enzymes by interaction with the active center.[14,15] This means that the complex of thrombin with α_2-macroglobulin, although incapable to attack proteins (fibrinogen, factor V, etc.) retains activity towards small molecular weight substrates (tetrapeptides and smaller ones). This is why in serum an important amidolytic activity is found that is due to thrombin, but does not have the biological functions of thrombin. Patients with a reduced level of AT III (50%), either congenital or acquired, show a serious thrombosis tendency.[35] This stresses the importance of thrombin inhibition for natural thrombosis prevention.

IX. THE NEGATIVE FEEDBACK PHASE

The negative feedback phase of thrombin formation is not or hardly observed when blood clots outside the body. This may be why it is a relatively recent discovery. In 1976, Stenflo[36] described a vitamin K-dependent protein without knowing the function in coagulation: protein C. In 1981, Esmon and Owen[37] showed that thrombin passing through the vascular system of a perfused heart endowed the system with the capacity to convert protein C into an enzyme that destructs factors V_a and VIII_a. In fact, thrombin adsorbs onto thrombomodulin, a protein on the surface of the endothelial cell. The complex thrombin-thrombomodulin retains the proteolytic activity of thrombin, but with a profound change in specificity. It no longer clots fibrinogen or activates factors V and VIII. It does, however, turn protein C into an enzyme that degrades factors V_a and VIII_a.

Thus, thrombin, when present in a vessel wall, eventually has a negative influence on its own formation rate. In the absence of endothelium, i.e., in the cavity of a wound, this mechanism will not play a role. It appears that the action of activated protein C is enhanced by the presence of protein S, another vitamin K-dependent protein of blood plasma.[38-40] The fact that only partial congenital deficiencies of proteins C and S have been found (>40%) and that these patients suffer from serious thrombotic disease indicates that the negative feedback mechanism is essential in the natural prevention of thrombosis.

The fact that factors C and S are vitamin K-dependent factors implicates that the plasma levels are reduced during oral anticoagulant treatment. This is probably why "moderate" oral anticoagulant treatment does not reduce the risk of thrombosis and may even increase it. At a level of 25 to 50%, the procoagulant factors still can function adequately, whereas proteins C and S are in a concentration range that can bring about serious thrombosis. The beneficial effect of oral anticoagulation is not seen until the vitamin K-dependent factors are in the range of 12 to 35%.[41,42]

The last remark illustrates one of the main fascinations of blood coagulation biochemistry; the insights gained may eventually help in the struggle against thrombotic diseases such as coronary infarction, thrombotic stroke, etc., that at this moment are the number one killers in Western society.

REFERENCES

1. **Buchanan, A.,** Original communications on the coagulation of the blood and other fibrinigenous liquids, *London Med. Systems. Gaz.*, 27, 617, 1845.
2. **Selkov, E. E.,** Nonlinearity of multienzyme systems, in *Analysis and Simulation of Biochemical Systems*, Hemker, H. C. and Hess, B., Eds., Elsevier/North-Holland, Amsterdam, 1972, 145.
3. **Hemker, H. C. and Zwaal, R. F. A.,** Heterogeneous biocatalysis in the generation of thrombin, *TIBS*, 7, 378, 1982.
4. **Pekelharing, C. A.,** Over de betrekking van het fibrineferment van het bloedserum tot de nucleoproteide van het bloedplasma, *Versl. Kon. Acad. Wetensch.(Amsterdam)*, 3, 272, 1895.
5. **Owen, W. G., Esmon, C. T., and Jackson, C. M.,** The conversion of prothrombin to thrombin. I. Characterization of the reaction products formed during the activation bovine prothrombin, *J. Biol. Chem.*, 249, 594, 1974.
6. **Esmon, C. T., Owen, W. G., and Jackson, C. M.,** The conversion of prothrombin to thrombin. II. The factor X_a-catalyzed activation of prothrombin, *J. Biol. Chem.*, 249, 606, 1974.
7. **Esmon, C. T. and Jackson, C. M.,** The conversion of prothrombin to thrombin. III. The factor X_a-catalyzed activation of prothrombin, *J. Biol. Chem.*, 249, 7782, 1974.
8. **Esmon, C. T. and Jackson, C. M.,** The conversion of prothrombin to thrombin. IV. The function of the fragment 2 region during activation in the presence of factor V, *J. Biol. Chem.*, 249, 7791, 1974.
9. **Esmon, C. T., Owen, W. G., and Jackson, C. M.,** The conversion of prothrombin to thrombin. V. The activation of prothrombin by factor X_a in the presence of phospholipid, *J. Biol. Chem.*, 249, 7798, 1974.

10. **Esmon, C. T., Owen, W. G., and Jackson, C. M.**, A plausible mechanism for prothrombin activation by factor X_a, factor V_a, phospholipid and calcium ions, *J. Biol. Chem.*, 249, 8045, 1974.
11. **Nesheim, M. E. and Mann, K. G.**, Thrombin-catalyzed activation of single chain bovine factor V, *J. Biol. Chem.*, 254, 1326, 1979.
12. **Suzuki, K., Dahlbäck, B., and Stenflo, J.**, Thrombin-catalyzed activation of human coagulation factor V, *J. Biol. Chem.*, 257, 6556, 1982.
13. **Hemker, H. C.**, *Handbook of Synthetic Substrates*, Martinus Nijhoff, Boston, 1983.
14. **Harpel, P. C.**, Studies of human plasma α_2-macroglobulin enzyme interactions. Evidence for proteolytic modification of the subunit chain structure, *J. Exp. Med.*, 138, 508, 1973.
15. **Rinderknecht, H., Feling, R. M., and Geokas, M. C.**, Effect of α_2-macroglobulin in some kinetic parameters of trypsin, *Biochim. Biophys. Acta*, 377, 150, 1975.
16. **Hendrix, H., Lindhout, T., Mertens, K., Engels, W., and Hemker, H. C.**, Activation of human prothrombin by stoichiometric levels of staphylocoagulase, *J. Biol. Chem.*, 258, 3637, 1983.
17. **Hemker, H. C. and Hemker, P. W.**, The kinetics of enzyme cascade systems. General kinetics of enzyme cascades, *Proc. R. Soc., Ser. B*, 173, 411, 1969.
18. **Josso, F. and Prou-Wartelle, O.**, Interaction of tissue factor and factor VII at the earliest phase of coagulation, *Thromb. Diath. Haemorr.*, Suppl. 17, 35, 1965.
19. **Marlar, R. A. and Griffin, J. H.**, Alternative pathways of thromboplastin-dependent activation of human factor X in plasma, *Ann. N.Y. Acad. Sci.*, 370, 325, 1981.
20. **Nemerson, Y.**, Regulation of the initiation of coagulation by Factor VII, *Haemostasis*, 13, 150, 1983.
21. **Østerud, B. and Rapaport, S. I.**, Activation of factor IX by the reaction product of tissue factor and factor VII: additional pathway for initiating blood coagulation, *Proc. Natl. Acad. Sci. U.S.A.*, 74, 5260, 1977.
22. **Van Trotsenburg, L.**, Neurological complications of haemophilia, in *Handbook of Hemophilia*, Brinkhous, K. M. and Hemker, H. C., Eds., Excerpta Medica, Amsterdam, 1975, 389.
23. **Biggs, R. and Macfarlane, R. G.**, *Human Blood Coagulation and Its Disorders*, Blackwell Scientific, Oxford, 1953.
24. **Nesheim, M. E., Eid, S., and Mann, K. G.**, Assembles of the prothrombinase complex in the absence of prothrombin, *J. Biol. Chem.*, 256, 9874, 1981.
25. **Rosing, J., Tans, G., Govers-Riemslag, J. W. P., Zwaal, R. F. A., and Hemker, H. C.**, The role of phospholipids and factor V_a in the prothrombinase complex, *J. Biol. Chem.*, 255, 274, 1980.
26. **van Rijn, J. L. M. L., Govers-Riemslag, J. W. P., Zwaal, R. F. A., and Rosing, J.**, Kinetic studies of prothrombin activation: effect of factor V_a and phospholipids on the formation of the enzyme-substrate complex, *Biochemistry*, 23, 4557, 1984.
27. **Hermens, W.**, personal communications.
28. **Tans, G., van Zutphen, H., Comfurius, P., Hemker, H. C., and Zwaal, R. F. A.**, Lipid phase transitions and procoagulant activity, *Eur. J. Biochem.*, 95, 449, 1979.
29. **Béguin, S.**, personal communications.
30. **Sixma, J., Wester, J., Geuze, J. J., and Van der Veen, J.**, Morphology of the early hemostasis in human skin wounds. Influence of acetylsalicylic acid, *J. Clin. Lab. Invest.*, 39, 298, 1978.
31. **Mann, K. G., Nesheim, M. E., and Tracy, P. B.**, Nonenzymatic cofactors: factor V, *New Compr. Biochem.*, 13, 15, 1986.
32. **Fay, P. J., Chavin, S. I., Meyer, D., and Marder, V. J.**, Nonenzymatic cofactors: factor VIII, *New Compr. Biochem.*, 13, 35, 1986.
33. **Hurlet-Birk Jensen, A., Béguin, S., and Josso, F.**, Factor V and VIII activation "in vivo" during bleeding, evidence of thrombin formation at the early stage of hemostasis, *Pathol. Biol.*, 24, 6, 1976.
34. **Hemker, H. C., Willems, G., and Béguin, S.**, A computer assisted method to obtain the prothrombin activation velocity in whole plasma independent of thrombin decay processes, *Thromb. Haemostasis*, 56, 9, 1986.
35. **Egeberg, O.**, Inherited antithrombin deficiency causing thrombophilia, *Thromb. Diath. Haemorrh.*, 13, 516, 1965.
36. **Stenflo, J.**, A new vitamin K-dependent purification from bovine plasma and preliminary characterization, *J. Biol. Chem.*, 251, 355, 1976.
37. **Esmon, C. T. and Owen, W. G.**, Identification of an endothelial cofactor for thrombin-catalyzed activation of protein C, *Proc. Natl. Acad. Sci. U.S.A.*, 78, 2249, 1981.
38. **Walker, F. J.**, Regulation of activated protein C by a new protein. A possible function for bovine protein S, *J. Biol. Chem.*, 255, 5521, 1980.
39. **Walker, F. J.**, Regulation of bovine activated protein C by protein S: the role of the cofactor protein in species specificity, *Thromb. Res.*, 22, 321, 1981.
40. **Walker, F. J.**, Regulation of activated protein C by protein S. The role of phospholipid in factor V_a inactivation, *J. Biol. Chem.*, 256, 11128, 1981.

41. **Loeliger, E. A.,** The sixty plus reinfarction study research group. A double-blind trial to assess long-term oral anticoagulant therapy in elderly patients after myocardial infarction, *Lancet,* II, 989, 1980.
42. **Loeliger, E. A.,** Second report of the sixty plus reinfarction study research group. Risks of long-term oral anticoagulant therapy in elderly patients after myocardial infarction, *Lancet,* I, 64, 1982.

Chapter 2

INTRODUCTION TO MEMBRANE PHOSPHOLIPIDS: STRUCTURE, ORGANIZATION, AND FUNCTION

Ben Roelofsen and Jos A. F. Op den Kamp

TABLE OF CONTENTS

I. INTRODUCTION

It is generally accepted that the structural backbone of most, if not all, biological membranes is provided by a (phospho)lipid bilayer. As a consequence of their amphiphilic character, provided by a hydrophilic polar headgroup attached to a hydrophobic moiety which consists of two long aliphatic carbon chains, most phospholipids will spontaneously adopt a bilayer structure when dispersed in water; the acyl chains of the phospholipids forming the core of the bilayer, whereas the polar headgroups face the aqueous environments at either side of it. The occurrence of such a lipid bilayer was for the first time suggested as early as 1925 by the Dutch pediatricians Gorter and Grendel.[1] They noted that, when a lipid extract from red cell membranes is spread at an air-water interface, the total surface area occupied by such a monomolecular lipid film is about twice as large as the total surface area of the membranes from which the extract had been derived.

Although a number of alternatives has been proposed, experimental information accumulating in the late 1960s and early 1970s led to a revival of the lipid bilayer concept, finally resulting in the ''fluid mosaic'' model.[2] This model proposes a biological membrane as a fluid lipid bilayer in which integral proteins are dispersed and to which peripheral proteins are attached. In general, both these classes of proteins experience — similar to the lipids — a considerable degree of lateral diffusion in the plane of the membrane.

In this chapter we shall review some structural features of membrane phospholipids, their organization and dynamics in the bilayer, and how these parameters are controlled. Attention will be paid also to some specific functions of those molecules, particularly in relation to membrane proteins. The discussion will be focused mainly on the mammalian erythrocyte, because its membrane has been characterized in greater detail than any other membrane system. Although some care may be due in extrapolating conclusions derived from studies on the erythrocyte membrane to other (in particular, nonplasma) membrane systems, it may be argued that this membrane may still have some features in common with the plasma membranes of other types of blood cells.

II. CHEMICAL STRUCTURE AND PROPERTIES OF PHOSPHOLIPIDS

A. Phospholipid Classes

The vast majority of phospholipids found in natural membranes comprises that of the *glycero*-phospholipids, all having a glycerol molecule as the common structural feature (Figure 1). Long chain fatty acids are esterified to the hydroxyl groups at, respectively, the 1 and 2 position of the glycerol skeleton. The hydroxyl group at the 3 position, on the other hand, is linked via an ester bond to phosphate. This provides the most simple phospholipid known, e.g., 1,2-diacyl-*sn*-glycero-3-phosphate, which is usually called phosphatidic acid (PA) or phosphatidate. Since the two remaining valences of the phosphate group exhibit pK values for dissociation of protons of approximately 3.5 and 8, the molecule will carry a strong negative charge at physiological pH. The most abundant glycerophospholipid classes are those in which the second valence of the phosphate group is esterified to either ethanolamine, serine, or choline, resulting in, respectively, 1,2-diacyl-*sn*-glycero-3-phosphoethanolamine, -serine, or -choline (Figure 1). These are usually denoted as phosphatidyle-

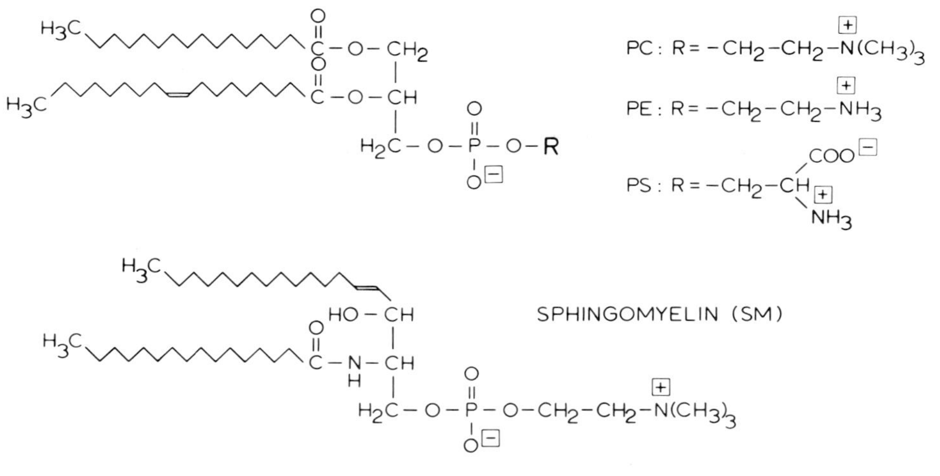

PC : $R = -CH_2-CH_2-\overset{+}{N}(CH_3)_3$

PE : $R = -CH_2-CH_2-\overset{+}{N}H_3$

PS : $R = -CH_2-CH(COO^-)(\overset{+}{N}H_3)$

SPHINGOMYELIN (SM)

FIGURE 1. Chemical structure of four major membrane phospholipids. Abbreviations: PC, PE, and PS, phosphatidylcholine, -ethanolamine, and -serine, respectively.

thanolamine (PE), -serine (PS), and -choline (PC), respectively. Under physiologic conditions, the NH_2 groups of both PE and PS will be protonated. Since PS also carries two negative charges at the phosphate and carboxyl group, respectively, the net charge will be negative at pH 7, such in contrast to the zwitterionic PE in which the positive charge on its protonated NH_2 group will be compensated for by the negative one on the phosphate moiety (Figure 1). Similarly, the zwitterionic PC will have a net neutral charge at physiologic pH values. Mono- and dimethyl PE may be present in minute quantities as intermediates in the metabolic pathway that converts PE into PC.[3] 1,2-Diacyl-*sn*-glycero-3-phosphoinositol (phosphatidylinositol, PI) and the two phosphorylated derivatives, phosphatidylinositol 4-phosphate (PIP) and 4,5-bisphosphate (PIP_2), usually comprise only a few percent of the total phospholipid complement in plasma membranes. These highly negatively charged phospholipids play an important role in membrane signal transduction (see Section V.B). Two other negatively charged phospholipids are phosphatidylglycerol (PG) and diphosphatidylglycerol (DPG) or cardiolipin. PG is not normally found in mammalian plasma membranes, whereas high concentrations of DPG are specifically present in the inner mitochondrial membrane.[4] Lyso-, or 1-monoacyl-glycerophospholipids, which lack the fatty acid at the 2 position of the glycerol backbone, may be present in small amounts as metabolic intermediates.

Another major phospholipid constituent of plasma membranes is sphingomyelin (SM), a nonglycerophospholipid. The polar headgroup, phosphocholine, is identical to that in PC. The hydrophobic part of the molecule is formed by the aliphatic tail of sphingosine plus a long chain fatty acid, which is coupled to the NH_2 group of the sphingosine via an amide bond (Figure 1).

Depending on the chemical structure, which governs the molecular geometry, the above-mentioned phospholipids may adopt either of the following three different phases when dispersed in a pure form in an aqueous buffer: (1) the micellar phase, (2) the bilayer phase, or (3) the hexagonal H_{II} phase (Figure 2). The average diameter of the polar headgroup of a lysophospholipid is larger than that of the single fatty acyl chain, thus resulting in a molecular shape corresponding with an inverted cone (Figure 2). Consequently, lysophospholipids will easily form micellar structures. PC and SM, on the other hand, have a cylindrical shape which gives rise to the formation of bilayers, irrespective of temperature, pH, ionic strength, or the presence of divalent cations. Similarly, PS, PI, PG, PA, and DPG (cardiolipin) will also give rise to the formation of bilayers, provided the buffer is not acidic

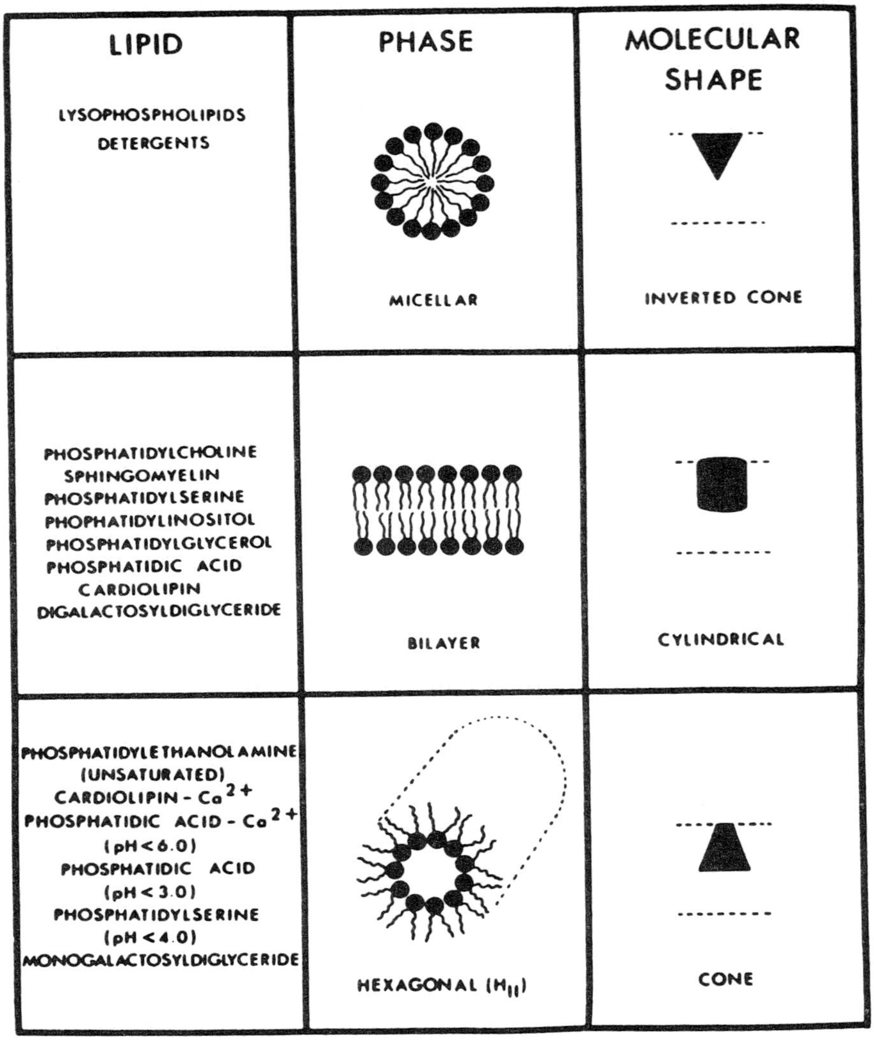

LIPID	PHASE	MOLECULAR SHAPE
LYSOPHOSPHOLIPIDS DETERGENTS	MICELLAR	INVERTED CONE
PHOSPHATIDYLCHOLINE SPHINGOMYELIN PHOSPHATIDYLSERINE PHOPHATIDYLINOSITOL PHOSPHATIDYLGLYCEROL PHOSPHATIDIC ACID CARDIOLIPIN DIGALACTOSYLDIGLYCERIDE	BILAYER	CYLINDRICAL
PHOSPHATIDYLETHANOLAMINE (UNSATURATED) CARDIOLIPIN - Ca^{2+} PHOSPHATIDIC ACID - Ca^{2+} ($pH < 6.0$) PHOSPHATIDIC ACID ($pH < 3.0$) PHOSPHATIDYLSERINE ($pH < 4.0$) MONOGALACTOSYLDIGLYCERIDE	HEXAGONAL (H_{II})	CONE

FIGURE 2. Polymorphic phases and corresponding molecular shapes of various lipids. (From Cullis, P. R., Hope, M. J., de Kruijff, B., Verkleij, A. J., and Tilcock, C. P. S., *Phospholipids and Cellular Regulation,* Vol. 1, Kuo, J. F., Ed., CRC Press, Boca Raton, Fla., 1985, 1. With permission.)

and free of calcium ions. However, at acidic pH values and/or the presence of Ca^{2+}, the bilayers formed by either of these phospholipids may convert into a hexagonal H_{II} phase (Figure 2). This phase consists of hexagonally packed cylinders in which aqueous channels are formed by the polar head groups. Such a phase will be also formed by PEs containing unsaturated fatty acids, which render this phospholipid with a relatively small polar head group a cone shape. For more detailed information on the polymorphism of phospholipids, the influence of proteins on it, the possible occurrence of inverted micelles, and the significance in membrane fusion phenomena, the reader is referred to some recent reviews.[6-8]

B. Fatty Acyl Constituents

The fatty acyl constituents of phospholipids largely determine the physical characteristics, and thereby various membrane parameters such as fluidity[8,9] and permeability.[8-10] The chain

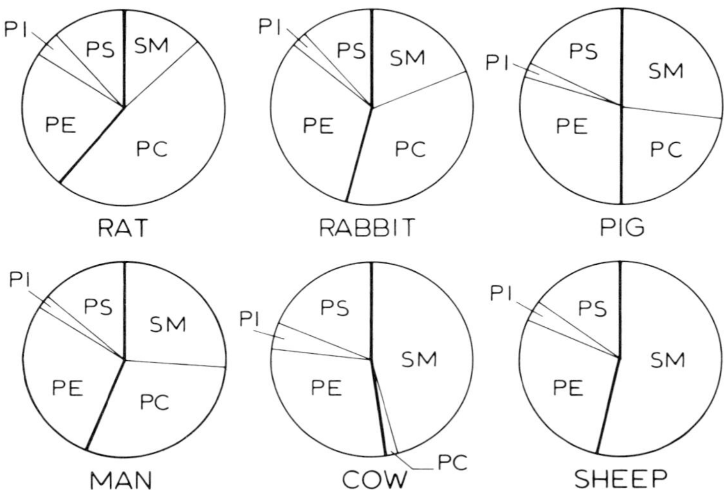

FIGURE 3. Phospholipid composition of erythrocytes from various mammalian species. Abbreviations: as in Figure 1 and PI — phosphatidylinositol.

length of human red cell membrane fatty acids ranges from 16 to 26 carbon atoms. The vast majority of the fatty acids found in the glycerophospholipids (75 to 85% of the total) is formed by those having 16, 18, or 20 carbons, i.e., the saturated palmitic (16:0) and stearic (18:0) acid and the unsaturated oleic (18:1), linoleic (18:2), and arachidonic (20:4) acid.[11-13] SM, on the other hand, is highly enriched in fatty acids with 20 to 26 carbon atoms, which comprise approximately 60% of the total.[11,14] Virtually all double bonds in the unsaturated fatty acids, found in mammalian red cell and other membranes, occur in the *cis*-configuration. Both PE and PS contain, relative to PC, more of the polyunsaturated fatty acids, 18:2 and 20:4.[11,12] The great variety in fatty acyl constituents gives rise to over 20 different molecular species within each phospholipid class. The most abundant type of species are those which have a saturated fatty acid at the 1 and an unsaturated fatty acid at the 2 position. Detailed analyses on molecular species composition have been mainly performed on PC from the human erythrocyte.[15,16]

Next to fatty acids, part of the hydrophobic moiety of a glycerophospholipid may be formed by fatty aldehydes, which are attached via a vinyl ether linkage to the 1 position of the glycerol backbone. In the (human) red cell membrane, these so-called plasmalogens are almost exclusively found in PE[11,17] and account for 35 to 40% of this fraction. Red cell membrane phospholipids, in particular PC, may be subject to a certain degree of metabolism taking place via two different pathways: first, a reacylation of lysophospholipids,[18-20] exclusively occurring in the cytoplasmic half of the membrane,[21-23] and, second, an exchange of intact molecules with those in the serum lipoproteins[20,24,25] and therefore involving the phospholipid in the outer leaflet of the membrane bilayer.[22,23]

III. PHOSPHOLIPID COMPOSITION OF ERYTHROCYTES FROM VARIOUS MAMMALIAN SPECIES

It is a well-known phenomenon that a great many different cell types show a considerable degree of tissue specificity in phospholipid composition, which is largely independent of the mammalian species. Contrastingly, erythrocytes are rather unique in that the composition of the phospholipids varies markedly from one mammalian species to another[26] (Figure 3). This variation mainly concerns the two choline-containing phospholipids, PC and SM. The sum of these two is, in all cases, between 48 and 60% of the total phospholipid, but the relative amounts vary considerably from one species to another. The most extreme situation is found in erythrocytes from ruminants, in which most, if not all, of the PC is replaced by SM. This is striking since the serum lipoproteins in ruminants, as in all other mammalian species, contain not less than 70% of the phospholipids in the form of PC which is subject to a continuous exchange with the red cell membranes (see Section II.B). In order to maintain this typical difference in composition, the ruminant erythrocyte membrane appears to be exclusively equipped with a phospholipase A_2 that has a relatively high specificity for PC, the active center of this enzyme being located on the external surface of the membrane.[27-29] While this accounts for low PC levels in the erythrocyte of ruminants, the intriguing question remains as to what special function may be served by this high SM content in the membranes of those cells.

IV. ORGANIZATION OF MEMBRANE PHOSPHOLIPIDS

A. Transbilayer Distribution and Dynamics

Since either side of any biological membrane is in contact with milieus that are entirely different in chemical composition and physiological functions, one may expect a specific asymmetry in the transverse distribution of the membrane constituents. Indeed, it is generally recognized that proteins exhibit an absolute asymmetry in both their transmembrane localization (peripheral proteins) and orientation (integral proteins). However, it was only in the early 1970s when it was for the first time proposed that phospholipids might also be distributed over both halves of a membrane bilayer in an asymmetric fashion. In his pioneering studies, Bretscher[30,31] observed that treatment of intact erythrocytes with nonpenetrating NH_2 group-specific reagents did not result in the labeling of appreciable quantities of the aminophospholipids, PE and PS, whereas these phospholipids reacted extensively when open ghost membranes were exposed to those reagents. Hence, it was concluded that the majority of the aminophospholipids is located in the inner leaflet of the red cell membrane, and consequently that the other two major phospholipid classes, PC and SM, should be present predominantly in the outer monolayer. Since then, such studies involving a great variety of different probes have been extended to many other membrane systems, but unfortunately not always as successful as in case of that of the erythrocyte. This section will discuss briefly the various techniques that are used nowadays to determine the transbilayer localization and dynamics of phospholipids (Section IV.A.1) and the results and conclusions derived from such studies on normal and abnormal erythrocytes (Section IV.A.2 to 4), as well as the platelet plasma membrane (Section IV.A.5). For more detailed information, the reader is referred to some recent reviews.[32-34]

1. Techniques

The general strategy to determine transbilayer phospholipid distributions is straightforward and simple. Intact cells or sealed membrane vesicles are exposed to the action of a suitable probe, and the results thus obtained are compared with those derived from identical treatments of open membranes. The approach assumes that when intact cells or vesicles are exposed to the reagent, only those phospholipid molecules will react which are located in the exterior half of the membrane. This strategy implies a number of highly essential prerequisites which are discussed in detail elsewhere.[32-34] Furthermore, it is important to emphasize that conclusive results can be obtained only when a number of different probes is used, since each of them has specific pros and cons.[32-34]

a. Chemical Reagents

A variety of chemical reagents has been developed which specifically react with free NH_2 groups, thus limiting the application to the localization of aminophospholipids such as PE

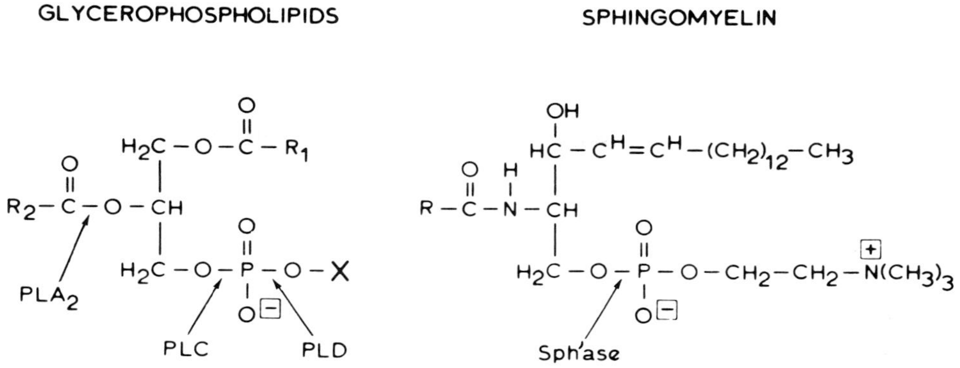

FIGURE 4. Mode of action of various phospholipases on phospholipid molecules. Abbreviations: PLA_2, PLC, and PLD — phospholipase A_2, C, and D, respectively; Sphase C — sphingomyelinase C, X represents various groups such as choline, ethanolamine, serine, etc.

and PS. The molecular size of those reagents is relatively small, so that the absence of permeation through the membrane studied should be checked carefully. For instance, the widely used trinitrobenzene sulfonic acid was believed not to permeate through the membrane of intact erythrocytes.[35] More recently, however, it was observed that this reagent actually permeates through the red cell membrane very rapidly.[36] Another serious problem inherent to NH_2 group-specific reagents is that they introduce a rather bulky group in both lipids and proteins. This may give rise to a considerable degree of sterical hindrance,[37] which causes the reaction to be self-quenching. Many examples are known which show incomplete reactions between such probes and aminophospholipids in biological membranes.[32]

Although this disadvantage may also apply to fluorescamine, this reagent has the marked advantage in that it reacts with free NH_2 groups within a couple of seconds, any excess of it being destroyed by aqueous hydrolysis within half a minute. Due to this property, fluorescamine could be successfully applied to localize PE in the plasma membrane of Friend erythroleukemic cells, despite that this membrane appeared to be permeable for the probe.[38] An additional advantage of fluorescamine is that, in contrast to the aqueous hydrolysis product, the product formed by reaction with an NH_2 group is a fluorophor which enables a direct and sensitive quantitative determination.

b. Phospholipases

The application of phospholipases in localization studies requires some additional prerequisites, discussed in detail elsewhere.[34] Due to differences in the mode of action (Figure 4) and substrate specificities,[34] phospholipases represent the most versatile group of probes.

The selection of the phospholipase(s) to be used is governed not only by the phospholipid composition, but also by a number of other intrinsic properties of the membrane to be studied — for instance, the packing of the lipids.[39] Furthermore, it should be noted that even in case a particular phospholipase can be applied on one type of cell without disturbing the structural integrity of the membrane, it may cause considerable lysis when used on another cell species.[32,34] For instance, nonspecific phospholipases C have been used in localization studies on a number of cell membranes, but appeared to be unsuccessful when applied on intact erythrocytes.[40-45] On the other hand, the use of phospholipase $A_2(PLA_2)$, from either bee or *Naja naja* venom, in combination with *Staphylococcus aureus* sphingomyelinase C(SMase C), appeared to be most successful to assess the transbilayer distribution of phospholipids in mammalian erythrocytes.[44-46]

It is essential to emphasize that a complete picture is obtained only when intact cells are exposed to the action of this combination of phospholipases. The action of either of the above-mentioned two PLA_2s towards the intact human red cell ceases before all substrates in the outer monolayer have been degraded to completion.[44-46] This is due to an increase in lateral surface pressure in the outer membrane leaflet, caused by the generation of the two split products, free fatty acids and 1-acyl lysoderivatives herein.[34,39,45,47] This PLA_2-induced increase in lateral surface pressure, specifically taking place in the outer monolayer, causes the morphology of the cell to change from the smooth discoid shape into that of a (sphero)echinocyte.[48] Treatment of intact cells with SMase C has the opposite effect, resulting in the formation of stomatocytes.[48] This is ascribed to a selective decrease in lateral surface pressure in the outer monolayer, as a consequence of the complete removal of the polar headgroup from the SM molecules present in that layer.[44-46] This decrease in lateral surface pressure in the outer monolayer, induced by this treatment, appears to be sufficient for the *N. naja* (or bee venom) PLA_2 to complete the degradation of the substrates herein.[45,46] It should be added, however, that the cells must be treated with PLA_2 first, SMase C being added some 60 min thereafter. For reasons which are not yet fully understood, addition of these enzymes simultaneously or in reversed order will inevitably lead to complete lysis of the cells.[45]

Free fatty acids and lysophospholipids are well-known membrane-perturbing agents. It seems surprising, therefore, that the functioning of the red cell membrane as a permeability barrier remains intact despite the complete replacement of the diacyl glycerophospholipids in the outer monolayer by these compounds. This may at least partly be due to the notably high cholesterol content of the erythrocyte membrane, which may stabilize the lysocompounds in a bilayer configuration. This view is supported by ^{31}P nuclear magnetic resonance (NMR) studies which showed that, even after treatment of open ghost membranes with the above phospholipases, the residual phospholipids still maintain a bilayer phase.[49]

c. Phospholipid Transfer Proteins

Compared to both phospholipases and chemical reagents, phospholipid transfer proteins provide more gentle and elegant tools for assessing membrane phospholipid distributions.[32-34,50-52] The molecular size of those proteins (20,000 to 30,000 daltons) is such that they will not permeate through a membrane. Furthermore, disruption of the membrane studied will be minimal, particularly in case the transfer protein used mediates a one-for-one exchange of phospholipid molecules, thereby not disturbing the native lipid composition of the membrane either qualitatively or quantitatively. Hence, only those phospholipid molecules which are present at the side of the membrane that is exposed to the medium containing the transfer protein will be available to take part in the exchange process.

In practice, intact cells or sealed membranes to be studied (acceptor membranes) are incubated, in the presence of transfer protein, with a suitable donor system (usually rat liver microsomes or small sonicated lipid vesicles) containing radiolabeled phospholipid(s) of known specific radioactivity. The time course of the protein mediated transfer of radioactive phospholipid from the donor to the acceptor membrane is determined either by recording the decrease in specific radioactivity of the phospholipid in the donor, the increase in the acceptor, or both. Studying this time course provides information not only as to the size of the phospholipid pools at either side of the membrane, but also regarding the absence or presence of relatively fast transmembrane movements (flip-flop) of phospholipid molecules. The following three different situations regarding the exchange of a particular phospholipid class may be distinguished:

1. Only a certain fraction of the lipid can be exchanged, which is not increased during prolonged incubations. (Flip-flop is very slow or even absent.)
2. One fast exchangeable pool is followed by a second one which exhibits a slower exchange rate. (Flip-flop occurs in the membrane at a rate which is relatively slow compared to that of the exchange process.)

3. All of the lipid is exchanged as one single pool. (The lipid is either entirely located in one half of the membrane bilayer or experiences flip-flop at a rate which exceeds that of the exchange process.)

Comparing the exchange rates for the two pools of a phospholipid in a particular membrane (the above case 2) provides an estimation of the half-time value for the flip-flop process experienced by this phospholipid. This parameter can be determined more directly and accurately by following the fate of a radiolabeled phospholipid which has been introduced exclusively into one of the two halves of the lipid bilayer. (Details of this technique, introduced by Van Meer and Op den Kamp[53] to study transbilayer movements of PC in intact human erythrocytes and involving the insertion of radioactive PC into the outer membrane leaflet by means of a PC-specific transfer protein [PC-TP] from beef liver, are described elsewhere.[54]) In brief, the protocol is as follows: after insertion of the [*methyl*-^{14}C]PC into the outer membrane leaflet of the intact cells and subsequent removal of the PC-TP and ^{14}C-PC donor system, the cells are incubated to enable the ^{14}C-PC to equilibrate between the two halves of the bilayer. At timed intervals, samples are taken and the cells treated under nonlytic conditions with PLA_2 and SMase C, thereby exclusively converting all of the PC in the outer monolayer into the lysoderivative (see Section IV.A.1.a above). The rate of transbilayer movement of the previously inserted PC can be easily calculated from the time-dependent decay in specific radioactivity of the lyso-PC thus formed, which is a genuine representative of the PC in the outer monolayer.[53,54] It may be clear that, although special experimental prerequisites should be fulfilled,[54] this technique also can be used to determine flip-flop rates of individual molecular species of PC.[55]

Since the PC-TP mediates a genuine one-for-one exchange of PC molecules, it has been most widely and successfully used both for assessing inner and outer pools of PC in a variety of membranes, as well as to determine transbilayer mobility.[32-34,50-55] The application of nonspecific lipid transfer proteins (ns-LTPs) in such studies, however, requires particular care, because those proteins can mediate the transfer of almost all phospholipids and cholesterol.[50,51] Moreover, a ns-LTP may even facilitate a net transfer of both phospholipids and cholesterol, thereby not only altering the composition but also the total amount of lipids in a membrane.[56] Nevertheless, ns-LTP has been used under appropriate experimental conditions to determine the distribution and transbilayer movement of PC, PE, PS, and SM in intact erythrocytes.[57,58]

d. Physical Techniques

The NMR technique has been used successfully to study the transbilayer distribution of phospholipids in small, unilamellar, lipid vesicles, but application on biological membranes encounters some technical problems as a consequence of the complexity and large dimensions of such membranes.[32,33,59] However, NMR has been shown to be a powerful technique to study the various phases (bilayer/nonbilayer) in which phospholipids may occur in a membrane,[7,8,60,61] and which may have important consequences for both distribution and dynamics of those membrane components.[62] Valuable information on phospholipid polymorphism can be also obtained by other structural techniques such as X-ray[63,64] and neutron[65,66] diffraction, as well as by freeze-fracture electron microscopy.[6]

Transbilayer distribution and, in particular, transbilayer mobility of phospholipids can be also studied by electron spin resonance (ESR).[67] Nitroxide spin-labeled phospholipid analogues are introduced into the outer membrane leaflet of an intact cell. Subsequent reduction of the nitroxide group by treatment of the (intact) cell with ascorbate, thereby destroying paramagnetism and consequently the ESR signal, enables a discrimination of the fraction of probe molecules still present in the outer membrane layer from the fraction that has been translocated to the inner one.

e. Lysophospholipids

A third method to determine the transbilayer mobility of phospholipids in erythrocyte membranes has been introduced recently.[68,69] The procedure involves the use of radiolabeled lysophospholipids as probe molecules. Those compounds can be easily incorporated into the red cell membrane by incubating intact cells for a short period in a buffer containing a low concentration of the lysophospholipid. During a subsequent incubation, the reporter molecules thus introduced into the outer membrane leaflet are enabled to equilibrate between the two halves of the bilayer. Samples are taken at timed intervals and the cells treated with a 1.5% (w/v) solution of fat-free bovine serum albumin, thereby selectively extracting the lysophospholipid still present in the *outer* monolayer. The distribution of the probe molecules over both halves of the bilayer can be determined this way, from which data the rate of the transbilayer equilibration can be easily calculated. Although the simplicity of this method is a great advantage by itself, it should be noted that in the red cell membrane lysophospholipids may be subject to either acylation to form diacyl glycerophospholipids or deacylation resulting in glycerylphosphorylcholine. Both these processes take place specifically in the *inner* membrane leaflet[70] (see also Section II.B) and may therefore interfere in the transbilayer equilibration of those probe-molecules. Furthermore, it should be realized that lysophospholipids, like the spin-labeled phospholipid analogues mentioned in Section IV.A.1.d, are structurally different from the naturally occurring glycerophospholipids which have two fatty acyl chains of 16 or more carbon atoms. Although these probe molecules may provide valuable information when used in comparative studies,[68-73] they cannot be used to determine the actual rate of transbilayer movement experienced by the native membrane phospholipids. The only option for studying this aspect is to use the procedure described in Section IV.A.1.c.

2. Normal Erythrocytes

Soon after publication of the pioneering studies[30,31,74] which, on basis of chemical labeling experiments, indicated a preferential localization of the aminophospholipids in the inner membrane leaflet, the use of purified phospholipases provided a complete picture of the distribution of the main phospholipid classes in human,[44-46,75] rat,[22,75] pig,[75] and rabbit[75] erythrocytes. Although some criticism has been raised regarding the reliability of experiments involving phospholipases,[77-80] the results have appeared to be in perfect agreement with those derived from studies using phospholipid transfer proteins.[57,81-83] Hence, it is nowadays generally accepted that the phospholipids in the red cell membrane show a considerable degree of asymmetry in the transbilayer distribution; i.e., the choline-containing phospholipids (SM and PC) dominate the outer membrane layer, whereas the aminophospholipids (PE and PS), as well as PI,[84] are predominantly (PE and PI) or even exclusively (PS) found in the cytoplasmic half of the lipid bilayer.[32-34] Focused on the human erythrocyte, the outside/inside distribution is as follows: SM — 85/15, PC — 76/24, PE — 20/80, and PS — 0/100.

As mentioned earlier in Section II.B, the phospholipids in the red cell membrane comprise a great many different molecular species, differing in fatty acyl constituents. For PC, for instance, over 20 different molecular species have been found.[15,16] In view of the topological asymmetry in metabolism (see Section II.B), one might expect that the outer and inner pools of the PC in the erythrocyte membrane are composed of different molecular species. This appears not to be the case.[21] The observed ''random'' distribution of molecular species can be explained only when those molecules experience transbilayer movements with half-time values which are relatively short when compared to the average lifetime of the cell. The existence of such a flip-flop process has indeed been established in both the human[53,83] and rat[22,25,57,76,81,83,85] erythrocyte, and the actual rates of flip-flop of four individual molecular species of PC in the human red cell membrane have been determined very recently.[55]

Table 1
HALFTIMES OF TRANSBILAYER MOVEMENT OF INDIVIDUAL MOLECULAR SPECIES OF PHOSPHATIDYLCHOLINE IN THE HUMAN ERYTHROCYTE MEMBRANE

PC species	Halftime (hr)
1,2-Dipalmitoyl	26.3 + 4.4
1,2-Dioleoyl	14.4 + 3.5
1-Palmitoyl,2-linoleoyl	2.9 + 1.7
1-Palmitoyl,2-arachidonoyl	9.7 + 1.6

Note: ^{14}C-labeled molecular species of PC were introduced into the outer membrane leaflet of intact human erythrocytes, using a PC-TP from beef liver. Cells were subsequently incubated at 37°C (up to 8 hr) to allow the [^{14}C]PC to equilibrate over both halves of the bilayer. At various time intervals, cells were treated with *Naja naja* PLA_2 and *Staphylococcus aureus* SMase C to convert the PC in the outer monolayer into lyso-PC. Specific radioactivity of the lyso-PC was determined after extraction and thin-layer chromatographic separation of the lipids. Halftime values of transbilayer movement (means +SD) were derived from the best linear fit calculated for a semilogarithmic plot of duplicate determinations of the relative specific radioactivities of the (lyso-)PC in the outer monolayer at the various time points of sampling and obtained from a series of independent experiments.

From Middelkoop, E., Lubin, B. H., Op den Kamp, J. A. F., and Roelofsen, B., *Biochim. Biophys. Acta,* 855, 421, 1986. With permission.

In agreement with previous studies, it appeared that species containing one or two unsaturated fatty acids experience transbilayer movements at higher rates than a completely saturated species, such as dipalmitoyl-PC (Table 1). It is of interest to note that the flip-flop rate of (1-palmitoyl,2-linoleoyl)PC is about five times as fast as that of (1,2-dioleoyl)PC, despite the fact that both species have the same degree of overall unsaturation. That the flip-flop rates of PC molecules in the red cell membrane are not strictly proportional to their degree of unsaturation, as has been suggested before, is also obvious from the rather surprising observation that the transbilayer movement of (1-palmitoyl,2-arachidonoyl)PC proceeds at a rate that is three times slower than that of (1-palmitoyl,2-linoleoyl)PC (Table 1). Further studies will be necessary to gain insight into the actual reasons for these differences in transbilayer dynamics of the individual molecular species.

In contrast to PC, the other choline-containing phospholipid, SM, appeared to show a significant degree of asymmetry in the composition of molecular species at either side of the red cell lipid bilayer.[14] Some 70% of the *outer* SM pool is composed of species bearing fatty acyl chains with 16 or 18 carbon atoms, whereas the species containing fatty acids with 20 to 24 carbon atoms account for over 70% of the pool in the *inner* half of the bilayer. This strongly suggests that, in contrast to PC, SM does not experience transbilayer movements, which is supported by recent studies involving a spin-labeled analogue.[86]

3. Erythroblasts and Reticulocytes

One of the intriguing questions related to the pronounced asymmetric phospholipid distribution in the erythrocyte membrane concerns its biogenesis. The erythrocyte represents the end product of a complicated series of cell differentiations.[87] This process starts in the bone marrow, and within a couple of days erythropoietic-committed pluripotential stem cells differentiate via the proerythroblast, basophilic erythroblast, and polychromatophilic erythroblast stage, into a normoblast. After subsequent enucleation, a reticulocyte is formed which enters the bloodstream to mature within another 2 to 3 days into an erythrocyte.

Human (pro)erythroblasts are, for obvious reasons, not easily accessible for experimental purposes. However, infection of mice with the Friend virus complex results in the accumulation of erythroid cells which closely resemble the proerythroblast stage. These so-called Friend erythroleukemic cells (Friend cells) are blocked in the differentiation, but still possess the ability of proliferation and, after isolation from the spleens, can be taken into culture under appropriate conditions.[88] In culture, those cells can be induced to differentiate up to a normoblast-like stage by a variety of chemicals, among which is dimethyl sulfoxide (DMSO).[87]

Phospholipid distributions in the plasma membrane of Friend cells have been studied by using various independent techniques, i.e., nonlytic treatments with phospholipases A_2 and C, SMase C, chemical labeling with fluorescamine, and protein-mediated exchange of PC. The results derived from such studies have been compared with those obtained from similar experiments on mature murine erythrocytes. In contrast to the mature red cell, the Friend cell contains a great variety of subcellular membrane systems, which introduces an additional experimental problem. Comparison of phospholipid compositions in extracts derived from treated and nontreated cells will not provide the desired information. On the other hand, isolation of pure plasma membrane fractions is usually very laborious and therefore not suitable to be performed in great numbers of routine analyses. This problem can be elegantly circumvented by a procedure developed by Chap and colleagues[89] when they studied the phospholipid distribution in the platelet surface membrane.[89] Application of this procedure, and using either SMase C[90] or fluorescamine,[38] made it possible to assess the relative amount of each phospholipid class present in the plasma membrane of the Friend cell. Once this information was available, all subsequent analyses and calculations regarding the phospholipid distribution in this plasma membrane could be performed on lipid extracts derived from whole cells.

The results derived from the comparative studies[91] on Friend cells and mature murine erythrocytes are depicted in Figure 5. The distribution of SM in the plasma membrane of the Friend cell, 85% of it being located in the outer monolayer, is identical to that in the murine erythrocyte. Also, PS shows already a considerable extent of asymmetry in distribution in the plasma membrane of the erythroid precursor, i.e., 90% in the inner monolayer vs. all of it in the cytoplasmic leaflet of the mature erythrocyte. PC, PE, and PI, on the other hand, are still randomly distributed over both halves of the proerythroblast plasma membrane, while the distribution is clearly asymmetric in the membrane of the mature cell.

Similar symmetric orientations of PC and PE are found in both DMSO-differentiated Friend cells[92] and colony-forming unit erythroid cells.[93] However, an asymmetric distribution of these phospholipids is observed in murine reticulocytes.[92] This suggests that the ultimate phospholipid asymmetry may be constituted during the enucleation process or immediately thereafter.

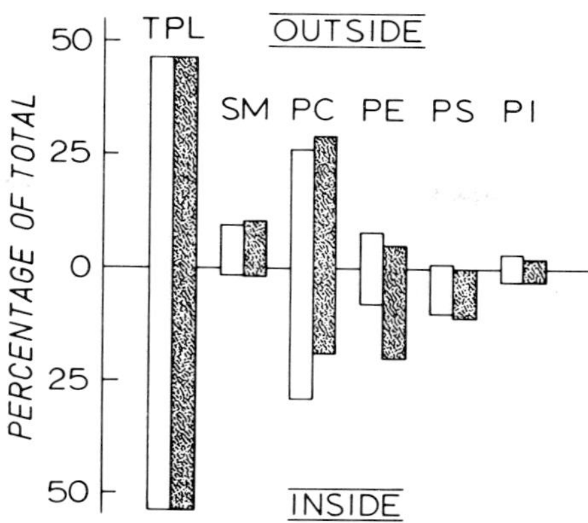

FIGURE 5. Phospholipid composition and transbilayer distribution in plasma membranes of Friend erythroleukemic cells (open bars) and mature mouse erythrocytes (solid bars). Abbreviations: as in Figures 1 and 3 and TPL — total phospholipid. (Rawyler, A., van der Schaft, P. H., Roelofsen, B., and Op den Kamp, J. A. F., reprinted with permission from *Biochemistry,* 24, 1777. Copyright 1985 American Chemical Society.)

4. Abnormal Erythrocytes

Recent studies on abnormal erythrocytes, either chemically modified or naturally occurring, provided interesting information concerning the factors that may be involved in stabilization of the lipid bilayer and the asymmetric localization of the (glycero)phospholipids herein.

a. Chemically Modified Cells

Treatment of intact human erythrocytes with either diamide or tetrathionate causes an oxidative cross-linking of spectrin,[94] one of the major constituents of the protein skeleton that underlies the cytoplasmic half of the membrane.[95-97] This cross-linking of spectrin appears to cause an appreciable enhancement of transbilayer dynamics in the lipid bilayer. Increased flip-flop rates in diamide/tetrathionate treated erythrocytes are observed, not only for exogenously added lysophospholipids,[68,72] but also for the endogenous PC molecules in the membrane.[98] Treatment of intact human erythrocytes with these oxidizing agents also caused drastic changes in the accessibility of the aminophospholipids for exogenous probes, most specifically phospholipase A_2.[94,99] For instance, exposure of such treated cells to bee venom phospholipase A_2 resulted in the nonlytic hydrolysis of not less than 50% of the PE and 30% of the PS, whereas in native erythrocytes only 5% of the PE and none of the PS can be digested by this enzyme.[99,100] It is of interest to note, however, that the chemically induced cross-linking of spectrin does not at all affect the accessibility of SM to SMase C,[94] once again illustrating the special position this phospholipid occupies with respect to organization in the lipid bilayer (also compare Sections IV.A.2 and 3).

The most obvious and unequivocal interpretation from the above observations seemed to be that spectrin plays a key role in maintaining the asymmetric distribution of the *glycero*-phospholipids in the red cell membrane.[72,94,101] The exposure of considerable fractions of PS in the outer membrane leaflet of the intact erythrocyte should be easily detectable by the prothrombinase assay, which is a specific and sensitive method to probe the presence of PS in a lipid surface[102,103] (also compare Chapter 7). However, the response of this system towards diamide-treated human red cells is absolutely negative,[104] which raises some serious doubts against the *in situ* occurrence of an altered phospholipid asymmetry in those cells. In this context, it is relevant to recall (see above) that chemically induced cross-linking of spectrin in the intact erythrocyte results in enhanced transbilayer mobilities of *glycero*-phospholipids. Hence, the question was raised whether the treatment with phospholipase A_2, which requires relatively lengthy incubations, could induce transbilayer reorientations of substrates in those destabilized membranes. In a very recent study,[99] it was shown that no more than 15% of the PE in intact diamide-treated cells can be labeled with the rapidly reacting fluorescamine, which result is identical to that obtained with control cells. Moreover, this value is in reasonable agreement with the 20% of this phospholipid that can be degraded when intact native cells are exposed to phospholipase A_2 in the presence of SMase C.[45,46] From the above, it can be concluded that diamide-induced oxidative cross-linking of spectrin in the intact human erythrocyte does not necessarily result in an immediate loss of phospholipid asymmetry. However, such a structural modification of the membrane skeleton causes a destabilization of the lipid bilayer, as expressed by an enhanced transmembrane mobility of the PC molecules,[99] which may enable particular agents — such as phospholipases — to induce transbilayer reorientations of *glycero*-phospholipids. As will be discussed below (Sections IV.A.4.c and d), accelerated PC flip-flop is also observed in pathologic erythrocytes which have an established structural defect in the skeletal network or in the interaction of this skeleton with the lipid bilayer. Hence, it may be concluded that this protein network plays an important role in stabilizing the lipid bilayer in the red cell membrane.

b. ATP-Depleted Cells

ATP-depletion of intact human erythrocytes causes an enhanced reactivity of PE towards trinitrobenzene sulfonate,[105] and this observation had been suggested to be indicative of a translocation of part of the inner pool of PE to the outer membrane leaflet. However, subsequent studies involving phospholipase A_2 showed no changes in the asymmetric distribution of the phospholipids in those cells.[106] These observations, therefore, once again demonstrate that results obtained from labeling experiments with trinitrobenzene sulfonate should be considered with some care (compare Section IV.A.1.a). Indeed, the absence of ATP as such appears to have no consequences as to the transverse distribution of phospholipids in the red cell membrane, as is clearly demonstrated by the fact that phospholipid asymmetry is completely preserved in erythrocyte ghosts, resealed in the absence of ATP.[45,107,108] It should be added, however, that resealing of such ghosts in the presence of 5 to 10 μM Ca^{2+} may abolish lipid asymmetry, as probed by either phospholipase A_2 digestion or merocyanine 540 staining.[108]

Recently, Seigneuret and Devaux[109] observed that spin-labeled analogues of PC, PE, and PS, when added to suspensions of human erythrocytes, are readily incorporated into the outer membrane leaflet of the cells. In fresh erythrocytes, the labeled PC molecules remained mainly in the outer layer, such in contrast to both aminophospholipids which underwent a rapid translocation to the cytoplasmic half of the membrane. The latter effect was not observed in erythrocytes previously depleted of ATP. Experiments with resealed ghosts showed the same phenomenon, i.e., a rapid translocation of both spin-labeled PE and PS in favor of the inner monolayer, taking place only in case the ghosts had been resealed in the presence of Mg-ATP.

Essentially identical results were obtained by Daleke and Huestis,[110] using either dilauroyl or dimyristoyl species of PE and PS. Translocation of these short-chain aminophospholipids from the outer to the inner membrane leaflet appeared again to be dependent on intracellular Mg-ATP concentrations. Very recently, the above observations could be confirmed by Tilley and colleagues,[58] who used radiolabeled derivatives of naturally occurring SM, PC, PE, and PS of which trace amounts were introduced into the outer membrane layer of fresh and ATP-depleted human erythrocytes, using a nonspecific phospholipid transfer protein (compare Section IV.A.1.c). It appeared that in fresh erythrocytes, 95% of the PS and 75 to 85% of the PE had been translocated to the inner monolayer within 1 and 6 hr, respectively. The choline phospholipids, on the other hand, approached an equilibrium distribution strongly favoring the outer layer, in which 75% of the PC and 90% of the SM was found after 21 hr of incubation at 37°C. Once the labeled aminophospholipids had adopted the inner monolayer positions, subsequent depletion of intracellular ATP did not result in appreciable changes in the highly asymmetric distribution.[58] This observation may lend support to the view that the aminophospholipids are retained in the inner leaflet by (specific) interactions with the membrane skeleton.[62,95] However, when the radiolabeled phospholipids were introduced into the outer monolayer of erythrocytes, previously depleted of the ATP content, not only the choline-, but also the aminophospholipids largely remained in the outer membrane leaflet.[58] Hence, these studies with naturally occurring phospholipid species strongly support the suggestions derived from the above mentioned experiments involving either spin-labeled analogues[86,109] or short-chain phospholipids,[110] namely, that the red cell membrane is equipped with an energy-dependent transfer system which translocates the aminophospholipids from the outer to the inner half of the lipid bilayer. Finally, it is worth noting that, in contrast to the diacyl derivative,[58] exogenous lyso-PS still accumulates in the inner membrane layer of resealed ghosts, not containing ATP.[73] Another striking difference between the lyso- and diacyl derivatives of PS concerns the translocation rates in fresh erythrocytes. The accumulation of 80% of exogenous lyso-PS in the inner membrane layer requires not less than 15 hr at 37°C,[69] whereas at the same temperature it takes only 1 hr to translocate over 90% of the diacyl derivative from the outer to the inner monolayer.[58] These differences illustrate again (see also Section IV.A.1.e) that lysophospholipids are not very suitable probes to gain information about the actual transbilayer movements of diacyl glycerophospholipids in the red cell membrane.

c. Sickle Cells

The primary abnormality of the sickle erythrocyte concerns hemoglobin. As a consequence of a single amino acid substitution in the β chain, sickle cell hemoglobin (HbS) polymerizes to form bundles of long, winding cylinders upon deoxygenation, which cause the cell to adopt the typical sickled morphology.[111] In addition to this primary defect, other abnormalities have been also documented for the sickle cell, a variety of them concerning the membrane[112,113] and, in particular, the skeletal network.[114,115] Also, the organization of phospholipids in the sickle cell membrane has attracted considerable attention.

It has been observed that the accessibility of both aminophospholipids, PE and PS, for chemical probes[116,117] as well as phospholipase A_2[118] is increased, not only in irreversibly sickled cells (ISCs) but also in deoxygenated (sickled) reversibly sicklable cells (RSCs), when compared to both normal erythrocytes or oxygenated (discoid) RSCs. With regard to the deoxygenated RSCs, it is worth noting that both the morphology of the cells, as well as the altered accessibility of PE and PS to exogenous probes, revert to the normal situation upon unsickling of the cells by reoxygenation. These observations have been interpreted in terms of appreciable changes in membrane phospholipid asymmetry in the sickled erythrocyte.[116-118] This view, and particularly as far as it concerns PS, found support in the observation that in a modified Russell's viper venom assay system those cells accelerated clotting only when they were present in the sickled form.[119] Subsequent studies[103,120] demonstrated that deoxygenation (sickling) of RSCs induces a marked acceleration in transbilayer movement of PC molecules, a process which again appeared to be completely reversible in that the normal flip-flop rate is restored immediately upon reoxygenation of the cells. Similarly, as in the case of the above-discussed diamide-treated normal erythrocytes (Section IV.A.4.a), accelerated flip-flop of PC points to a destabilization of the lipid bilayer also occurring in the sickled erythrocyte. This destabilization not only explains that, unlike native

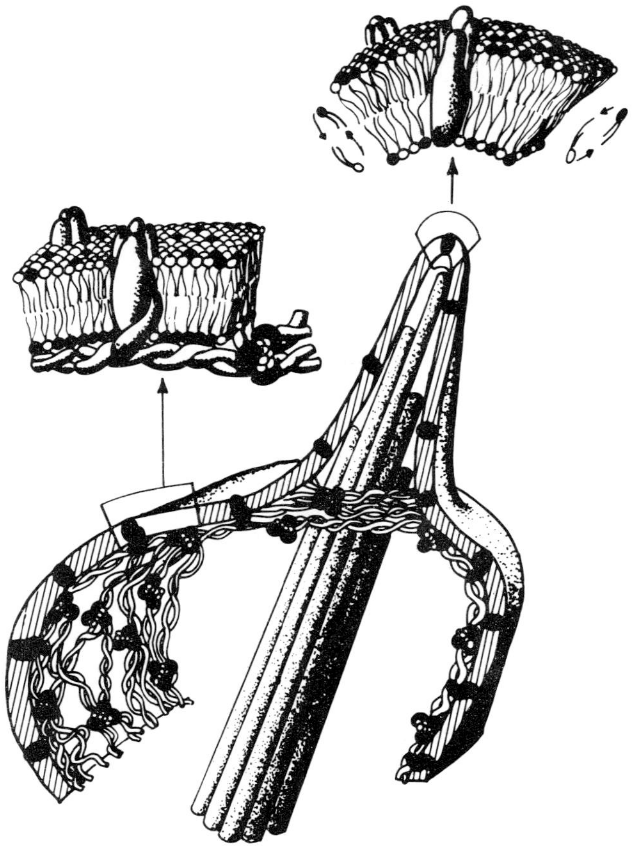

FIGURE 6. Spicule formation in sickled erythrocytes. During the process of sickling, hemoglobin S molecules polymerize into fibers and align with other fibers to bundles. These bundles of polymerized hemoglobin protrude through the membrane skeletal network, thereby breaking the interaction between the membrane bilayer and the membrane skeleton, which results in the formation of the long terminal spicules of the sickled cell. In those areas of the membrane where the bilayer and membrane skeleton are uncoupled, the phospholipids no longer experience the constraints of the skeletal protein network and an enhanced transbilayer mobility may ultimately occur, resulting in an altered distribution of phospholipids over both halves of the bilayer. (From Op den Kamp, J. A. F., Roelofsen, B., and van Deenen, L. L. M., *Trends Biochem. Sci.*, 10, 320, 1985. With permission.)

normal erythrocytes, sickled RSCs exhibit almost complete hemolysis when exposed to the combined action of phospholipase A_2 and SMase C,[118] but it also implies that, again in similarity with the diamide-treated erythrocyte, great care must be exercised when using phospholipases to assess the transbilayer distribution of phospholipids in the sickled cell. Indeed, deoxygenated RSCs showed virtually no response when they were applied in the prothrombinase assay system,[103] indicating that the localization of PS in the membranes deviates not appreciably from the normal situation, in contrast to earlier observations.[116-119]

Further studies[103] have been performed on free spicules (Figure 6), which can be released from RSCs by repeated sickling/unsickling,[121] as well as on remnant despiculated cells. The latter appeared to have a normal composition and localization of the phospholipids. More important, however, was the observation that PC flip-flop in those cells is very similar to that in normal cells, even when they were studied under hypoxic conditions.[103] Also, the free spicules had the same lipid composition as the native cell, but were, in agreement with earlier studies,[121] essentially devoid of membrane skeletal proteins. Those spicules appeared to be highly sensitive to various phospholipases.[103] In agreement with their behavior in the Russell's viper venom assay,[122] free spicules were found to be most active when probed with the prothrombinase assay system.[103] Although a recent study[123] with phospholipase A_2 claimed the contrary, the latter observation does not seem to leave much room for any conclusion other than that an appreciable fraction of the PS is exposed at the outer surface of those spicules.

The above observations led to the conclusion that the abnormal organization of the lipid bilayer in the sickled RSC is confined to those areas of the membrane that are in spicular form, areas where this bilayer is uncoupled from the membrane skeleton (Figure 6). This is in support of the view that a proper interaction with an intact skeletal network is essential for the stabilization of the lipid bilayer. When this interaction is broken, as is obviously the case in the spicules of the sickled RSC, enhanced transbilayer dynamics may eventually lead to some changes in the transverse distribution of the glycerophospholipids, changes which may even affect the localization of PS. It is important to add, however, that such an externalization of PS in the deoxygenated RSC involves only marginal amounts of this phospholipid as long as the cell does not suffer a considerable degree of energy deprivation. Very recently, and in analogy to earlier studies on normal erythrocytes,[58] experiments have been undertaken in which trace amounts of radiolabeled PS were introduced into the outer membrane leaflet of both fresh and ATP-depleted intact RSCs, using the nonspecific lipid transfer protein from beef liver.[211] The fate of this newly introduced PS was monitored by subsequent treatment of the cells with phospholipase A_2 at timed intervals. Introduction of this probe molecule into RSCs, previously depleted of the ATP, showed that about 90% of this PS remained available to phospholipase A_2-induced hydrolysis after 2 hr of incubation of the cells under either oxygenating or deoxygenating conditions. This is in agreement with similar observations with normal erythrocytes (compare Section IV.A.2.b) and shows again that due to a lack of ATP, the aminophospholipid translocation system was not operating and the newly introduced PS remained in the outer monolayer.

Again, in agreement with the previous studies on normal erythrocytes[58] was the observation that within 1 hr after its insertion into fresh RSCs no more than 10% of the labeled PS appeared to be accessible to phospholipase A_2, indicating that 90% of it had been rapidly translocated to the inner monolayer. Subsequent deoxygenation of these RSCs caused only a small enhancement in the phospholipase A_2-induced hydrolysis of both the newly introduced as well as the endogenous PS. The latter effect had been previously observed.[118] As discussed above, it has been suggested that only in the spicular areas of the membrane of the sickled RSC, where the membrane skeleton has been uncoupled from the lipid bilayer, conditions are fulfilled to allow translocation of PS from the inner to the outer monolayer. As there seems to be no reason to suppose that the ATP-dependent translocation of aminophospholipids would have been arrested in the (fresh) deoxygenated RSCs, those PS molecules which have flipped from the inner to the outer monolayer in the spicular areas of the membrane will be rapidly retranslocated back to the inner leaflet by this energy-dependent system. This view is supported by the observation that treatment of ATP-depleted RSCs with phospholipase A_2 caused significantly enhanced hydrolysis of both newly introduced (radiolabeled) as well as endogenous PS, *only* when these cells were subjected to a prolonged incubation under nitrogen.[211] This effect, not observed upon prolonged deoxygenation of ATP-containing RSCs, demonstrates a time-dependent increase in the accessibility of PS in the outer membrane surface of the deoxygenated ATP-depleted RSC. In other words, increasing amounts of PS tend to migrate from the inner to the outer membrane leaflet when the cell is forced to maintain the sickled morphology.

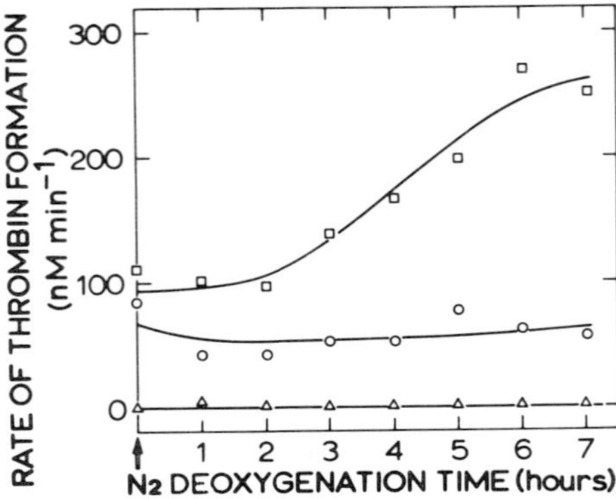

FIGURE 7. Effect of prolonged deoxygenation on the prothrombinase activity of fresh (○) and ATP-depleted RSCs (□), as well as of ATP-depleted normal erythrocytes (△). ATP depletion was achieved by incubating the cells for 24 hr at 37°C in a glucose-free buffer. Suspensions of cells were incubated under nitrogen and, at the time points indicated, samples were taken to determine the prothrombinase activity of the cells. (From Middelkoop, E., Lubin, B. H., Bevers, E. M., Op den Kamp, J. A. F., Comfurius, P., Chiu, D. T.-Y., Zwaal, R. F. A., van Deenen, L. L. M., and Roelofsen, B., *Biochim. Biophys. Acta*, 937, 281, 1988. With permission.)

In view of the above critical comments concerning the use of phospholipase A_2 as a probe for phospholipid localization under those conditions (see also Section IV.A.4.a), the prothrombinase assay has been also applied to confirm this phenomenon.[211] The results thus obtained showed that prolonged deoxygenation of ATP-depleted normal erythrocytes does not result in the exposure of PS in the outer surface of the intact cell (Figure 7). This is in agreement with the notion that the interaction of the membrane skeleton with the lipid bilayer is preserved under these conditions, which retains all of the PS in the inner half of the bilayer. Incubation of ATP-depleted RSCs under deoxygenating conditions, on the other hand, induced a time-dependent appearance of appreciable amounts of PS in the outer monolayer, as monitored by the prothrombinase assay (Figure 7). The explanation of this phenomenon is obvious. The broken interaction between the membrane skeleton and the lipid bilayer, which is found in the spicules protruding from the sickled cell (Figure 6), gives the PS the freedom of being translocated to the exofacial half of the membrane. Once arrived here, the PS molecules will be rapidly spread out over the entire membrane surface as a consequence of the lateral movements experienced by the lipid molecules. At the same time, the PS that has disappeared from the inner monolayer of the spicular membrane will be replenished from the surrounding areas of that leaflet. In the absence of ATP, the PS in the outer monolayer will not be retranslocated to the inner one. Hence, the net result will be a continuous increase in the amount of PS in the outer membrane leaflet until equilibrium is reached. This view is supported by the observation that deoxygenated fresh (ATP containing) RSCs induce only a slow rate of thrombin formation which does not depend on the duration of deoxygenation (Figure 7). Once diffused from the inner to the outer monolayer in the spicular areas of the membrane, the PS molecules will be retranslocated to the inner one by the ATP-dependent system. When this occurs in those areas of the membrane where the interaction with the membrane skeleton is preserved, these PS molecules will be retained in the cytoplasmic monolayer until they again reach the spicular areas of the membrane by means of lateral diffusion. In the latter case, they will have another chance to translocate to the outer monolayer again. Consequently, these mechanisms maintain a steady state of only small amounts of PS being present in the outer membrane layer of the sickled fresh RSC, which is exactly what is observed (Figure 7). The above studies on fresh and ATP-depleted RSCs provide experimental evidence that the asymmetric distribution of PS (and possibly also PE) in the erythrocyte membrane is maintained by two independent mechanisms, i.e., the energy-dependent translocation towards the inner half of the lipid bilayer and the interaction with the membrane skeleton.

Obviously, the exposure of PS at the exofacial leaflet of the membrane renders the cell procoagulant activity. Although, as discussed above, it is unlikely that at any time point appreciable quantities of PS will be present at the outer surface of the sickled RSC, unless the cell has been deprived of the energy source, it seems conceivable that such a situation may indeed occur in vivo during prolonged deoxygenation accompanying a vaso-occlusive crisis. In that case, appreciable amounts of PS may remain in the outer half of the membrane bilayer. The hypercoagulable state observed in sickle cell disease[212] may also be attributed to the free spicules released from the RSCs, since these vesicles also have been shown to possess a marked degree of procoagulant activity (see above). Furthermore, the exposure of PS at the outer surface of both free spicules and ATP-depleted RSCs may provide the basis for interactions with monocytes,[126,213] macrophages,[213,214] and endothelial cells,[124,125,215,216] which represents another contribution to the clinical manifestations of this disease.[217]

d. Hereditary Pyropoikylocytes

Further experimental evidence for the hypothesis that an intact membrane skeleton is essential for stabilizing the lipid bilayer in the erythrocyte membrane comes from recent studies[127] on hereditary pyropoikylocytosis (HPP). HPP is a congenital hemolytic anemia due to an abnormality in the membrane skeleton, more specifically an impaired ability of the spectrin dimers to self-associate into tetramers.[114,128,129] This defect causes an enhanced thermal sensitivity of this protein network. In normal erythrocytes, the skeletal network undergoes irreversible structural changes at 49°C, whereas in HPP a similar disintegration is observed already at 46°C. But even at 37°C, HPP cells show increased osmotic fragility, abnormal morphology, and a clear tendency to vesiculation. Although no abnormalities were found in either composition or distribution of the phospholipids, it appeared that in HPP cells PC flip-flop is more than two times as fast as in normal erythrocytes.[127] Increasing the incubation temperature causes a gradual enhancement of PC flip-flop in both normal and HPP cells. However, sudden and considerable accelerations in this process are observed at 44 and 46°C in case of HPP and normal erythrocytes, respectively.[127] Since in both these cases those temperatures are only a few degrees below the corresponding transition temperature of spectrin in those cells, it seems evident that the marked accelerations in PC flip-flop reflect early major changes in the structural integrity of the membrane skeleton.

e. Red Cells Lacking Particular Antigens

Recently, studies have been performed on erythrocytes which are deficient in particular integral membrane proteins, representing different antigens. The results from those studies, involving four different phenotypes, may be summarized as follows:

1. The absence of glycophorin A in En(a-) cells appears to have no consequences for either cell morphology, osmotic fragility, or organization of the lipid bilayer.[130]
2. A normal membrane lipid organization is also observed in the Leach phenotype,[131] despite the absence of minor sialoglycoproteins, elliptocytic morphology, and increased osmotic fragility of the cells.

3. Acanthocytic McLeod cells, on the other hand, show an appreciably enhanced transbilayer mobility of PC, but the phospholipid asymmetry is identical to that in normal red cells.[131]
4. Rh_{null} erythrocytes, which lack particular integral proteins that are bound to the membrane skeleton, have a stomatocytic morphology, increased osmotic fragility, and exhibit not only accelerated PC flip-flop, but also an abnormal transverse distribution of PE.[132]

Although it is too early to draw definite conclusions, the above studies seem to indicate that particular integral proteins may contribute, either directly or indirectly, to maintain the correct phospholipid organization in the red cell membrane.

5. The Platelet Plasma Membrane

A few years after the successful application of purified phospholipases to establish the distribution of phospholipids in the red cell membrane (see Section IV.A.2), those probes proved suitable again when used to study phospholipid sidedness in the platelet surface membrane.[89] Phospholipids in the human platelet plasma membrane do not differ considerably from those in the human erythrocyte, either in composition or in transbilayer distribution. It should be added, however, that the latter applies only to the platelet in a resting (nonactivated) state. Activation of platelets induces considerable changes in the transverse distribution of the phospholipids in the plasma membrane, most notably an increased exposure of PS on the outer surface.[102] Since those features of the blood platelet, the asymmetric distribution of the phospholipids in the plasma membrane, and the significance in hemostasis have been reviewed recently[133,134] and will be subject to ample discussions in Chapters 8 and 9 of this volume; they will not be dealt with here. However, in the context of the above-discussed relationship that appears to exist between the skeletal protein network and phospholipid organization in the red cell membrane (see Sections IV.A.4.a, c, and d), it may be relevant yet to note that a similar phenomenon has been observed in the platelet.[135] Stimulation of platelets induces alterations in the organization of the cytoskeleton, which may be considered as the key event leading to reorientations of (amino)phospholipids in the plasma membrane. Hence, it was concluded that those alterations in the cytoskeleton play a regulatory role in the expression of platelet procoagulant activity.

B. Lateral Distribution and Dynamics

The question of whether, in a biological membrane, phospholipids are homogeneously distributed in the plane of each bilayer half or, alternatively, might be arranged (partly) in a heterogeneous manner so as to form distinct lateral domains, is still subject to much debate. Using various biophysical techniques such as ESR, fluorescence polarization, fluorescence recovery after photobleaching, and DSC, lateral inhomogeneities in phospholipid distribution have been demonstrated to occur in lipid vesicles composed of binary or ternary mixtures. The occurrence of lateral phase separations strongly depends on the composition of such mixtures, both with respect to polar headgroups and fatty acyl constituents, as well as on the temperature. Furthermore, such lateral heterogeneities may be largely influenced by the pH of the medium and for the presence of Ca^{2+} and (poly)peptides. For detailed discussions on this topic, the reader is referred to some recent reviews.[6,8,67,136] Since the formation of distinct domains of phospholipids may induce local disturbances leading to nonbilayer configurations, the significance for physiologically important phenomena such as exo- or endocytosis and cell fusion will be obvious.[6,8]

Although the *in situ* occurrence of lipid domains in biological membranes has been reported in some cases,[137-140] conclusive evidence of the existence in native red cell membranes has not been produced yet. The differential action of two phospholipase A_2 isoenzymes from

Agkistrodon halys blomhoffii, which has been interpreted to be indicative of different domains of PC in that membrane,[141] may equally well reflect differences in the molecular species specifity of these isoenzymes.

Possibly with the exception of those phospholipids which experience relatively long-lived interactions with membrane proteins (boundary or annular lipids),[67] the molecules present in the lipid bulk of the membrane exhibit a rapid lateral mobility. In a fluid lipid vesicle, the diffusion coefficient of phospholipid molecules is on the order of 2 to $6 \cdot 10^{-8}$ cm^2/sec, when determined at 25°C.[95,142,143] The presence of proteins reduces the lateral mobility of the phospholipids in a protein concentration-dependent manner, both in artificial and biological membranes.[139] For red cell phospholipids, lateral diffusion coefficients are $2.4 \cdot 10^{-8}$ and $0.5 \cdot 10^{-8}$ cm^2/sec (at 25°C) in red cell lipid vesicles and native membranes, respectively.[95] Although not concerning phospholipids themselves, it is of interest to note that the diffusion coefficients of a great many different proteins incorporated in lipid vesicles are of the same order of magnitude.[143] The situation in the biological membrane, however, may be very different, as has been shown for the band 3 protein of the erythrocyte membrane. When determined at 37°C, the diffusion coefficient in a lipid vesicle is $1.6 \cdot 10^{-8}$ cm^2/sec, whereas it is only $4.6 \cdot 10^{-11}$ cm^2/sec in the native membrane.[95] No doubt this considerable reduction in mobility is due to the interaction with the membrane skeleton.

V. FUNCTIONAL ASPECTS OF MEMBRANE PHOSPHOLIPIDS

The primary and most important function of membrane (phospho)lipids obviously is to provide an efficient permeability barrier between two completely different aqueous compartments. The great variety of different lipid molecules present in a given membrane — a number of 400 different species seems a fair estimate for the red cell — is of great importance, not only to accomodate proteins in such a way that the membrane remains properly sealed, but also because it provides the means for regulation of a great many other functions such as the activity of membrane-bound enzymes or signal transduction. In many cases, those functions are dependent on (phospho)lipid-protein interactions.

A. Phospholipid-Protein Interactions

Phospholipid-protein interactions are of mutual importance: particular proteins may govern the phospholipid organization which serves at best the specific structural and functional requirements of a given membrane, whereas phospholipids in turn may play an essential role in the regulation of specific functions of membrane proteins.

1. Lipoproteins

A very special example of (phospho)lipid-protein interactions is found in lipoproteins. Strictly speaking, lipoproteins are entirely different from biological membranes, but as those lipid-protein complexes play a most essential role in lipid transport through the body, they also will be relevant to plasma membranes, not at least for those of blood cells. Mainly according to their density, plasma lipoproteins can be subdivided in four major classes. Chylomicrons, produced by the intestine, transport dietary cholesterol and triglycerides to peripheral tissues. Very low density lipoproteins (VLDL) mediate the transport of those neutral lipids from the liver and are usually metabolized in the plasma, a process involving lipases and lecithin-cholesterol acyltransferase, to form low-density lipoproteins (LDL). The removal of LDL from the bloodstream, a process important to keep plasma cholesterol levels within an acceptable range so as to limit the risk of atherosclerosis and heart attacks, has been described recently.[144] High-density lipoproteins (HDL) can be released from both liver and intestine. They can mediate the transport of cholesterol from peripheral tissues back to the liver,[145] and have been suspected of playing a negative role in vascular diseases.[145]

Although the different classes may vary considerably in lipid and protein composition, they all have a common structure, i.e., an apolar core of triglycerides and cholesterolesters, covered by a monomolecular layer of cholesterol, phospholipids, and apoproteins. Those proteins, of which at least eight different types have been characterized, fulfill a number of important functions, among which is the regulation of lipoprotein metabolism.[147]

Similar to the outer monolayers of the plasma membranes of both erythrocytes and platelets (compare Sections IV.A.2 and 5, respectively), PC and SM are the predominant phospholipids present in the surface coat of plasma lipoproteins. Not only cholesterol, which exchanges very rapidly between plasma lipoproteins and blood cells, but also PC and SM take part in this process, although an efficient exchange of SM with erythrocytes may be questionable.[14] A variety of inborn errors have been described which concern abnormalities in the composition of plasma lipoproteins and the total lipid content, as well as the relative proportions of cholesterol and phospholipids present. In view of the above-mentioned exchange of those components with cellular membranes, it is not surprising that such abnormalities may drastically affect the concentration and composition of lipids, particularly cholesterol/phospholipid ratios, in red cells and platelets. Such changes, in turn, may have considerable consequences for the proper functioning of those cells. More detailed surveys on plasma lipoprotein metabolism and the effect on cell membranes and cellular function have been published recently.[148,149]

2. *Phospholipid-Protein Interactions in Membranes*

The characterization of phospholipid-protein interactions is of paramount importance to gain insight into membrane functioning. Such studies, which involve a great variety of (bio)chemical and physical techniques, give rise to a continuous and still growing flow of review articles and even complete volumes. In the context of this chapter, it will not therefore be possible to cover this topic in any detail. The selection of items discussed below is rather arbitrary and meant mainly to illustrate the complexity of the problems and the possibilities and limitations of some experimental approaches.

a. Techniques

One of the main targets in studies on phospholipid-protein interactions concerns membrane-bound enzymes. The first question to be answered, then, is whether or not a given enzyme requires the presence of phospholipids to maintain activity. A positive answer immediately raises a second question concerning a possible specificity in lipid requirement. Answers to both these questions are usually derived from studies involving (1) a modification of endogenous phospholipids present in the membrane and/or (2) reconstitution of the isolated protein in artificial membrane systems composed of well-defined lipids. Physical techniques (3) are mainly applied to characterize the nature of phospholipid-protein interactions on a molecular level.

i. Modification of Endogenous Phospholipids

A first indication as to whether a particular membrane-bound enzyme requires (phospho)lipids to maintain activity can be derived from experiments involving delipidation of the membrane. In the "early days", organic solvents were used for this purpose, but soon it was recognized that in most cases they caused an irreversible denaturation of proteins. The use of detergents, on the other hand, may give rise to trivial results, due to either incomplete delipidation or to the fact that the detergent may mimic the function of the lipid in maintaining enzyme activity. This leaves phospholipases, provided they are highly purified, about the only tools of choice. Particularly when using a combination of those enzymes with broad substrate specificities, a complete delipidation can be efficiently achieved. Moreover, phospholipases are most powerful tools to induce well-defined modifications in the endogenous phospholipid composition of membranes, particularly since the enzymes of different sources exhibit different modes of action (Figure 4) and substrate specificities.[34] These features made it possible not only to assess the minimal lipid requirement of a membrane-bound enzyme, i.e., the (Na^+ + K^+)-ATPase, but also to characterize the endogenous lipidic activator (compare Section V.A.2.b). However, as is the case also in phospholipid localization studies, (see Section IV.1.b and Reference 34) the use of phospholipases requires a number of essential prerequisites. The fact that in a number of studies the negligence of (some of) those prerequisites has resulted in erroneous results and conflicting conclusions[150] may be the reason that the application of phospholipases in such studies is remarkably limited yet, despite the fact that a great variety of those enzymes is nowadays commercially available in a purified form.

An elegant technique to achieve a direct replacement of endogenous (phospho)lipids was developed in the early 1970s,[151,152] in the first instance to study the lipid requirement of the Ca^{2+}-ATPase from sarcoplasmic reticulum (SR). The method involves the treatment of a (detergent) solubilized protein with a large excess of exogenous (phospho)lipid in the presence of cholate, which is subsequently removed by discontinuous sucrose density-gradient centrifugation. Strictly speaking, the technique represents a special kind of reconstitution. More important to note, however, is that it also represents one of the most dramatic examples of the potential danger inherent to the use of detergents in such studies (see Section V.A.2.b).

ii. Reconstitution

The simplest variant of reconstitution concerns experiments which attempt to reactivate the enzyme in previously delipidated membranes by the addition of dispersions of well-defined phospholipids. Usually, however, the term "reconstitution" refers to studies in which a previously isolated protein is incorporated into artificial (phospho)lipid bilayers. To that end, a variety of techniques has been developed, such as detergent-dialysis, detergent-dilution, sonication (with or without freeze-thawing), incorporation into preexisting liposomes (with or without the use of detergents), fusion, direct transfer of protein-lipid complexes from native membranes in ether or pentane, followed by sonication of the complex in the apolar solvent with aqueous buffer and subsequent solvent evaporation under reduced pressure, etc. Detailed descriptions of these methods and discussions of the pros and cons can be found elsewhere.[153-157] It is worthwhile to emphasize again that particular care should be exercised when applying those methods involving detergents, the complete removal of which may be a difficult task to achieve.[158] One of the newly added methods involves a temporary immobilization of the protein to be incorporated on a gel matrix.[159]

Reconstitution experiments not only enable a study of the effects that the surrounding lipid matrix exerts on the incorporated protein and functioning,[155,157] but conversely also the influence the protein has on the properties of the lipid bilayer. One of the many examples of the latter type of studies concerns the major glycoprotein of the red cell membrane, glycophorin.[160]

iii. Physical Techniques

During the last 2 decades, a variety of (bio)physical, mainly spectroscopic, techniques has been developed to study the specificity in membrane (phospho)lipid-protein interactions on a molecular level, both in artificial and biological membranes. Very recently, a number of excellent comprehensive reviews has been published on the application of ESR,[67,161] ^{13}C- and ^{1}H-NMR,[67,162,163] ^{2}H-NMR,[67,162,164] various fluorescence techniques (fluorescence-quenching, -energy transfer, -polarization, and -recovery after photobleaching),[67] Fourier-transform infrared spectroscopy,[162,165] and photoreactive phospholipids.[166]

The answer to the question as to whether long-lived (specific) interactions between membrane proteins and surrounding phospholipids exist appears to depend largely on the technique used, in particular on the time scales involved. For instance, motions that appear to be fast on the NMR time scale may be slow on that of ESR.[162,164] The latter technique has been applied successfully to assess the specificity of several membrane proteins in the ability to select particular phospholipids from the bulk lipid matrix, as well as to determine the number of phospholipid molecules that are motionally restricted this way.[161] This could be done despite the fact that the lipid exchange rates at the boundary of intrinsic membrane proteins are as high as 10^6 to 10^7/sec.[161,162] Hence, in contrast to what had been believed about one decade ago, there appear to exist no long-lived lipid molecules surrounding such proteins.

b. Lipid-Requirement of Cation-Transporting ATPases

The lipoprotein nature of the (Na^+ + K^+)-ATPase in the human erythrocyte membrane was recognized for the first time by Schatzmann[167] as early as 1962. The period of more than a decade following thereafter was characterized by many conflicting results and conclusions concerning the actual (phospho)lipid requirement of this enzyme in the red cell and other membrane systems.[150] Those controversies became acute to the question of whether or not the system requires the presence of negatively charged phospholipids for proper functioning. Studies propagating the view that negatively charged phospholipids are not essential invariably involved the use of negatively charged detergents and/or the use of phospholipases under inadequate conditions.[150] However, reactivation experiments with membranes, previously delipidated by exhaustive phospholipase treatments and subsequent removal of digestion products, demonstrated an absolute requirement for negatively charged phospholipids.[150,168,169] This effect may be mimicked by a cationic detergent in the presence of a neutral phospholipid, such as PC,[150,169] which illustrates the potential danger of using those detergents in such studies. Since membranes usually contain more than one class of anionic phospholipids, the question was raised as to which of them is the actual endogenous activator in a particular membrane. The answer came from studies in which endogenous phospholipids were modified in various manners using highly purified phospholipases. It appeared that in the red cell membrane, the (Na^+ + K^+)-ATPase activity is maintained by PS,[150,168] whereas in rabbit kidney microsomal membranes this role is fulfilled by PI.[150,169,170] In both cases, only a minor fraction of the total amount of the activating phospholipid appeared to be directly involved.[168,170] The strong preference of the (Na^+ + K^+)-ATPase for acidic phospholipids has been confirmed more recently by reconstitution[171] and spin-label experiments.[172,173]

In contrast to the (Na^+ + K^+)-ATPase, the (Ca^{2+} + Mg^{2+})-ATPase in the red cell membrane appeared to be less specific in the lipid requirement. The activity of this enzyme appeared to be directly proportional to the total amount of (intact) diacyl *glycero*-phospholipids (PC + PE + PS) present in the *inner* half of the bilayer;[150,174] no particular preference for either of these three glycerophospholipids could be detected. It should be added, however, that the above-described lipid requirement of the (Ca^{2+} + Mg^{2+})-ATPase in the red cell membrane refers to the situation *in situ*, i.e., in the presence of calmodulin.[150] Indeed, in the presence of calmodulin, even the isolated enzyme shows full activity in the presence of PC.[175,176] However, in the absence of this Ca^{2+}-modulating protein, the enzyme is fully active only in the presence of acidic phospholipids such as PS.[176,177] The (Ca^{2+} + Mg^{2+})-ATPase activity in human platelets, on the other hand, has been recently shown to be dependent of negatively charged phospholipids.[178]

Among the cation-pumps found in various membranes, the Ca^{2+}-activated one from SR appears to be the least demanding as to the type of lipid by which it has to be surrounded. In fact, early studies on this enzyme once more illustrate the care to be exercised when using detergents for that purpose. Based on lipid substitutions involving cholate, it was generally accepted that the minimal lipid requirement of this pump should be fulfilled by an "annulus" of 30 (zwitterionic) phospholipid molecules directly interacting with the protein.[179] However, later studies learned that the enzyme retains full activity, even when solubilized by particular nonionic detergents which had replaced essentially all of the endogenous phospholipids.[180] Nevertheless, in the native SR membrane, the Ca^{2+}-ATPase is surrounded by a matrix of phospholipids. The nature and physical state of those lipids — as in case of the $(Na^+ + K^+)$-ATPase in other membranes[181-183] — have a direct effect on its functioning.[184-186] Conversely, the protein influences the organization of the phospholipids at its immediate vicinity.[184,187-190]

Finally, it is of interest to note that the activity of both the $(Na^+ + K^+)$- and $(Ca^{2+} + Mg^{2+})$-ATPases are affected by the thickness of the lipid bilayer in which they are incorporated.[191,192]

c. *Interactions with the Red Cell Membrane Skeleton*

Phospholipid-protein interactions not only involve integral membrane proteins, but also the peripheral ones. A typical example to be discussed here concerns the erythrocyte membrane skeleton. This two-dimensional protein network, which is composed of heterodimers of α- and β-spectrin chains, actin, and two proteins denoted as bands 4.1 and 4.9 (according to the nomenclature of Steck), underlies the cytoplasmic side of the membrane bilayer and is believed to govern the shape and flexibility of the cell.[95-97] This skeletal network is coupled to the membrane via ankyrin, which provides the link between the β-spectrin chain and the cytoplasmic domain of the major integral membrane protein, band 3.

Studies on membrane model systems, both liposomes and monomolecular lipid films, showed preferential interactions of spectrin with PS (reviewed in Reference 95). Such interactions, possibly including PE, also appear to exist in the native erythrocyte and are believed to play an important role in the maintenance of phospholipid asymmetry in the membrane,[95,113] thereby contributing to the stability of the lipid bilayer (see the above Sections IV.A.4.a, c, and d). However, it has been argued that those interactions may be rather weak.[193]

In addition to the above-mentioned interactions between the red cell membrane and skeleton, the existence of a glycophorin-protein 4.1 association, regulated by a polyphosphoinositide, has been demonstrated recently.[194] Indeed, a PI-4-phosphate kinase appears to be associated with the skeletal network in human erythrocytes,[195] whereas the maintenance of cell morphology has been attributed to polyphosphoinositide metabolism.[196,197]

B. The Phosphatidylinositol Cycle

One of the highlights in biochemical research of today concerns the metabolism of polyphosphoinositides, usually referred to as the PI-cycle, and its function in membrane signal transduction. During the past 10 years, this interesting field has been subject to an explosive development which makes it impossible to discuss it here in any detail. Hence, for more information, the interested reader is referred to some comprehensive reviews that have been published recently.[198-201]

PI, one of the minor phospholipid constituents of plasma membranes, where it is located in the inner half of the bilayer, can be sequentially phosphorylated at the 4- and 5-positions of the inositol ring, resulting in PI-4-phosphate (PIP) and PI-4,5-bisphosphate (PIP_2), respectively. These phosphorylations involve corresponding kinases, the phosphate groups being derived from ATP. In response to a great variety of external stimuli, of which thrombin, collagen, and platelet-activating factor may be mentioned here because of the relevance in platelet activation, PIP_2 is hydrolyzed by a membrane-bound phosphodiesterase (PDE) to form the hydrophobic diacylglycerols (DG) and the highly hydrophilic inositol triphosphate (IP_3). The transduction of the external signal to the PDE, causing activation, is mediated by a so-called G protein which is phosphorylated by GTP. Both split products, DG and IP_3, function as second messengers. The water-soluble IP_3 immediately leaves the membrane and is believed to induce the release of Ca^{2+} from the endoplasmic reticulum. Ca^{2+}, a second messenger by itself, may in turn activate particular (calmodulin mediated) protein kinases in the cytosol. DGs, on the other hand, remain in the membrane where they can activate (membrane-bound) protein kinase C. These two signal pathways can, but do not necessarily have to, act synergistically to elicit full physiological responses, as has been shown, for instance, in studies on platelets.[198] To close the cycle, DG and IP_3 are recycled to form PI again. To that end, DG is first phosphorylated, involving DG-kinase and ATP, to form phosphatidic acid (PA). PA is subsequently converted into phosphatidyl-cytosine-monophosphate, which reacts with the (stepwise) dephosphorylated IP_3 (myoinositol) to produce PI.

Finally, it is worth mentioning that the DGs, produced in a stimulated platelet after activation of the PDE, can also serve as a source of arachidonic acid which may be further metabolized to thromboxane A_2. This may cause a cascade of activations of other platelets, since also thromboxane A_2 is one of the stimuli for the G-protein-mediated activation of PDE[198] (see Chapter 3).

C. Molecular Species Heterogeneity

As was mentioned earlier in this chapter (Section II.B), membrane phospholipids comprise an impressive number of different molecular species. Obviously, this heterogeneity serves important functional parameters, as, for instance, the regulation of membrane-bound enzymes.[202,203] In addition, it has been noticed recently that this heterogeneity also has significant structural implications. It appeared that the human red cell membrane tolerates only limited changes in the fatty acid composition of the PC.[204] Studies have been carried out in which the endogenous PC molecules in the outer membrane layer of intact cells were replaced by exogenous PC species of well-defined fatty acid composition. This was achieved by incubation of the cells, in the presence of a phosphatidylcholine specific transfer protein (PC-TP) from beef liver, together with sonicated lipid vesicles composed of equimolar amounts of cholesterol and the PC species of choice. Due to the specific feature of the PC-TP to mediate a genuine one-for-one exchange of PC molecules,[205] neither the total amount nor the composition of the membrane lipids is altered this way.[204,206] (The most important results of such studies are listed in Table 2.) Up to 75% of the total PC complement of the human erythrocyte membrane, comprising all of the PC in the outer monolayer (see Section IV.A.2), can be replaced by either (1-palmitoyl,2-oleoyl)PC or (1-palmitoyl,2-linoleoyl)PC without affecting cellular parameters such as K^+ permeability, osmotic fragility, or morphologic appearance.[204,207] It should be remembered that these two species are major PC constituents of the human erythrocyte.[15] Similarly, no changes in the above-mentioned parameters are observed when all of the PC in the outer monolayer is replaced by egg-PC (Table 2), of which the molecular species composition closely resembles that of the human red cell PC.

Entirely different situations are created, however, when the endogenous PC is retailored with either a disaturated or diunsaturated PC (Table 2). When the relative amount of (1,2-dipalmitoyl)PC is increased from 6% to 25%, no changes are observed as to the permeability characteristics of the membrane, but the shape of the cell changes from a discocyte to an echinocyte.[207] A further increase in (1,2-dipalmitoyl)-PC content up to 40% causes a marked destabilization of the cell, as expressed by an enhanced osmotic fragility,[204] whereas the shape further deforms to that of a spheroechinocyte.[207] Increasing this replacement beyond 40% of the total cellular PC causes complete hemolysis.

The double unsaturated (1,2-dilinoleoyl)PC is a species not normally found in the human erythrocyte. Replacement of the endogenous PC for up to 40% by this species has most dramatic consequences for the stability of the cell as, following this retailoring, osmotic fragility gradually increases as does the permeability of the membrane for K^+.[204] The

Table 2
EFFECT OF CHANGES IN PHOSPHATIDYLCHOLINE SPECIES COMPOSITION IN THE OUTER MEMBRANE LEAFLET OF INTACT HUMAN ERYTHROCYTES

Species	Increase in erythrocyte membrane (% of total PC)	K^+ leakage[a]	Osmotic fragility	Cell shape
16:0/18:1	23[b] }			
16:0/18:2	27[b] } → 75	Normal	Normal	Discocyte
Egg-PC	— }			
16:0/16:0	6[b] → 25	Normal	Normal	Echinocyte
	25 → 40	Normal	Increased	Sphero-echinocyte
	>40	—	Hemolysis	—
18:2/18:2	— → 40	Increased	Increased	Stomatocyte
	>40	—	Hemolysis	—

Note: Native PC in the outer membrane leaflet of intact erythrocytes was replaced by incubation of the cells in the presence of a PC-TP from beef liver, together with sonicated vesicles containing equimolar amounts of cholesterol and the PC species indicated.

[a] K^+ leakage from the cells was determined under isotonic conditions.
[b] Concentration of the species (% of total PC) in the native erythrocyte.

Adapted from Kuypers, F. A., Roelofsen, B., Op den Kamp, J. A. F., and van Deenen, L. L. M., *Biochim. Biophys. Acta,* 769, 337, 1984; Kuypers, F. A., Roelofsen, B., Berendsen, W., Op den Kamp, J. A. F., and van Deenen, L. L. M., *J. Cell Biol.,* 99, 2260, 1984.

morphology of the cell is converted to that of a so-called stomatocyte.[207] Replacement of more than 40% of the native PC by the 1,2-dilinoleoyl species again results in lysis of the cells (Table 2). Since abnormalities in the erythrocyte are, in some cases, already detectable upon retailoring of the native PC to an extent which accounts for only 0.5 to 1% of the total lipid content of the cell, it is quite clear that this membrane tolerates only very limited changes in the fatty acid composition of the PC.[204]

The changes in cell morphology induced by retailoring of PC species, i.e., echinocytes and stomatocytes in case of replacement by (1,2-dipalmitoyl)PC and (1,2-dilinoleoyl)PC, respectively, have been proposed to result from differences in geometry of the individual PC molecules.[207] A working model that tries to explain how differences in geometry of individual PC molecules may induce those marked changes in cell morphology has been presented recently.[208]

It is noteworthy to add that studies with rabbit and horse erythrocytes showed that replacement of no more than 20% of native PC by (1,2-dipalmitoyl)PC gives rise to a drastic decrease in the in vivo survival time after reinjection of those modified cells into the same animal.[209] At 30% replacement with this disaturated PC species, clearance from circulation occurred even within 24 hr. On the other hand, experiments with erythrocytes in which not less than 40% of the PC had been replaced by (1-palmitoyl,2-linoleoyl)PC showed that the in vivo survival time cannot be distinguished from that of unmodified control cells.[209] These observations obviously indicate that the in vivo existing repair mechanisms, particularly the exchange of intact PC molecules with the serum lipoproteins (see Section II.B), are insufficient to cope with the drastic changes in the erythrocyte membrane that are induced by replacing an appreciable fraction of native PC by the dipalmitoyl species.

VI. CONCLUDING REMARKS

This chapter has presented an overview of the major characteristics of phospholipids, as well as the organization, dynamics, and functional roles in biological membranes. Attention has been paid also to a number of techniques that are nowadays available to study those parameters. It should be emphasized again, however, that for obvious reasons this treatise is far from complete. This even applies in the case of the erythrocyte membrane, which has been frequently used as a model in the above discussions. Hence, it may be useful to recall that more detailed information on the structure and function of phospholipids in biological membranes can be found in a variety of comprehensive reviews. Those published during the last 5 years are listed under References 6 to 8, 33, 34, 50 to 52, 59, 61, 62, 67, 95, 133, 134, 136, 138, 142, 143, 149, 150, 155 to 157, 161 to 166, 198 to 203, and 210.

ACKNOWLEDGMENT

The authors are most grateful to Mrs. Eva A. M. Bouabbas-Donkerbroek for skillful typing of the manuscript.

REFERENCES

1. **Gorter, E. and Grendel, F.,** On bimolecular layers of lipids on the chromatocytes of the blood, *J. Exp. Med.*, 41, 439, 1925.
2. **Singer, S. J. and Nicolson, G. L.,** The fluid mosaic model of the structure of cell membranes, *Science,* 175, 720, 1972.
3. **Hirata, F. and Axelrod, J.,** Enzymatic synthesis and rapid translocation of phosphatidylcholine by two methyltransferases in erythrocyte membranes, *Proc. Natl. Acad. Sci. U.S.A.*, 75, 2348, 1978.
4. **Krebs, J. J. R., Hauser, H., and Carafoli, E.,** Asymmetric distribution of phospholipids in the inner membrane of beef heart mitochondria, *J. Biol. Chem.*, 254, 5308, 1979.
5. **Van den Bosch, H.,** Phosphoglyceride metabolism, *Annu. Rev. Biochem.*, 43, 243, 1974.
6. **Verkleij, A. J.,** Lipidic intramembranous particles, *Biochim. Biophys. Acta,* 779, 43, 1984.
7. **Gruner, S. M., Cullis, P. R., Hope, M. J., and Tilcock, C. P. S.,** Lipid polymorphism: the molecular basis of non-bilayer phases, *Annu. Rev. Biophys. Biophys. Chem.*, 14, 211, 1985.
8. **Cullis, P. R., Hope, M. J., de Kruijff, B., Verkleij, A. J., and Tilcock, C. P. S.,** Structural properties and functional roles of phospholipids in biological membranes, in *Phospholipids and Cellular Regulations,* Vol. 1, Kuo, J. F., Ed., CRC Press, Boca Raton, Fla., 1985, 1.
9. **Stubbs, C. D. and Smith, A. D.,** The modification of mammalian membrane polyunsaturated fatty acid composition in relation to membrane fluidity and function, *Biochim. Biophys. Acta,* 779, 89, 1984.
10. **Deuticke, B.,** Properties and structural basis of simple diffusion pathways in the erythrocyte membrane, *Rev. Physiol. Biochem. Pharmacol.*, 78, 1, 1977.
11. **Dodge, J. T. and Phillips, G. B.,** Composition of phospholipids and of phospholipid fatty acids and aldehydes in human red cells, *J. Lipid Res.*, 8, 667, 1967.
12. **Manku, M. S., Horrobin, D. F., Huang, Y.-S., and Morse, N.,** Fatty acids in plasma and red cell membranes in normal humans, *Lipids,* 18, 906, 1983.
13. **Alexander, L. R. and Justice, J. B.,** Fatty acid composition of human erythrocyte membranes by capillary gas chromatography-mass spectrometry, *J. Chromatogr.*, 342, 1, 1985.
14. **Boegheim, J. P. J., van Linde, M., Op den Kamp, J. A. F., and Roelofsen, B.,** The sphingomyelin pools in the outer and inner layer of the human erythrocyte membrane are composed of different molecular species, *Biochim. Biophys. Acta,* 735, 438, 1983.
15. **Van Golde, L. M. G., Tomasi, V., and van Deenen, L. L. M.,** Determination of molecular species of lecithin from erythrocytes and plasma, *Chem. Phys. Lipids,* 1, 282, 1967.

16. **Marai, L. and Kuksis, K.,** Molecular species of lecithins from erythrocytes and plasma of man, *J. Lipid Res.*, 10, 141, 1969.
17. **Antoku, Y., Sakai, T., and Iwashita, H.,** Fatty acid analysis of phosphatidylethanolamine subclasses of human erythrocyte membranes by high-performance liquid chromatography, *J. Chromatogr.*, 342, 359, 1985.
18. **Mulder, E. and van Deenen, L. L. M.,** Metabolism of red cell lipids. I. Incorporation in vitro of fatty acids into phospholipids from mature erythrocytes, *Biochim. Biophys. Acta,* 106, 106, 1965.
19. **Shohet, S. B. and Nathan, D. G.,** Incorporation of phosphatide precursors from serum into erythrocytes, *Biochim. Biophys. Acta,* 202, 202, 1970.
20. **Mulder, E. and van Deenen, L. L. M.,** Metabolism of red cell lipids. III. Pathways for phospholipid renewal, *Biochim. Biophys. Acta,* 106, 348, 1965.
21. **Renooij, W., van Golde, L. M. G., Zwaal, R. F. A., Roelofsen, B., and van Deenen, L. L. M.,** Preferential incorporation of fatty acids at the inside of human erythrocyte membranes, *Biochim. Biophys. Acta,* 363, 287, 1974.
22. **Renooij, W., van Golde, L. M. G., Zwaal, R. F. A., and van Deenen, L. L. M.,** Topological asymmetry of phospholipid metabolism in rat erythrocyte membranes. Evidence for flip-flop of lecithin, *Eur. J. Biochem.*, 61, 53, 1976.
23. **Renooij, W. and van Golde, L. M. G.,** Asymmetry in the renewal of molecular classes of phosphatidylcholine in the rat-erythrocyte membrane, *Biochim. Biophys. Acta,* 558, 314, 1979.
24. **Reed, C. F.,** Phospholipid exchange between plasma and erythrocytes in man and the dog, *J. Clin. Invest.*, 47, 749, 1968.
25. **Renooij, W. and van Golde, L. M. G.,** The exchange of phospholipids between rat erythrocytes and plasma, and the translocation of phosphatidylcholine across the red cell membrane, are temperature dependent processes, *FEBS Lett.*, 71, 321, 1976.
26. **Nelson, G. J.,** Lipid composition of erythrocytes in various mammalian species, *Biochim. Biophys. Acta,* 144, 221, 1967.
27. **Zwaal, R. F. A., Flückiger, R., Moser, S., and Zahler, P.,** Lecithinase activities at the external surface of ruminant erythrocyte membranes, *Biochim. Biophys. Acta,* 373, 416, 1974.
28. **Frei, E. and Zahler, P.,** Phospholipase A_2 from sheep erythrocyte membranes. Ca^{2+} dependence and localization, *Biochim. Biophys. Acta,* 550, 450, 1979.
29. **Jimeno-Abendano, J. and Zahler, P.,** Purified phospholipase A_2 from sheep erythrocyte membrane. Preferential hydrolysis according to polar groups and 2-acyl chains, *Biochim. Biophys. Acta,* 573, 266, 1979.
30. **Bretscher, M. S.,** Phosphatidylethanolamine: differential labelling in intact cells and ghosts of human erythrocytes by a membrane-impermeable reagent, *J. Mol. Biol.*, 71, 523, 1972.
31. **Bretscher, M. S.,** Asymmetrical lipid bilayer structure for biological membranes, *Nat. New Biol.*, 236, 11, 1972.
32. **Op den Kamp, J. A. F.,** Lipid asymmetry in membranes, *Annu. Rev. Biochem.*, 48, 47, 1979.
33. **Etemadi, A. H.,** Membrane asymmetry. A survey and critical appraisal of the methodology. II. Methods for assessing the unequal distribution of lipids, *Biochim. Biophys. Acta,* 604, 423, 1980.
34. **Roelofsen, B.,** Phospholipases as tools to study the localization of phospholipids in biological membranes. A critical review, *J. Toxicol. Toxin Rev.*, 1, 87, 1982.
35. **Gordesky, S. E., Marinetti, G. V., and Love, R.,** The reaction of chemical probes with the erythrocyte membrane, *J. Membr. Biol.*, 20, 111, 1975.
36. **Haest, C. W. M., Kamp, D., and Deuticke, B.,** Penetration of 2,4,6-trinitrobenzene sulfonate into human erythrocytes. Consequences for studies on phospholipid asymmetry, *Biochim. Biophys. Acta,* 640, 535, 1981.
37. **Bishop, D. G., Bevers, E. M., van Meer, G., Op den Kamp, J. A. F., and van Deenen, L. L. M.,** A monolayer study of the reaction of trinitrobenzene sulfonic acid with aminophospholipids, *Biochim. Biophys. Acta,* 551, 122, 1979.
38. **Rawyler, A., Roelofsen, B., and Op den Kamp, J. A. F.,** The use of fluorescamine as a permeant probe to localize phosphatidylethanolamine in intact Friend erythroleukaemic cells, *Biochim. Biophys. Acta,* 769, 330, 1984.
39. **Demel, R. A., Geurts van Kessel, W. S. M., Zwaal, R. F. A., Roelofsen, B., and van Deenen, L. L. M.,** Relation between various phospholipase actions on human red cell membranes and the interfacial phospholipid pressure in monolayers, *Biochim. Biophys. Acta,* 406, 97, 1975.
40. **Roelofsen, B., Zwaal, R. F. A., Comfurius, P., Woodward, C. B., and van Deenen, L. L. M.,** Action of pure phospholipase A_2 and phospholipase C on human erythrocytes and ghosts, *Biochim. Biophys. Acta,* 241, 925, 1971.
41. **Bowman, M. H., Ottolenghi, A. C., and Mengel, C. E.,** Effects of phospholipase C on human erythrocytes, *J. Membr. Biol.*, 4, 156, 1971.

42. **Woodward, C. B. and Zwaal, R. F. A.,** The lytic behavior of pure phospholipase A_2 and C towards osmotically swollen erythrocytes and resealed ghosts, *Biochim. Biophys. Acta,* 274, 272, 1972.
43. **Colley, C. M., Zwaal, R. F. A., Roelofsen, B., and van Deenen, L. L. M.,** Lytic and non-lytic degradation of phospholipids in mammalian erythrocytes by pure phospholipases, *Biochim. Biophys. Acta,* 307, 74, 1973.
44. **Zwaal, R. F. A., Roelofsen, B., and Colley, C. M.,** Localization of red cell membrane constituents, *Biochim. Biophys. Acta,* 300, 159, 1973.
45. **Zwaal, R. F. A., Roelofsen, B., Comfurius, P., and van Deenen, L. L. M.,** Organization of phospholipids in human red cell membranes as detected by the action of various purified phospholipases, *Biochim. Biophys. Acta,* 406, 83, 1975.
46. **Verkleij, A. J., Zwaal, R. F. A., Roelofsen, B., Comfurius, P., Kastelijn, D., and van Deenen, L. L. M.,** The asymmetric distribution of phospholipids in the human red cell membrane. A combined study using phospholipases and freeze-etch electron microscopy, *Biochim. Biophys. Acta,* 323, 178, 1973.
47. **Roelofsen, B., Sibenius Trip, M., Verheij, H. M., and Zevenbergen, J. L.,** The action of cobra venom phospholipase A_2 isoenzymes towards intact human erythrocytes, *Biochim. Biophys. Acta,* 600, 1012, 1980.
48. **Fujii, T. and Tamura, A.,** Asymmetric manipulation of the membrane lipid bilayer of intact human erythrocytes with phospholipases A, C or D induces a change in cell shape, *J. Biochem.,* 86, 1345, 1979.
49. **Van Meer, G., de Kruijff, B., Op den Kamp, J. A. F., and van Deenen, L. L. M.,** Preservation of bilayer structure in human erythrocytes and erythrocyte ghosts after phospholipase treatment. A ^{31}P-NMR study, *Biochim. Biophys. Acta,* 596, 1, 1980.
50. **Bloj, B. and Zilversmit, D. B.,** Lipid transfer proteins in the study of artificial and natural membranes, *Mol. Cell. Biochem.,* 40, 163, 1981.
51. **Zilversmit, D. B.,** Lipid transfer proteins, *J. Lipid Res.,* 25, 1563, 1984.
52. **Wirtz, K. W. A., Op den Kamp, J. A. F., and Roelofsen, B.,** Phosphatidylcholine transfer protein: properties and applications in membrane research, in *Progress in Protein-Lipid Interactions,* Vol. 2, Watts, A. and de Pont, J. J. H. H. M., Eds., Elsevier, Amsterdam, 1986, 221.
53. **Van Meer, G. and Op den Kamp, J. A. F.,** Transbilayer movement of various phosphatidylcholine species in intact human erythrocytes, *J. Cell Biochem.,* 19, 193, 1982.
54. **Op den Kamp, J. A. F. and Roelofsen, B.,** Determination of transbilayer mobility of phosphatidylcholine in the red blood cell, in *Methods in Enzymology,* Fleischer, S. and Fleisher, B., Eds., Academic Press, New York, in press.
55. **Middelkoop, E., Lubin, B. H., Op den Kamp, J. A. F., and Roelofsen, B.,** Flip-flop rates of individual molecular species of phosphatidylcholine in the human red cell membrane, *Biochim. Biophys. Acta,* 855, 421, 1986.
56. **Franck, P. F. H., de Ree, J. M., Roelofsen, B., and Op den Kamp, J. A. F.,** Modification of the erythrocyte membrane by a non-specific lipid transfer protein, *Biochim. Biophys. Acta,* 77, 405, 1984.
57. **Crain, R. C. and Zilversmit, D. B.,** Two non-specific phospholipid exchange proteins from beef liver. II. Use in studying the asymmetry and transbilayer movement of phosphatidylcholine, phosphatidylethanolamine, and sphingomyelin in intact rat erythrocytes, *Biochemistry,* 19, 1440, 1980.
58. **Tilley, L., Cribier, S., Roelofsen, B., Op den Kamp, J. A. F., and van Deenen, L. L. M.,** ATP-dependent translocation of amino phospholipids across the human erythrocyte membrane, *FEBS Lett.,* 194, 21, 1986.
59. **Krebs, J. J. R.,** The topology of phospholipids in artificial and biological membranes, *J. Bioenerg. Biomembr.,* 14, 141, 1982.
60. **Cullis, P. R. and de Kruijff, B.,** Lipid polymorphism and the functional roles of lipids in biological membranes, *Biochim. Biophys. Acta,* 559, 399, 1979.
61. **De Kruijff, B., Cullis, P. R., and Verkleij, A. J.,** Non-bilayer lipid structures in model and biological membranes, *Trends Biochem. Sci.,* 5, 79, 1980.
62. **Van Deenen, L. L. M.,** Topology and dynamics of phospholipids in membranes, *FEBS Lett.,* 123, 3, 1981.
63. **Luzatti, V.,** X-ray diffraction studies of lipid-water systems, in *Biological Membranes,* Chapman, D., Ed., Academic Press, London, 1968, 71.
64. **Blaurock, A. E.,** Evidence of bilayer structure and of membrane interactions from X-ray diffraction analysis, *Biochim. Biophys. Acta,* 650, 167, 1982.
65. **Buldt, G., Gally, H. U., Seelig, J., and Zaccai, G.,** Neutron diffraction studies on phosphatidylcholine model membranes. I. Head group conformation, *J. Mol. Biol.,* 134, 673, 1979.
66. **Zaccai, G., Buldt, G., Seelig, A., and Seelig, J.,** Neutron diffraction studies on phosphatidylcholine model membranes. II. Chain conformation and segmental disorder, *J. Mol. Biol.,* 134, 693, 1979.
67. **Devaux, P. F. and Seigneuret, M.,** Specificity of lipid-protein interactions as determined by spectroscopic techniques, *Biochim. Biophys. Acta,* 822, 63, 1985.
68. **Mohandas, N., Wyatt, J., Mel, S. F., Rossi, M. E., and Shohet, S. B.,** Lipid translocation across the human erythrocyte membrane. Regulatory factors, *J. Biol. Chem.,* 257, 6537, 1982.

69. **Bergmann, W. L., Dressler, V., Haest, C. W. M., and Deuticke, B.,** Reorientation rates and asymmetry of distribution of lysophospholipids between the inner and outer leaflet of the erythrocyte membrane, *Biochim. Biophys. Acta,* 772, 328, 1984.
70. **Fujii, T., Tamura, A., and Yamane, T.,** Trans-bilayer movement of added phosphatidylcholine and lysophosphatidylcholine species with various acyl chain lengths in plasma membrane of intact human erythrocytes, *J. Biochem.,* 98, 1221, 1985.
71. **Dressler, V., Schwister, K., Haest, C. W. M., and Deuticke, B.,** Dielectric breakdown of the erythrocyte enhances transbilayer mobility of phospholipids, *Biochim. Biophys. Acta,* 732, 304, 1983.
72. **Bergmann, W. L., Dressler, V., Haest, C. W. M., and Deuticke, B.,** Cross-linking of SH-groups in the erythrocyte membrane enhances transbilayer reorientation of phospholipids. Evidence for a limited access of phospholipids to the reorientation sites, *Biochim. Biophys. Acta,* 769, 390, 1984.
73. **Dressler, V., Haest, C. W. M., Plasa, G., Deuticke, B., and Erusalimsky, J. D.,** Stabilizing factors of phospholipid asymmetry in the erythrocyte membrane, *Biochim. Biophys. Acta,* 775, 189, 1984.
74. **Gordesky, S. E. and Marinetti, G. V.,** The asymmetric arrangement of phospholipids in the human erythrocyte membrane, *Biochem. Biophys. Res. Commun.,* 50, 1027, 1973.
75. **Kahlenberg, A., Walker, C., and Rohrlick, R.,** Evidence for an asymmetric distribution of phospholipids in the human erythrocyte membrane, *Can. J. Biochem.,* 52, 803, 1974.
76. **Renooij, W.,** Renewal of Erythrocyte Phospholipids. Evidence for a Metabolic Membrane Asymmetry, Ph.D. thesis, State University of Utrecht, The Netherlands, 1977.
77. **Adamich, M. and Dennis, E. A.,** Exploring the action and specificity of cobra venom phospholipase A_2 toward human erythrocytes, ghost membranes and lipid mixtures, *J. Biol. Chem.,* 253, 5121, 1978.
78. **Adamich, M. and Dennis, E. A.,** *Progress in Clinical and Biological Research,* Vol. 30, Lux, S. E., Marchesi, V. T., and Fox, C. F., Eds., Alan R. Liss, New York, 1979, 515.
79. **Shukla, S. D. and Hanahan, D. J.,** Differences in the pattern of attack of acidic, neutral, and basic phospholipases A_2 of A. halys blomhoffii on human erythrocyte membranes: problems in interpretation of phospholipid localization, *Arch. Biochem. Biophys.,* 209, 668, 1981.
80. **Martin, J. K., Luthra, M. G., Wells, M. A., and Hanahan, D. J.,** Phospholipase A_2 as a probe of phospholipid distribution in erythrocyte membranes. Factors influencing the apparent specificity of the reaction, *Biochemistry,* 14, 5400, 1975.
81. **Bloj, B. and Zilversmit, D. B.,** Asymmetry and transposition rates of phosphatidylcholine in rat erythrocyte ghosts, *Biochemistry,* 15, 1277, 1976.
82. **Kramer, R. M. and Branton, D.,** Retention of lipid asymmetry in membranes on polylysine-coated beads, *Biochim. Biophys. Acta,* 556, 219, 1979.
83. **Van Meer, G., Poorthuis, B. J. H. M., Wirtz, K. W. A., Op den Kamp, J. A. F., and van Deenen, L. L. M.,** Transbilayer distribution and mobility of phosphatidylcholine in intact erythrocyte membranes. A study with phosphatidylcholine exchange protein, *Eur. J. Biochem.,* 103, 283, 1980.
84. **Low, M. G. and Finean, J. B.,** Modification of erythrocyte membranes by a purified phosphatidylinositol-specific phospholipase C (Staphylococcus aureus), *Biochem. J.,* 162, 235, 1977.
85. **Renooij, W. and van Golde, L. M. G.,** The transposition of molecular classes of phosphatidylcholine across the rat erythrocyte membrane and their exchange between the red cell membrane and plasma lipoproteins, *Biochim. Biophys. Acta,* 470, 465, 1977.
86. **Zachovsky, A., Fellman, P., and Devaux, P. F.,** Absence of transbilayer diffusion of spin-labeled sphingomyelin in human erythrocytes. Comparison with the diffusion of several spin-labeled glycerophospholipids, *Biochim. Biophys. Acta,* 815, 510, 1985.
87. **Mark, P. A. and Rifkind, R. A.,** Erythroleukaemic differentiation, *Annu. Rev. Biochem.,* 47, 419, 1978.
88. **Friend, C., Scher, W., Holland, J. G., and Sato, T.,** Hemoglobin synthesis in murine virus-induced leukemic cells in vitro: stimulation of erythroid differentiation by dimethyl sulfoxide, *Proc. Natl. Acad. Sci. U.S.A.,* 68, 378, 1971.
89. **Chap, H. J., Zwaal, R. F. A., and van Deenen, L. L. M.,** Action of highly purified phospholipases on blood platelets. Evidence for an asymmetric distribution of phospholipids in the surface membranes, *Biochim. Biophys. Acta,* 467, 146, 1979.
90. **Rawyler, A. J., Roelofsen, B., Op den Kamp, J. A. F., and van Deenen, L. L. M.,** Isolation and characterization of plasma membranes from Friend erythroleukaemic cells. A study with sphingomyelinase C, *Biochim. Biophys. Acta,* 730, 130, 1983.
91. **Rawyler, A. J., van der Schaft, P. H., Roelofsen, B., and Op den Kamp, J. A. F.,** Phospholipid localization in the plasma membrane of Friend erythroleukaemic cells and mouse erythrocytes, *Biochemistry,* 24, 1777, 1985.
92. **Van der Schaft, P. H., Roelofsen, B., and Op den Kamp, J. A. F.,** unpublished data, 1986.
93. **Nijhof, W., van der Schaft, P. H., Wierenga, P. K., Roelofsen, B., Op den Kamp, J. A. F., and van Deenen, L. L. M.,** The transbilayer distribution of phosphatidylethanolamine in erythroid plasma membranes during erythropoiesis, *Biochim. Biophys. Acta,* 862, 273, 1986.

94. **Haest, C. W. M., Plasa, G., Kamp, D., and Deuticke, B.,** Spectrin as a stabilizer of the phospholipid asymmetry in the human erythrocyte membrane, *Biochim. Biophys. Acta,* 509, 21, 1978.
95. **Haest, C. W. M.,** Interactions between membrane skeleton proteins and the intrinsic domain of the erythrocyte membrane, *Biochim. Biophys. Acta,* 694, 331, 1982.
96. **Marchesi, V. T.,** The red cell membrane skeleton: recent progress, *Blood,* 61, 1, 1983.
97. **Bennett, V.,** The membrane skeleton of human erythrocytes and its implications for more complex cells, *Annu. Rev. Biochem.,* 54, 273, 1985.
98. **Franck, P. F. H., Roelofsen, B., and Op den Kamp, J. A. F.,** Complete exchange of phosphatidylcholine from intact erythrocytes after protein cross-linking, *Biochim. Biophys. Acta,* 687, 105, 1982.
99. **Franck, P. F. H., Op den Kamp, J. A. F., Roelofsen, B., and van Deenen, L. L. M.,** Does diamide treatment of intact human erythrocytes cause a loss of phospholipid asymmetry?, *Biochim. Biophys. Acta,* 857, 127, 1986.
100. **Haest, C. W. M. and Deuticke, B.,** Possible relationship between membrane proteins and phospholipid asymmetry in the human erythrocyte membrane, *Biochim. Biophys. Acta,* 436, 353, 1976.
101. **Williamson, P., Bateman, J., Kozarsky, K., Mattocks, K., Hermanowicz, N., Choe, H. R., and Schlegel, R. A.,** Involvement of spectrin in the maintenance of phase-state asymmetry in the erythrocyte membrane, *Cell,* 30, 725, 1982.
102. **Bevers, E. M., Comfurius, P., and Zwaal, R. F. A.,** Changes in membrane phospholipid distribution during platelet activation, *Biochim. Biophys. Acta,* 736, 57, 1983.
103. **Franck, P. F. H., Bevers, E. M., Lubin, B. H., Comfurius, P., Chiu, D. T.-Y., Op den Kamp, J. A. F., Zwaal, R. F. A., van Deenen, L. L. M., and Roelofsen, B.,** Uncoupling of the membrane skeleton from the lipid bilayer. The cause of accelerated phospholipid flip-flop leading to an enhanced procoagulant activity of sickled cells, *J. Clin. Invest.,* 75, 183, 1985.
104. **Zwaal, R. F. A. and Bevers, E. M.,** personal communication, 1985.
105. **Haest, C. W. M. and Deuticke, B.,** Experimental alteration of phospholipid-protein interactions within the human erythrocyte membrane. Dependence on glycolytic metabolism, *Biochim. Biophys. Acta,* 401, 468, 1975.
106. **Haest, C. W. M., Plasa, G., Kamp, D., and Deuticke, B.,** Protein-lipid interactions in the erythrocyte membrane: relevance for structural properties, in *Membrane Transport in Erythrocytes,* Lassen, U. V., Ussing, H. H., and Wieth, J. O., Eds., Munksgaard, Copenhagen, 1980, 108.
107. **Marinetti, G. V. and Crain, R. C.,** Topology of amino-phospholipids in the red cell membrane, *J. Supramol. Struct.,* 8, 191,1978.
108. **Williamson, P., Algarin, L., Bateman, J., Choe, H.-R., and Schlegel, R. A.,** Phospholipid asymmetry in human erythrocyte ghosts, *J. Cell Physiol.,* 123, 209, 1985.
109. **Seigneuret, M. and Devaux, P. F.,** ATP-dependent asymmetric distribution of spin-labeled phospholipids in the erythrocyte membrane: relation to shape changes, *Proc. Natl. Acad. Sci. U.S.A.,* 81, 3751, 1984.
110. **Daleke, D. L. and Huestis, W. H.,** Incorporation and translocation of aminophospholipids in human erythrocytes, *Biochemistry,* 24, 5406, 1985.
111. **Noguchi, C. T. and Schechter, A. N.,** Sickle hemoglobin polymerization in solution and in cells, *Annu. Rev. Biophys. Biophys. Chem.,* 14, 239, 1985.
112. **Luer, C. A. and Wong, P. A.,** Altered erythrocyte membrane proteins in sickle cell patients associated with the severity of the disease, *Biochem. Med.,* 19, 95, 1978.
113. **Wagner, C. M., Schwartz, R. S., Chiu, D. T.-Y., and Lubin, B. H.,** Membrane phospholipid organization and vesiculation of erythrocytes in sickle cell anemia, *Clin. Haematol.,* 14, 183, 1985.
114. **Lux, S. E.,** Spectrin-actin membrane skeletons of normal and abnormal red blood cells, *Semin. Hematol.,* 16, 21, 1979.
115. **Platt, O. S., Falcone, J. F., and Lux, S. E.,** Molecular defect in the sickle erythrocyte skeleton. Abnormal spectrin binding to sickle inside-out vesicles, *J. Clin. Invest.,* 75, 266, 1985.
116. **Gordesky, S. E., Marinetti, G. V., and Segel, G. B.,** Differences in the reactivity of phospholipids with FDNB in normal RBC, sickle cells and RBC ghosts, *Biochem. Biophys. Res. Commun.,* 47, 1004, 1972.
117. **Chiu, D., Lubin, B., and Shohet, S. B.,** Erythrocyte membrane lipid reorganization during the sickling process, *Br. J. Haematol.,* 41, 223, 1979.
118. **Lubin, B., Chiu, D., Bastacky, J., Roelofsen, B., and van Deenen, L. L. M.,** Abnormalities in membrane phospholipid organization in sickled erythrocytes, *J. Clin. Invest.,* 67, 1643, 1981.
119. **Chiu, D., Lubin, B., Roelofsen, B., and van Deenen, L. L. M.,** Sickled erythrocytes accelerate clotting in vitro: an effect of abnormal membrane lipid asymmetry, *Blood,* 58, 398, 1981.
120. **Franck, P. F. H., Chiu, D. T.-Y., Op den Kamp, J. A. F., Lubin, B., van Deenen, L. L. M., and Roelofsen, B.,** Accelerated transbilayer movement of phosphatidylcholine in sickled erythrocytes. A reversible process, *J. Biol. Chem.,* 258, 8435, 1983.
121. **Allan, D., Limbrick, A. R., Thomas, P., and Westerman, M. P.,** Release of spectrin-free spicules on reoxygenation of sickled erythrocytes, *Nature,* 295, 612, 1982.

122. **Westerman, M. P., Cole, E. R., and Wu, K.,** The effect of spicules obtained from sickle red cells on clotting activity, *Br. J. Haematol.,* 56, 557, 1984.
123. **Raval, P. J. and Allan, D.,** Sickling of sickle erythrocytes does not alter phospholipid asymmetry, *Biochem. J.,* 223, 555, 1984.
124. **Hebbel, R. P., Yamada, O., Moldow, C. F., Jacob, H. S., White, J. G., and Eaton, J. W.,** Abnormal adherence of sickle erythrocytes to cultured vascular endothelium. Possible mechanism for microvascular occlusion in sickle cell disease, *J. Clin. Invest.,* 65, 154, 1980.
125. **Mohandas, N. and Evans, E.,** Adherence of sickle erythrocytes to vascular endothelial cells: Requirement for both cell membrane changes and plasma factors, *Blood,* 64, 282, 1984.
126. **Schwartz, R. S., Tanaka, Y., Fidler, I. J., Chiu, D. T.-U., Lubin, B., and Schroit, A. J.,** Increased adherence of sickled and phosphatidylserine-enriched human erythrocytes to cultured human peripheral blood monocytes, *J. Clin. Invest.,* 75, 1965, 1985.
127. **Franck, P. F. H., Op den Kamp, J. A. F., Lubin, B., Berendsen, W., Joosten, P., Briët, E., van Deenen, L. L. M., and Roelofsen, B.,** Abnormal transbilayer mobility of phosphatidylcholine in hereditary pyropoikylocytosis reflects the increased heat sensitivity of the membrane skeleton, *Biochim. Biophys. Acta,* 815, 259, 1985.
128. **Liu, S. C., Palek, J., Prchal, J., and Castleberry, R. P.,** Altered spectrin dimer-dimer association and instability of erythrocyte membrane skeletons in hereditary pyropoikylocytosis, *J. Clin. Invest.,* 68, 597, 1981.
129. **Lawler, J., Liu, S. C., Palek, J., and Prchal, J.,** Molecular defects of spectrin in hereditary pyropoikylocytosis. Alterations in the trypsin-resistant domain involved in spectrin self-association, *J. Clin. Invest.,* 70, 1019, 1982.
130. **Van Meer, G., Gahmberg, C. G., Op den Kamp, J. A. F., and van Deenen, L. L. M.,** Phospholipid distribution in human En(a-) red cell membranes which lack the major sialoglycoprotein, glycophorin A, *FEBS Lett.,* 135, 53, 1981.
131. **Kuypers, F. A., van Linde-Sibenius Trip, M., Roelofsen, B., Op den Kamp, J. A. F., Tanner, M. J. A., and Anstee, D. J.,** The phospholipid organization in the membranes of McLeod and Leach phenotype erythrocytes, *FEBS Lett.,* 184, 20, 1985.
132. **Kuypers, F., van Linde-Sibenius Trip, M., Roelofsen, B., Tanner, M. J. A., Anstee, D. J., and Op den Kamp, J. A. F.,** Rh_{null} human erythrocytes have an abnormal membrane phospholipid organization, *Biochem. J.,* 221, 931, 1984.
133. **Zwaal, R. F. A. and Hemker, H. C.,** Blood cell membranes and haemostasis, *Haemostasis,* 11, 12, 1982.
134. **Zwaal, R. F. A. and Bevers, E. M.,** Platelet phospholipid asymmetry and its significance in hemostasis, in *Subcellular Biochemistry,* Roodyn, D. B., Ed., Plenum Press, New York, 1983, chap. 4.
135. **Comfurius, P., Bevers, E. M., and Zwaal, R. F. A.,** The involvement of cytoskeleton in the regulation of transbilayer movement of phospholipids in human blood platelets, *Biochim. Biophys. Acta,* 815, 143, 1985.
136. **Bergelson, L. D., Molotkovsky, J. G., and Manevich, Y. M.,** Lipid-specific fluorescent probes in studies of biological membranes, *Chem. Phys. Lipids,* 37, 165, 1985.
137. **Metcalf, T. N., III, Wang, J. L., and Schindler, M.,** Lateral diffusion of phospholipids in the plasma membrane of soybean protoplasts: evidence for membrane lipid domains, *Proc. Natl. Acad. Sci. U.S.A.,* 83, 95, 1986.
138. **Thompson, T. E. and Tillack, T. W.,** Organization of glycosphingolipids in bilayers and plasma membranes of mammalian cells, *Annu. Rev. Biophys. Biophys. Chem.,* 14, 361, 1985.
139. **Karnovsky, M. J., Kleinfeld, A. M., Hoover, R. L., and Klausner, R. D.,** The concept of lipid domains in membranes, *J. Cell Biol.,* 94, 1, 1982.
140. **Wolf, D. E. and Voglmayer, J. K.,** Diffusion and regionalization in membranes of maturing ram spermatozoa, *J. Cell Biol.,* 98, 1678, 1984.
141. **Shukla, S. D. and Hanahan, D. J.,** Identification of domains of phosphatidylcholine in human erythrocyte plasma membranes. Differential action of acidic and basic phospholipases A_2 from Agkistrodon halys blomhoffii, *J. Biol. Chem.,* 257, 2908, 1982.
142. **Vaz, W. L. C., Goodsaid-Zalduondo, F., and Jacobson, K.,** Lateral diffusion of lipids and proteins in bilayer membranes, *FEBS Lett.,* 174, 199, 1984.
143. **Clegg, R. M. and Vaz, W. L. C.,** Translational diffusion of proteins and lipids in artificial lipid bilayer membranes. A comparison of experiment with theory, in *Progress in Protein-Lipid Interactions,* Vol. 1, Watts, A. and de Pont, J. J. H. H. M., Eds., Elsevier, Amsterdam, 1985, 173.
144. **Goldstein, J. L., Brown, M. S., Andersen, R. G. W., Russell, D. W., and Schneider, W. J.,** Receptor mediated endocytosis, *Annu. Rev. Cell Biol.,* 1, 1, 1985.
145. **Mahley, R. W.,** Atherogenic hyperlipoproteinemia: the cellular and molecular biology of plasma lipoproteins altered by dietary fat and cholesterol, *Med. Clin. North Am.,* 66, 375, 1982.

146. **Heiss, G., Johnson, N. J., Reiland, S., Davis, C. E., and Tyroler, H. A.,** The epidemology of plasma high density lipoprotein cholesterol levels. The lipid research clinics program prevalence study. Summary, *Circulation,* 62, 116, 1980.
147. **Mahley, R. W., Innerarity, T. L., Rall, S. C., and Weisgraber, K. H.,** Plasma lipoproteins: apolipoprotein structure and function, *J. Lipid Res.,* 25, 1277, 1984.
148. **Owen, J. S. and McIntyre, N.,** Plasma lipoprotein metabolism and lipid transport, *Trends Biochem. Sci.,* 7, 95, 1982.
149. **Owen, J. S., McIntyre, N., and Gillett, M. P. T.,** Lipoproteins, cell membranes and cellular functions, *Trends Biochem. Sci.,* 9, 238, 1984.
150. **Roelofsen, B.,** The (non)specificity in the lipid-requirement of calcium- and (sodium plus potassium)-transporting adenosine triphosphatases, *Life Sci.,* 29, 2235, 1981.
151. **Warren, G. B., Toon, P. A., Birdsall, N. J. M., Lee, A. G., and Metcalfe, J. C.,** Complete control of the lipid environment of membrane-bound proteins: application to a calcium transport system, *FEBS Lett.,* 41, 122, 1974.
152. **Warren, G. B., Toon, P. A., Birdsall, N. J. M., Lee, A. G., and Metcalfe, J. C.,** Reversible lipid titrations of the activity of pure adenosine triphosphatase-lipid complexes, *Biochemistry,* 13, 5501, 1974.
153. **Racker, E.,** Reconstitution of membrane processes, *Methods Enzymol.,* 55, 699, 1979.
154. **Darszon, A., Vandenberg, C. A., Ellisman, M. H., and Montal, M.,** Incorporation of membrane proteins into large single bilayer vesicles. Application to rhodopsin, *J. Cell Biol.,* 81, 446, 1979.
155. **Hokin, L. E.,** Reconstitution of "carriers" in artificial membranes, *J. Membr. Biol.,* 60, 77, 1981.
156. **Eytan, G. D.,** Use of liposomes for reconstitution of biological functions, *Biochim. Biophys. Acta,* 694, 185, 1982.
157. **Levitzki, A.,** Reconstitution of membrane receptor systems, *Biochim. Biophys. Acta,* 822, 127, 1985.
158. **Allen, T. M., Romans, A. Y., Kercret, H., and Segrest, J. P.,** Detergent removal during membrane reconstitution, *Biochim. Biophys. Acta,* 601, 328, 1980.
159. **Darmon, A., Zangvill, M., and Cabantchik, Z. I.,** New approaches for the reconstitution and functional assay of membrane transport proteins. Application to the anion transporter of human erythrocytes, *Biochim. Biophys. Acta,* 727, 77, 1983.
160. **Van der Steen, A. T. M., Tarashi, T. F., Voorhout, W. F., and de Kruijff, B.,** Barrier properties of glycophorin-phospholipid systems prepared by different methods, *Biochim. Biophys. Acta,* 733, 51, 1983.
161. **Marsh, D.,** ESR spin label studies of lipid-protein interactions, in *Progress in Protein-Lipid Interactions,* Vol. 1, Watts, A. and de Pont, J. J. H. H. M., Eds., Elsevier, Amsterdam, 1985, 143.
162. **Chapman, D. and Hayward, J. A.,** New biophysical techniques and their application to the study of membranes, *Biochem. J.,* 228, 281, 1985.
163. **Deese, A. J. and Dratz, E. A.,** Carbon-13 and proton NMR studies of the interactions of lipids with membrane proteins, in *Progress in Protein-Lipid Interactions,* Vol. 2, Watts, A. and de Pont, J. J. H. H. M., Eds., Elsevier, Amsterdam, 1985, 45.
164. **Bloom, M. and Smith, I. C. P.,** Manifestations of lipid-protein interactions in deuterium NMR, in *Progress in Protein-Lipid Interactions,* Vol. 1, Watts, A. and de Pont, J. J. H. H. M., Eds., Elsevier, Amsterdam, 1985, 61.
165. **Mendelsohn, R. and Mantsch, H. H.,** Fourier transform infrared studies of lipid-protein interaction, in *Progress in Protein-Lipid Interactions,* Watts, A. and de Pont, J. J. H. H. M., Eds., Elsevier, Amsterdam, 1985, 103.
166. **Bisson, R. and Montecucco, C.,** Use of photoreactive phospholipids for the study of lipid-protein interactions, in *Progress in Protein-Lipid Interactions,* Vol. 1, Watts, A. and de Pont, J. J. H. H. M., Eds., Elsevier, Amsterdam, 1985, 259.
167. **Schatzmann, H. J.,** Lipoprotein nature of red cell adenosine triphosphatase, *Nature,* 196, 677, 1962.
168. **Roelofsen, B. and van Deenen, L. L. M.,** Lipid requirement of membrane-bound ATPase. Studies on human erythrocyte ghosts, *Eur. J. Biochem.,* 40, 245, 1973.
169. **Mandersloot, J. G., Roelofsen, B., and de Gier, J.,** Phosphatidylinositol as the endogenous activator of the (Na^+ + K^+)-ATPase in microsomes of rabbit kidney, *Biochim. Biophys. Acta,* 508, 478, 1978.
170. **Roelofsen, B. and van Linde-Sibenius Trip, M.,** The fraction of phosphatidylinositol that activates the (Na^+ + K^+)-ATPase in rabbit kidney microsomes is closely associated with the enzyme protein, *Biochim. Biophys. Acta,* 647, 302, 1981.
171. **Cornelius, F. and Skou, J. C.,** Reconstitution of (Na^+ + K^+)-ATPase in phospholipid vesicles with full recovery of its specific activity, *Biochim. Biophys. Acta,* 772, 357, 1984.
172. **Brotherus, J. R., Griffith, O. H., Brotherus, M. O., Jost, P. C., Silvius, J. R., and Hokin, L. E.,** Lipid-protein multiple binding equilibria in membranes, *Biochemistry,* 20, 5261, 1981.
173. **Zachowsky, A. and Devaux, P. F.,** Non-uniform distribution of phospholipids in (Na^+ + K^+)-ATPase-rich membranes from Torpedo Marmorata electric organ evidenced by spin-spin interactions between spin-labeled phospholipids, *FEBS Lett.,* 163, 245, 1983.

174. **Roelofsen, B. and Schatzmann, H. J.,** The lipid requirement of the (Ca^{2+} + Mg^{2+})-ATPase in the human erythrocyte membrane, as studied by various highly purified phospholipases, *Biochim. Biophys. Acta,* 464, 17, 1977.
175. **Gietzen, K., Tejcka, M., and Wolf, H. U.,** Calmodulin affinity chromatography yields a functional purified erythrocyte (Ca^{2+} + Mg^{2+})-dependent adenosine triphosphatase, *Biochem. J.,* 189, 81, 1980.
176. **Niggli, V., Adunyah, E. S., Penniston, J. T., and Carafoli, E.,** Purified (Ca^{2+} + Mg^{2+})-ATPase of the erythrocyte membrane. Reconstitution and effect of calmodulin and phospholipids, *J. Biol. Chem.,* 256, 395, 1981.
177. **Niggli, V., Penniston, J. T., and Carafoli, E.,** Purification of the (Ca^{2+} + Mg^{2+})-ATPase from human erythrocyte membranes using a calmodulin affinity column, *J. Biol. Chem.,* 254, 9955, 1979.
178. **De Metz, M., Lebret, M., Enouf, J., and Lévy-Tolédano, S.,** The phospholipid requirement of the (Ca^{2+} + Mg^{2+})-ATPase from human platelets, *Biochim. Biophys. Acta,* 770, 159, 1984.
179. **Hesketh, T. R., Smith, G. A., Houslay, M. D., McGill, K. A., Birdsall, N. J. M., Metcalfe, J. C., and Warren, G. B.,** Annular lipids determine the ATPase activity of a calcium-transport protein complexed with dipalmitoyllecithin, *Biochemistry,* 15, 4145, 1976.
180. **Dean, W. L. and Tanford, C.,** Properties of a delipidated, detergent-activated Ca^{2+}-ATPase, *Biochemistry,* 17, 1683, 1978.
181. **Yeagle, P. L.,** Cholesterol modulation of (Na^+ + K^+)-ATPase ATP hydrolyzing activity in the human erythrocyte, *Biochim. Biophys. Acta,* 727, 39, 1983.
182. **Harris, W. E.,** Modulation of (Na^+ + K^+)-ATPase activity by the lipid bilayer examined with dansylated phosphatidylserine, *Biochemistry,* 24, 2873, 1985.
183. **Marcus, M. M., Apell, H. J., Roudna, M., Schwendener, R. A., Weder, H. G., and Lauger, P.,** (Na^+ + K^+)-ATPase in artificial lipid vesicles: influence of lipid structure on pumping rate, *Biochim. Biophys. Acta,* 854, 270, 1986.
184. **Moore, B. M., Lentz, B. R., Hoechli, M., and Meissner, G.,** Effect of lipid membrane structure on the adenosine 5′-triphosphate hydrolyzing activity of the calcium-stimulated adenosine triphosphatase of sarcoplasmic reticulum, *Biochemistry,* 20, 6810, 1981.
185. **Navarro, J., Toivio-Kinnucan, M., and Racker, E.,** Effect of lipid composition on the calcium/adenosine 5′-triphosphate coupling ratio of the Ca^{2+}-ATPase of sarcoplasmic reticulum, *Biochemistry,* 23, 130, 1984.
186. **Almeida, L. M., Vaz, W. L. C., Zachariasse, K. A., and Madeira, V. M. C.,** Modulation of sarcoplasmic reticulum Ca^{2+}-pump activity by membrane fluidity, *Biochemistry,* 23, 4714, 1984.
187. **Lentz, B. R., Moore, B. M., Kirkman, C., and Meissner, G.,** Lipid-protein interactions in sarcoplasmic reticulum. A disrupted secondary lipid layer surrounds the Ca^{2+}-ATPase, *Biophys. J.,* 37, 30, 1982.
188. **Lentz, B. R., Clubb, K. W., Alford, D. R., Höchli, M., and Meissner, G.,** Phase behavior of membranes reconstituted from dipentadecanoylphosphatidylcholine and the Mg^{2+}-dependent, Ca^{2+}-stimulated adenosine-triphosphatase of sarcoplasmic reticulum: evidence for a disrupted lipid domain surrounding protein, *Biochemistry,* 24, 433, 1985.
189. **Seelinsky, B. S. and Yeagle, P. L.,** Two populations of phospholipids exist in sarcoplasmic reticulum and in recombined membranes containing Ca-ATPase, *Biochemistry,* 23, 2281, 1984.
190. **East, J. M., Melville, D., and Lee, A. G.,** Exchange rates and numbers of annular lipids for the calcium and magnesium ion dependent adenosine-triphosphatase, *Biochemistry,* 24, 2615, 1985.
191. **Johannsson, A., Smith, G. A., and Metcalfe, J. C.,** The effect of bilayer thickness on the activity of (Na^+ + K^+)-ATPase, *Biochim. Biophys. Acta,* 641, 416, 1981.
192. **Johannsson, A., Keightley, C. A., Smith, G. A., Richards, C. D., Hesketh, T. R., and Metcalfe, J. C.,** The effect of bilayer thickness and *n*-alkenes on the activity of the (Ca^{2+} + Mg^{2+})-dependent ATPase of sarcoplasmic reticulum, *J. Biol. Chem.,* 256, 1643, 1981.
193. **Farmer, B. T., Harmon, T. M., and Butterfield, D. A.,** ESR studies of the erythrocyte membrane skeletal protein network: influence of the state of aggregation of spectrin on the physical state of membrane proteins, bilayer lipids, and cell surface carbohydrates, *Biochim. Biophys. Acta,* 821, 420, 1985.
194. **Anderson, R. A. and Marchesi, V. T.,** Regulation of the association of membrane skeletal protein 4.1 with glycophorin by a polyphosphoinositide, *Nature,* 318, 295, 1985.
195. **Dale, G. L.,** Phosphatidylinositol 4-phosphate kinase is associated with the membrane skeleton in human erythrocytes, *Biochem. Biophys. Res. Commun.,* 133, 189, 1985.
196. **Ferrel, J. E. and Huestis, W. H.,** Phosphoinositide metabolism and the morphology of human erythrocytes, *J. Cell Biol.,* 98, 1992, 1984.
197. **Giraud, F., M'Zali, H., Chailley, B., and Mazet, F.,** Changes in morphology and in polyphosphoinositide turnover of human erythrocytes after cholesterol depletion, *Biochim. Biophys. Acta,* 778, 191,1984.
198. **Nishizuka, Y.,** Turnover of inositol phospholipids and signal transduction, *Science,* 225, 1365, 1984.
199. **Berridge, M. J.,** Inositol triphosphate and diacylglycerol as second messengers, *Biochem. J.,* 220, 345, 1984.
200. **Ashendel, C. L.,** The phorbol ester receptor: a phospholipid-regulated protein kinase, *Biochim. Biophys. Acta,* 822, 219, 1985.

201. **Hokin, L. E.,** Receptors and phosphoinositide-generated second messengers, *Annu. Rev. Biochem.*, 54, 205, 1985.
202. **Brenner, R. R.,** Effect of unsaturated acids on membrane structure and enzyme kinetics, *Prog. Lipid Res.*, 23, 69, 1984.
203. **Spector, A. A. and Yorek, M. A.,** Membrane lipid composition and cellular function, *J. Lipid Res.*, 26, 1015, 1985.
204. **Kuypers, F. A., Roelofsen, B., Op den Kamp, J. A. F., and van Deenen, L. L. M.,** The membrane of human erythrocytes tolerates only limited changes in the fatty acid composition of its phosphatidylcholine, *Biochim. Biophys. Acta,* 769, 337, 1984.
205. **Wirtz, K. W. A. and van Deenen, L. L. M.,** Phospholipid-exchange proteins: a new class of intracellular lipoproteins, *Trends Biochem. Sci.*, 2, 49, 1977.
206. **Lange, L. G., van Meer, G., Op den Kamp, J. A. F., and van Deenen, L. L. M.,** Haemolysis of rat erythrocytes by replacement of the natural phosphatidylcholine by various phosphatidylcholines, *Eur. J. Biochem.*, 110, 115, 1980.
207. **Kuypers, F. A., Roelofsen, B., Berendsen, W., Op den Kamp, J. A. F., and van Deenen, L. L. M.,** Shape changes in human erythrocytes induced by replacement of the native phosphatidylcholine with species containing various fatty acids, *J. Cell Biol.*, 99, 2260, 1984.
208. **Op den Kamp, J. A. F., Roelofsen, B., and van Deenen, L. L. M.,** Structural and dynamic aspects of phosphatidylcholine in the human erythrocyte membrane, *Trends Biochem. Sci.*, 10, 3206, 1985.
209. **Kuypers, F. A., Easton, E. W., van den Hoven, R., Wensing, T., Roelofsen, B., Op den Kamp, J. A. F., and van Deenen, L. L. M.,** Survival of rabbit and horse erythrocytes in vivo after changing fatty acyl composition of their phosphatidylcholine, *Biochim. Biophys. Acta,* 819, 170, 1985.
210. **Benga, G. and Holmes, R. P.,** Interactions between components in biological membranes and their implications for membrane function, *Prog. Biophys. Mol. Biol.*, 43, 195, 1984.
211. **Middelkoop, E., Lubin, B. H., Bevers, E. M., Op den Kamp, J. A. F., Comfurius, P., Chiu, D. T.-Y., Zwaal, R. F. A., van Deenen, L. L. M., and Roelofsen, B.,** Studies on sickled erythrocytes demonstrate that the asymmetric distribution of phosphatidylserine in the red cell membrane is maintained by both its ATP-dependent translocation to the inner monolayer and its interaction with the membrane skeleton, *Biochim. Biophys. Acta,* 937, 281, 1988.
212. **Richardson, S. G. N., Matthews, K. B., Stuart, J., Geddes, A. M., and Wilcox, R. M.,** Serial changes in coagulation and viscosity in sickle cell crisis, *Br. J. Haematol.*, 41, 95, 1979.
213. **Hebbel, R. P., Schwartz, R. S., and Mohandas, N.,** The adhesive sickle erythrocyte: cause and consequences of abnormal interactions with endothelium, monocytes/macrophages and model membranes, *Clin. Haematol.*, 14, 141, 1985.
214. **McEvoy, L., Williamson, P., and Schlegel, R. A.,** Membrane phospholipid asymmetry as a determinant of erythrocyte recognition by macrophages, *Proc. Natl. Acad. Sci. U.S.A.*, 83, 3311, 1986.
215. **Schlegel, R. A., Prendergast, T. W., and Williamson, P.,** Membrane phospholipid asymmetry as a factor in erythrocyte-endothelial interactions, *J. Cell. Physiol.*, 123, 215, 1985.
216. **Smith, B. D. and La Celle, P. L.,** Erythrocyte-endothelial cell adherence in sickle cell disorders, *Blood,* 68, 1050, 1986.
217. **Embury, S. H.,** The clinical pathophysiology of sickle cell disease, *Annu. Rev. Med.*, 37, 361, 1986.

Chapter 3

INTRODUCTION TO BLOOD PLATELETS

Jan Willem N. Akkerman

TABLE OF CONTENTS

I. INTRODUCTION

Platelets are small, disc-shaped cells that are extremely responsive to alterations in the surrounding medium. Under normal conditions the cells circulate in an inactive, dormant state until they are removed from circulation. The contact with components from the vessel wall, activated coagulation factors, immune complexes, and nonphysiological surfaces suddenly transforms them into dynamic units that within a few minutes change in shape, release a great number of vasoactive substances, and stick together. An important role in preventing platelet activation is played by the endothelial cells which cover the inner side of the vessel wall. These cells prevent the contact with subendothelial structures to which platelets are highly responsive, but also release substances that keep the platelets in an inactive state.

When a vessel wall is disrupted, the coagulation mechanism is activated and platelets are stimulated to form a hemostatic plug. One of the first steps in the formation of a platelet plug is the contact with collagen fibers in the subendothelium. Platelets stick to the fibers with the help of the von Willebrand Factor (vWF), a protein that circulates in a complex with coagulation factor VIII. Following adherence, the cells lose the disc shape, spread along the fibers, and form pseudopods which help them to stick to the fibers. Concurrently thrombin is formed, which, apart from many functions in the coagulation system, functions as a potent platelet activator. The activated platelets liberate chemical messengers that stimulate adjacent platelets to participate and stick together, forming aggregates that fill up the wound. The hemostatic plug is then strengthened by fibrin fibers and contracts, thereby effectively preventing further blood loss.

The formation of a hemostatic plug in the skin, as standardized in the Mielke bleeding time, takes less than 7 min. A shortage of circulating platelets seriously retards the cessation of bleeding and values of 20 min or more in thrombocytopenic patients are no exception. Prolonged bleeding times are also seen in patients with impaired platelet functions, indicating that a normal bleeding time requires normal numbers of well-functioning platelets. An exception is von Willebrand Disease, where an increased bleeding tendency is found due to a deficiency of the vWF, despite the fact that platelets are generally normal in number and behavior.

Although impaired platelet functions are a threat to life, overreacting platelets also form a risk factor. The slight but continuous alterations in the vessel wall leading to atherosclerosis are probably the sites where the hemostatic mechanism has been activated. The slight disturbances in the endothelial layer would permit the platelets to adhere and to secrete substances that penetrate into the vessel wall. The result is that smooth muscle cells are stimulated to migrate and proliferate, thereby decreasing the antihemostatic properties of the vessel wall. The thickening of the vessel wall is a further threat to blood circulation, which may be blocked completely when platelets release vasoconstricting substances. Thus, a platelet should maintain a balance between useful responsiveness to stimuli from a wound and unwanted overreaction to minor stimuli in the circulation. In the next sections a few aspects of this role will be discussed.

II. THROMBOPOIESIS

The first appearance of recognizable precursors of blood platelets is the formation of "blood islands" during the third week of human embryogenesis. These islands consist of mesenchymal cells and develop in two directions: (1) peripheral cells join and form a primitive vascular system and (2) central cells form yolk sac stem cells, some differentiating into primitive erythroblasts that do not reach maturation. During the 3rd month of gestation, these stem cells migrate to the liver, which then becomes the main site of blood cell production. In the 4th month, bone marrow hematopoiesis starts, which replaces the liver as the major source of blood cell production by the end of gestation.[1]

Hematopoiesis takes place in the marrow stroma. Matured hematopoietic cells gain access to sinusoids and release the blood cells. The first step in this process is the development of as yet poorly defined "stem cells", that are pluripotent and self-maintaining.[2] They form the basis of four cell lineages for the formation of erythrocytes, granulocytes-monocytes, lymphoid cells, and platelets. The next step is the formation of "committed stem cells", each type specific for one of the four cell lineages, and one being the precursor of the megakaryocytes. After a process of proliferation, maturation starts, in which endomitosis and cytoplasmic maturation occur in parallel, and megakaryoblasts are formed. The 2n stage develops into 4-, 8-, 16-, 32-, and even 64n stages. RNA production increases, filling the cytoplasm with polyribosomes, which give the cells a basophilic appearance. Finally, granules develop and maturation comes to completion.

Much new insight into this process has been gained since it became possible to grow megakaryocytes in culture.[3] The earliest recognizable form, called colony-forming unit for megakaryocytes (CFU-M), is probably close to the committed stem cell of the thrombopoietic lineage and develops into matured megakaryocytes in 2 to 3 weeks. Formation of colonies of megakaryocytes depends on at least two factors:[4-8] (1) a glycoprotein with an apparent molecular weight of 46,000 daltons called colony-stimulating factor (Meg-CSF), isolated from spleen, plasma, and certain cell lines that promotes the proliferation of the progenitor pool and may be closely related to Interleukin 3[6] and (2) a maturation promotor called thrombopoietin, present in urine and plasma from thrombopenic patients. Other factors may also be involved, such as erythropoietin and factors present in phytohemagglutinin-stimulated leukocyte-conditioned medium, which both promote megakaryocyte formation in vitro. Recently, an inhibitor of this process has been isolated from platelets, indicating that the mechanism of megakaryocyte production is subject to various control mechanisms.[2]

Several features that have so far been typical for platelets can be identified in megakaryocytes. Megakaryocytes contain platelet factor 4, β-thromboglobulin, and platelet-derived growth factor, and electron micrographs of more mature stages reveal the presence of dense-, α-, and lysosomal secretion granules.[9-11] The glycoproteins Ib and IIb-IIIa present in platelets are also located in megakaryocytes, together with fibrinogen, fibronectin, factor XIII, vWF, myosin, tubulin, and actin.[9-12] The cells have an active lipid, protein, and adenine nucleotide metabolism[13,14] and upon stimulation with platelet activating agents, they form prostaglandin metabolites such as thromboxane B_2, change in shape, and secrete the contents of the secretory granules.[15-17] Hence, many of the biochemical and functional characteristics of platelets are present in megakaryocytes.

It has been estimated that an adult person forms about 1.5×10^{11} platelets per day. Platelet formation occurs at any stage of megakaryocyte maturation, but the 16n stage contributes the major part, about 60%. There is a close coupling between mass (circulating platelets plus those present in the spleen) and the activity of the megakaryocytes, which respond to sudden stages of acute thrombocytopenia by an increase in number, ploidy, and volume and form platelets with a higher mean platelet volume than normal.[18] About 30% of the platelets is sequestered in the spleen, which accounts for the fact that only about 70% of reinfused labeled platelets can be recovered. The sequestered platelets are in dynamic equilibrium with the platelets in the circulation. Normally, the cells survive 8 to 10 days before being destructed in the reticuloendothelial system of the spleen, liver, and bone marrow. Platelet removal follows a pattern intermediate between an exponential disappearance curve, which is typical for random removal of young and old platelets, and a linear pattern, typical for senescent loss (multiple hit model).

III. MORPHOLOGY

A human platelet is a flat, discoid cell with numerous small openings at the cell surface. A transparent model of a platelet (Figure 1A) reveals that these openings are the exits of a

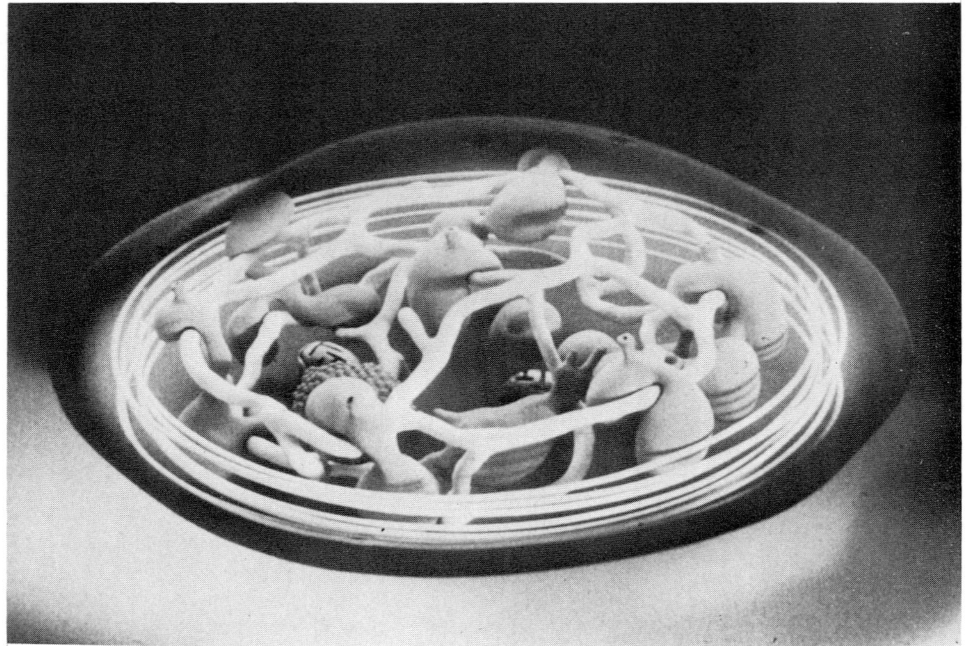

A

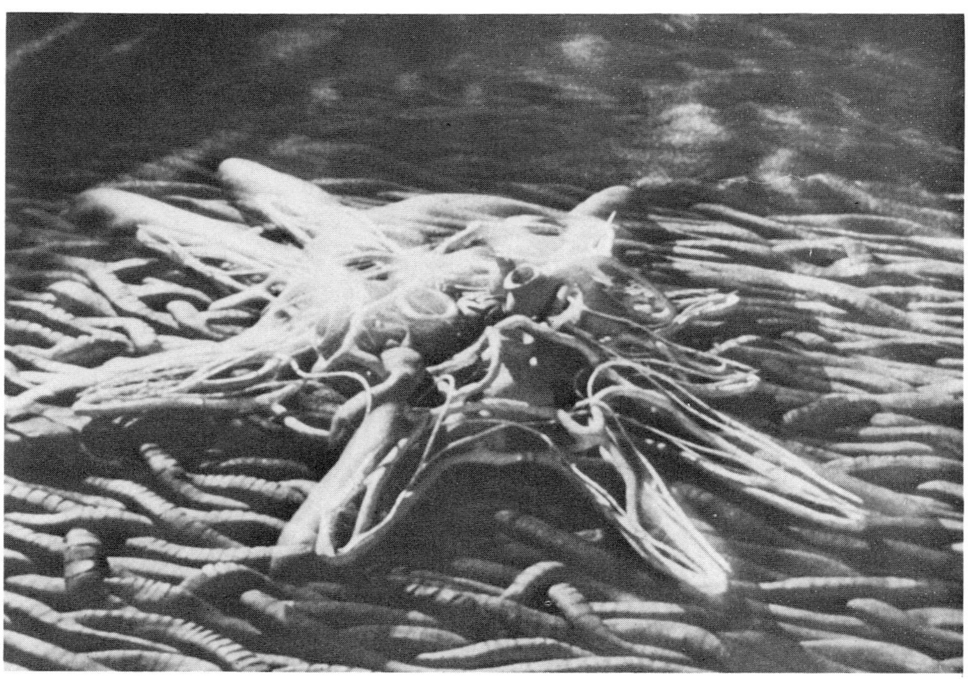

B

FIGURE 1. Model of a resting (A) and an activated (B) platelet. From the motion picture ''Blood Platelets. Fatal Effects of Their Function'' by Boehringer Ingelheim. (Reprinted with permission.)

branched canicular system surrounded by granules. Furthermore, a ring of microtubules is present, which preserves the disc shape, and areas with glycogen particles are seen together with a few mitochondria. When a platelet is activated (Figure 1B) the microtubules temporarily disappear and the cells lose the disc shape, forming long filopodia as well as broad-based pseudopodia filled up with microfilaments and microtubules. The secretion granules fuse with the canicular system, liberating the contents into the extracellular medium.

A more detailed structure is shown on transmission electron micrographs (Figure 2). According to the classification by White et al.,[19,20] four different compartments can be identified: the peripheral zone, the sol-gel zone, the organelle zone, and intracellular membrane systems. The peripheral zone contains the exterior coat or glycocalyx, an area on the membrane that is rich in glycoproteins and is the site of receptor and binding sites that are so important for processes such as adhesion and aggregation. The plasma membrane is a typical unit membrane with asymmetrically distributed phospholipids, which upon cell activation form the procoagulant activity described in detail elsewhere (Chapter 9). The area immediately beneath the membrane is never penetrated by organelles and appears to maintain the structure in which the signals generated by the receptors are translated to second messengers. The sol-gel zone constitutes the matrix of the cytoplasm and is built up of several fiber systems, including submembrane filaments, microtubules, and microfilaments, and provides the contractile system.

The organelle zone contains the secretion granules, peroxisomes, and mitochondria. Three different types of secretion granules can be identified: (1) the amine storage granules, or dense granules, named after the appearance as black dots on electron micrographs and containing several low molecular weight substances, (2) the α granules, which are the storage site of a great variety of proteins ranging from coagulation factors to platelet-specific proteins such as β-thromboglobulin, and (3) the lysosomal or acid hydrolase-containing granules, which in biochemical studies and congenital platelet abnormalities appear to exist in two subgroups. The peroxisomes are organelles specialized in oxidative reactions using molecular oxygen for the generation of H_2O_2. In addition to detoxification reactions, they catalyze the breakdown of fatty acids to acetyl CoA and contain the enzymes for synthesis of important ether phospholipids such as platelet-activating factor (PAF). The mitochondria contain the sequences for citric acid cycle, electron transport chain, synthesis, and catabolism of lipids, and form a major source of metabolic energy.

The membrane systems refer to two different structures. The surface-connecting open canalicular system (OCS) is the egress route for products from the secretion granules and originates from invaginations of the plasma membrane. The second structure, the dense tubular system (DTS), is analogous to the sarcoplasmatic reticulum of other cells and the site of Ca^{2+} sequestration and enzymes involved in prostanoid synthesis. Both membrane systems may form complexes.

IV. RECEPTORS AND BINDING SITES

The role of receptors and binding sites in the rapid cessation of bleeding requires that platelets be optimally responsive to external stimuli. Among the different platelet-activating substances are low molecular weight components such as ADP, proteins such as fibrillar collagen, but also substances normally not present in blood, e.g., immune complexes, glass surfaces, or air bubbles. For most of the physiological activators, specific receptors have been identified on the platelet plasma membrane.[21,22] The first step in receptor identification is binding studies with labeled ligands using intact cells and isolated membranes. Criteria for receptors are that binding of ligand is saturable, displacable, and specific. Receptor occupancy should affect cellular metabolism, thereby inducing or inhibiting certain responses. In platelets most of the receptors that have so far been identified only partly meet

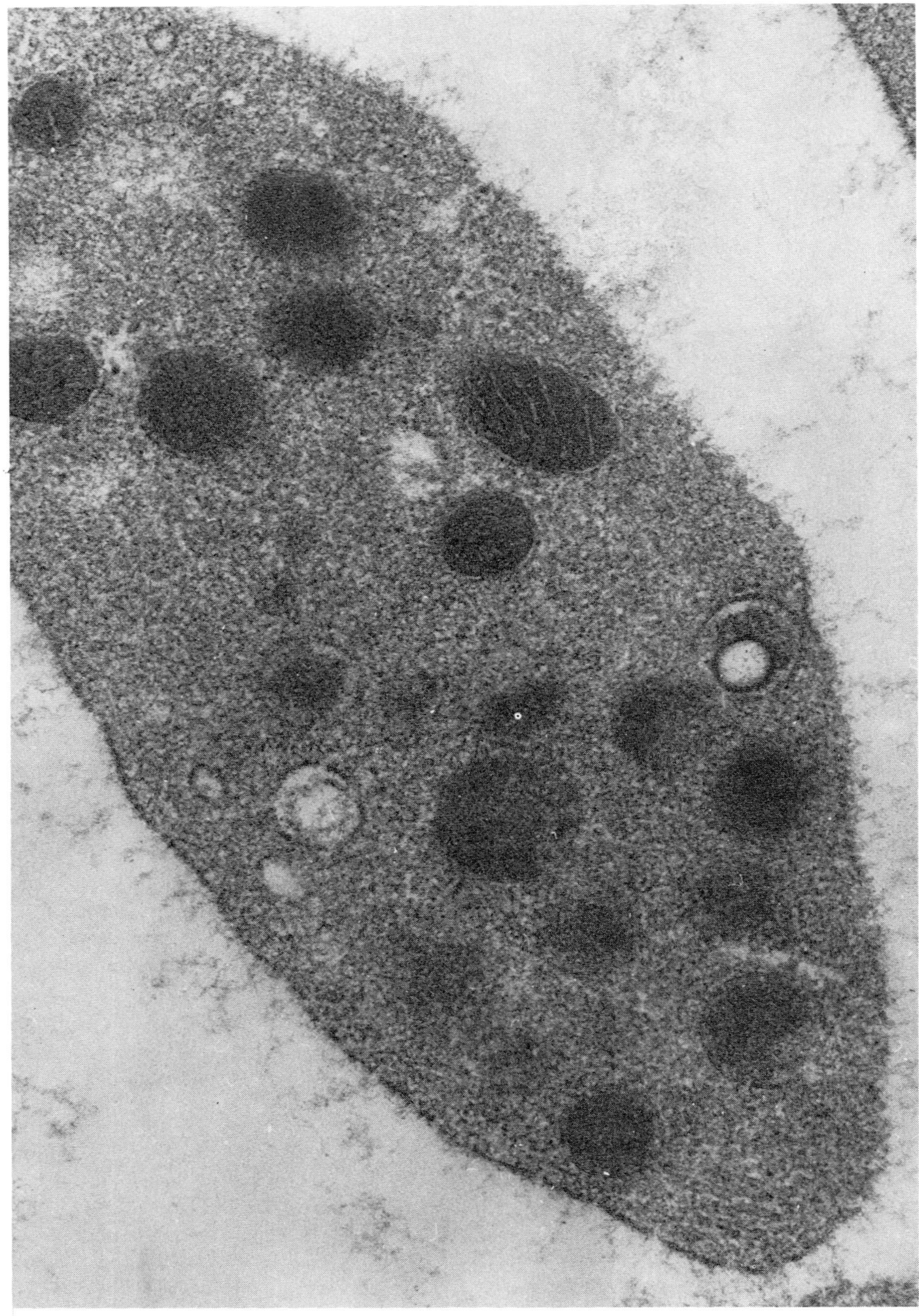

FIGURE 2. Transmission electron microscopy of a resting platelet. Magnification × 25,000. (Dr. J. J. Sixma, Department of Hematology, University Hospital Utrecht, The Netherlands.)

Table 1
RECEPTORS ON PLATELETS

First messenger	Numbers/ platelet	Kd	Properties	Ref.
ADP	30,000	5.5 μ*M*	Platelet activation	22—25
	500	100 n*M*	Coupled to AC (100 K; 61 K proteins?)	
Thrombin	50,000	100 n*M*	Binding ≠ activation	31, 32
	500	1 n*M*	(GPIb; GPV)	
Collagen	(600,000)	(1.7 μ*M*)	GPIa	38, 39
Adrenalin	200	1—4 n*M*	Binding + uptake coupled to AC (GP 64 K)	42—45
Serotonin	30—60	1 n*M*	Binding + uptake	48
PAF	240	0.06 n*M*	Binding + uptake (GP 180 K)	50—52
Vasopressin	15	1 n*M*	V1 (vascular) type coupled to Ca^{2+}_{in}	57—60
PGE_1-PGE_2-PGI_2	2,700	0.9 μ*M*	Coupled to AC	61—64
	90	3—12 n*M*		
PGD_2	210	53 n*M*	Coupled to AC	65, 66
Adenosine	—	—	Binding uptake	22
Fc	—	—	Latex + fibrinogen + IgG activation (GP IIIa)	70—72
vWF	—	—	GPIb	73
HDL	1,600	30 n*M*	Function uncertain	74, 75
LDL	7,100	40 n*M*	Coupled to AC (?)	74, 75
Insulin	570	3 n*M*	Function uncertain	77

these requirements. A major handicap is that binding studies are disturbed when the platelets aggregate, so they are, therefore, best carried out at 22°C in an unstirred suspension. In contrast, signal processing and the different functional responses are optimal at 37°C with stirring. Hence, comparisons between receptor-ligand interaction and platelet functions should be interpreted with caution.

Table 1 lists the properties of some of the most important receptors. Platelets contain at least two functionally different receptors for ADP. One type is involved in platelet activation while the other is coupled to adenylate cyclase, thereby inhibiting the formation of cyclic (c) AMP once the receptor is occupied. It has proven difficult to relate these different properties to the binding characteristics of ^{14}C-labeled ADP. An intact platelet binds about 30,000 molecules ^{14}C-ADP with a Kd of 5.5 μ*M*, which is close to the Km of shape change, suggesting that this type of binding is involved in platelet activation.[23] In contrast, 2-substituted derivatives, such as 2-azido ADP or 2-methylthio ADP, which also induce platelet functions, bind only at about 500 sites per platelet. This binding is inhibited by *p*-chloromercuribenzene sulfate, as is the activity of adenylate cyclase, suggesting that these sites are coupled to adenylate cyclase.[24,25] The receptor involved in platelet activation is specifically inhibited by 5′-*p*-fluorosulfonyl benzoyl-adenosine (FSBA), an effect that is antagonized by adrenaline.[26,27] Hence, the affinity of one receptor for the agonist can be increased by another receptor, making receptor-receptor interaction an important step in the regulation of cell activation.[28]

Binding studies with isolated membranes show that 200 to 1000 pmol ADP bind per milligram protein, but since many ADP binding proteins become accessible once the platelet is disrupted, components other than surface-oriented receptors such as actin and myosin may interfere. Despite these uncertainties, two ADP binding proteins with molecular weights of 100,000 and 61,000 daltons have been isolated and are possible candidates for either of the two classes of ADP-receptors.[21] Thrombin is one of the most potent platelet agonists, inducing aggregation and secretion in the nanomolar range. It is a crucial product of the coagulation cascade that not only forms fibrin clots, but also initiates platelet shape change, aggregation, secretion, contraction, and the generation of procoagulant activity. The well-known proteolytic activity is a requirement for platelet activation, as illustrated by the ineffectiveness of DIP-thrombin* and similar activating properties of other proteases. The mechanism by which thrombin activates platelets and, specifically, the role of proteolysis is poorly understood. Platelet-thrombin interaction is accompanied with proteolysis of a specific glycoprotein (GPV, M_r 82,000 daltons), thereby liberating a fragment designated GPV_{fl} (M_r 67,500 daltons).[29] Attempts to correlate the appearance of GPV_{fl} with platelet responses such as secretion, however, have been unsuccessful and a role for GPV in platelet activation is considered unlikely. A second candidate is glycoprotein Ib (M_r 160,000 daltons), which is partly deficient in platelets from patients with the Bernard-Soulier Syndrome. These platelets bind less ^{125}I-thrombin than normal cells. Under equilibrium conditions two types of binding can be found, differing about tenfold in affinity.[30-32] Although studies with purified glycoproteins confirm a role for GPIb as binding site, a function as a receptor is uncertain due to great discrepancies between binding properties and biological activities of a variety of thrombin derivatives. Using the technique of radiation inactivation, Harmon and Jamieson[33] identified three binding sites for thrombin. Two showed binding affinities beyond the range required for activation, but a 900,000-dalton binding site revealed a Kd (0.3 n*M*) that is more in the physiological range.

Studies with cholesterol-modified platelets[34] demonstrate a close correlation between the percentage of occupied thrombin receptors and platelet aggregation, suggesting that signal processing by the thrombin receptor follows the ''occupancy theory'', in which the degree of receptor occupancy determines the biological response. Similar findings have been obtained for insulin-induced α-aminoisobutyric acid influx in thymocytes,[35] in contrast with other receptors where the rate of agonist-binding is crucial for generating an effect. Bound thrombin can be neutralized by excess of hirudin, which rapidly abolishes secretion of dense, α-, and acid hydrolase granules. Hence, continuous receptor occupancy is required for normal secretion.[36,37]

Collagen fibers form a major constituent of the vessel wall. The localization immediately beneath the endothelial layer makes them a prime target for platelets when subendothelial layers become exposed. In combination with thrombin, collagen is a potent initiator of phosphatidylserine flip-flop leading to the generation of procoagulant activity of the plasma membrane (Chapter 8). Monomeric collagen consists of three polypeptide chains with a M_r of 100,000 daltons each, forming a triple helix. To date, eight different forms have been identified; with the exception of type II, all are present in the vessel wall. Collagen type I monomers, for instance, consist of two α1(I) and one α2(I) chain. Type III contains three α1(III) chains. Only the fibrillar insoluble forms have platelet-activating properties, forming an intrinsic difficulty for identifying collagen receptors by simple binding experiments. The few soluble forms which have retained some biological activity show a binding of 600,000 molecules per platelet.[38] This extremely high number is probably due to artifacts such as collagen-collagen interaction or implies that more than one type of glycoprotein may serve as a receptor.[21] Confusion exists regarding the nature of the collagen receptor, with studies showing a role for fibronectin (after exposure during α-granule secretion and subsequent binding to the plasma membrane), a M_r 65,000-dalton protein, or a glycosyl transferase.[21] Our recent discovery of a patient with a prolonged bleeding time, normal platelet responses towards all agonists except collagen, and complete failure to respond to collagen with signal processing, adhesion, aggregation, or secretion is therefore of special interest.[39] Those

* DIP: diisopropylphosphofluoridate.

platelets show a marked reduction in glycoprotein Ia, whereas other glycoproteins are normal. Hence, glycoprotein Ia may serve as a collagen receptor.

The receptor for adrenalin is a typical α-adrenergic receptor responding to catecholamines in the order adrenalin > noradrenalin > isoproterenol and which is antagonized by phentolamine, in contrast to β-adrenergic receptors which respond to isoproterenol > adrenalin > noradrenalin and are antagonized by propranolol. The adrenalin receptor is one of the few receptors that has been characterized in detail, including the mechanisms by which transmembrane signaling is carried out. The human platelet α-adrenergic receptor is a glycoprotein of M_r 64,000 daltons.[40] Receptor-ligand interaction induces a GTP-sensitive state, suggesting the involvement of GTP-sensitive proteins (G proteins) that mediate an activating (G_s) or inhibiting (G_i) signal to adenylate cyclase (see below). Depending on the nature of the ligand (the so-called "first messenger"), receptors coupled to G_s or to G_i proteins are activated, leading to an increase or decrease in cAMP, respectively. Since cAMP is an important modulator of other signal transducing mechanisms, activating signals can be inhibited or facilitated depending on the effect of the G proteins on adenylate cyclase. Reconstitution experiments using purified receptors, adenylate cyclase, G_s and G_i proteins, and liposomes show that receptor occupancy by adrenaline induces GTPase activity, an effect that is prevented by the α-adrenergic antagonist phentolamine via activation of the G_i-inhibitory protein.[41-45] Platelets are also susceptible to β-adrenergic agents and respond with the characteristics of cells possessing β2-adrenergic receptors.[46,47] Serotonin is mainly taken up and accumulated in the dense granules, although some degradation to indol acetic acid may occur by monoaminooxidase in the mitochondria. The few receptors identified on platelets are responsible for shape change and a slight, largely reversible aggregation.[48]

PAF, 1-*O*-alkyl-2-acetyl-sn-glycero-3-phosphocholine is one of the most potent platelet agonists, inducing shape change, aggregation, and secretion of dense-, α-, and acid hydrolase, containing granules at 0.1 to 1.0 n*M*.[49] Here, too, receptor studies are complicated by uptake and metabolism.[50-55] The receptors show a high affinity for the agonist and are presumably located on a M_r 180,000-dalton glycoprotein.[56] The rate with which PAF binds to the receptor determines the biological response.[51] Receptor affinity appears subject to control by Ca^{2+} channels[55] and can be differentiated into two subtypes on the basis of studies with inhibitors.

Vasopressin is a naturally occurring, hypothalamic peptide which controls free water clearance by the kidneys, increases glycogenolysis in hepatocytes, evokes a pressure response in arteriolar smooth muscle cells, and activates platelets. The platelet receptor is of the V1 type, which is coupled to Ca^{2+} translocation and induces the pressure response, in contrast to the V2 type, which is coupled to adenylate cyclase and takes part in the antidiuretic response.[57-60] The prostaglandins E_1, E_2, and especially I_2 (prostacyclin) are important inhibitors of platelet functions and raise cAMP via a common receptor, which shows two subtypes differing about tenfold in binding affinity.[61-65] Another inhibitor is PGD_2, which via a different receptor similarly inhibits platelet function.[66] Also, adenosine inhibits platelet activity via activation of adenylate cyclase.[22] Most of the adenosine is taken up and metabolized to ATP and ADP, making identification of a receptor difficult. The discrepancies between adenosine metabolism and the inhibition of platelet functions suggest that such a receptor must be present.

The activating properties of immune complexes (IgG) are mediated via binding to Fc-receptors,[67-71] probably located on glycoprotein IIIa.[72] The vWF circulates in a complex with coagulation factor VIII and is an essential adhesive protein in the adherence of platelets to subendothelial structures. It binds to glycoprotein Ib of activated platelets, through which further cell activation is mediated.[73] One of the results is the exposure of fibrinogen binding sites to which the vWF also couples, making quantitation of the role of PGIb difficult. Of specific interest is the binding of lipoproteins, in particular high-density lipoprotein (HDL) with antithrombotic properties, and low-density lipoprotein (LDL), which enhances thrombus formation.[74,75] LDL suppresses the increase in cAMP evoked by prostacyclin and at high concentrations induces platelet aggregation, but it is uncertain whether these are receptor-mediated responses.[76] A few reports describe the presence of insulin-binding sites on human platelets, but it is uncertain whether binding affects cell function.[77]

V. SIGNAL TRANSDUCTION

The coupling between an agonist and receptor triggers alterations in the plasma membrane that transfer the activating signals to the cytosol. This step is affected by the different physicochemical interactions of the membrane constituents that are generally summarized as membrane fluidity. Artificial enrichment of membrane cholesterol induces a more rigid membrane structure and enhances platelet responsiveness, leading to better aggregation and secretion.[78] This is accompanied by increased arachidonate mobilization and thromboxane B_2 formation.[79,80] In patients with hyperlipoproteinemia type IIa, a similar correlation between enhanced platelet functions and increased cholesterol content is seen.[81] When normal platelets interact with stimuli, changes in the anisotropy of lipophilic and protein-reactive fluorophores are seen, suggesting that rapid changes in the organization of the plasma membrane take place during the initial steps in platelet activation.[82] This may result in altered mobility of receptors and changes in the lateral pressure between enzymes and substrates, resulting in enhanced or diminished signal transduction.

A general scheme of current concepts on cell activation depicts a cAMP- and lipid/inositol-dependent pathway (Figure 3A and B). Both schemes start with binding of an agonist (the so-called first messenger) to the receptor, leading to the activation of transducing factors that modulate an amplifier capable of forming soluble second messengers from phosphorylated precursors. These second messengers transduce the signal from the plasma membrane to intracellular sites that are activated or inhibited either directly or after binding to internal effectors. In the cAMP-dependent pathway, the binding of a stimulatory or inhibitory first messenger to the specific receptors alters the conformation of specific transducers called G (or N) proteins, thereby making them susceptible to binding of GTP. This makes the proteins effectors of adenylate cyclase (''on reaction''), an effect that is terminated by the hydrolysis of GTP (''off reaction''). The result is activation or inhibition of adenylate cyclase, resulting in an increased or decreased cAMP content. A rise in cAMP inhibits platelet activation, whereas a decrease facilitates activation.

A great number of platelet receptors is coupled to adenylate cyclase (Table 1). This explains the strong inhibition of platelet functions by agents such as by prostaglandin E_1 and prostacyclin (PGI_2), which activate adenylate cyclase. On the other hand, adrenalin inhibits adenylate cyclase, and the receptors for PAF are also coupled to G_i proteins.[43,83] Inhibition of platelet activation by cAMP is mediated via the inhibitory effect on various steps in the activation mechanism, e.g., the liberation of arachidonate and the activation of actomyosin contractile activity. Although a low cAMP content facilitates platelet functions, a fall in cAMP alone is not a trigger for cell activation and the importance of the cAMP pathway lies predominantly in modulating the activation pathways evoked via other mechanisms.

In the lipid/inositol pathway membrane phospholipids, specifically phosphatidylinositol (PI) and the polyphosphates, are degraded upon receptor activation. As yet, no negative signals have been identified and the involvement of G proteins in this pathway in platelets is uncertain. Receptor activation leads to a rapid fall in PI, followed by reaccumulation above resting levels at later stages of activation.[84] This pattern clearly illustrates the activation of the PI-cycle (Figure 4).

More important than changes in PI is the formation of two intermediates in the cycle,

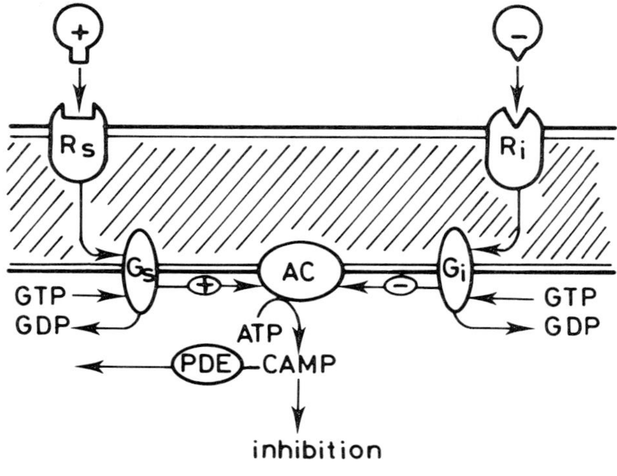

A

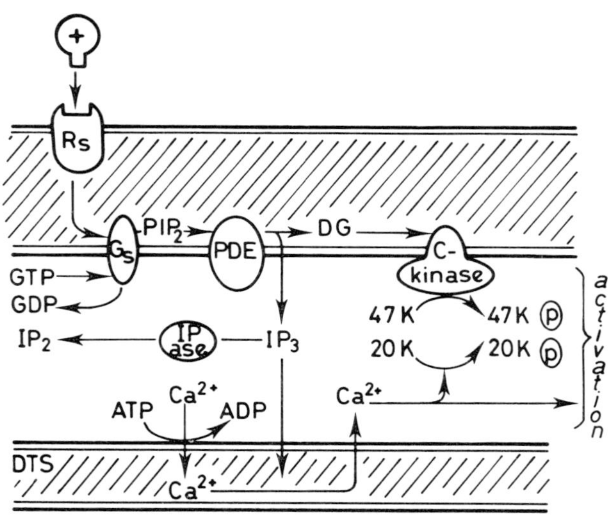

B

FIGURE 3. Stimulus response coupling in platelets. Shown are the cAMP pathway (A) and (B) the inositol/lipid pathway. Rs and Ri — receptors for stimulating or inhibitory signals, respectively, G proteins — GTP-sensitive proteins, AC — adenylate cyclase, PDE — phosphodiesterase, PIP_2 — phosphatidylinositolbisphosphate, DG — diacylglycerol, IPx — inositol phosphates, DTS — dense tubular system. (Adapted from Berridge, M. J., *Sci. Am.*, 253, 124, 1985.)

diacylglycerol and phosphatidic acid (PA). Diacylglycerol activates protein kinase C, leading to phosphorylation of a specific protein with M_r 47,000 daltons. The precise role is still uncertain, although phosphorylation appears essential for the secretion response.[85-87] PA has properties of a Ca^{2+}-ionophore and accumulation closely follows the formation of agonist-receptor complexes.[88] Receptor activation also triggers a rapid phosphodiesteratic cleavage of phosphatidylinositol 4,5-bisphosphate ($PI\text{-}P_2$), resulting in the formation of inositol 1,4,5 trisphosphate (IP_3). This soluble intermediate transduces the signal to the intracellular storage

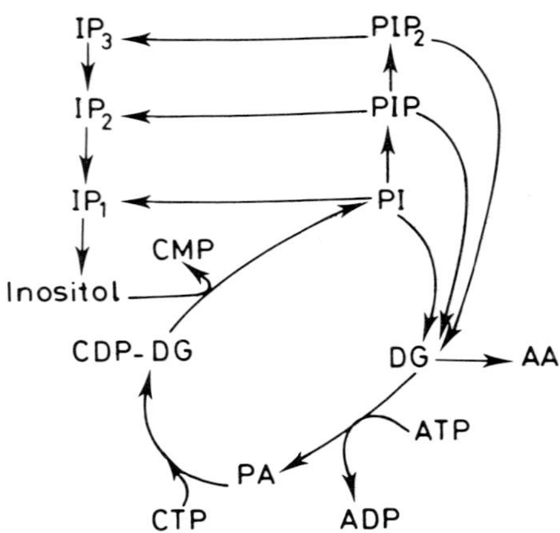

FIGURE 4. Phosphatidylinositol metabolism. Abbreviations as in Figure 3 and AA — arachidonate and PA — phosphatidic acid.

site for Ca^{2+} ions, the dense tubular system.[88,89] These membranes remove Ca^{2+} ions from the cytosol in an ATP-dependent process[90] and liberate them upon contact with IP_3.[91-94] This release is responsible for only part of the rise in cytosolic Ca^{2+} seen during activation (from about 10^{-7} to 10^{-6} *M*), the remainder being caused by influx of extracellular Ca^2 ions via — probably receptor-regulated — Ca^{2+} channels.[95,96] Cytosolic Ca^{2+}, either alone or after binding to calmodulin, plays a key role in platelet activation and has many and diverse effects, such as stimulation of arachidonate liberation via activation of phospholipase A_2, initiation of glycogen catabolism via glycogen phosphorylase, decreasing cAMP via activation of phosphodiesterase, and activation of contractile activity via the effect on myosin light chain kinase.[97-99] The concentration is under strict control by cAMP.[100]

Most of the steps discussed so far are probably more or less affected by changes in the cytosolic pH ($_pH_i$). Platelet activation is accompanied by an increase in $_pH_i$ as a result of efflux of protons in exchange for Na^+ via a specific antiporter.[101,102] This increase in $_pH_i$ greatly facilitates the influx of extracellular Ca^{2+}, as well as the mobilization of intracellular Ca^{2+}, thereby enhancing signal transduction.[102]

An important product of the PI cycle is arachidonic acid (Figure 5). This is the precursor of two important platelet activators, prostaglandin endoperoxides and thromboxane A2. The liberation is therefore an important step in signal transduction. About 90% of all arachidonate in the plasma membrane is located at the inner side, mainly in phosphatidylcholine (PC), phosphatidylethanolamine (PE), and PI. Liberation from PC and PE is mediated via phospholipase A2 in a Ca^{2+}-dependent reaction. In contrast, free arachidonate from PC and the PI cycle results from phospholipase C activity, which is less Ca^{2+} dependent.[103] Hence, the latter reaction may form the source of a small amount of arachidonate in the early phase of platelet activation when cytosolic Ca^{2+} is still low. Upon further activation, phospholipase A_2 may participate, forming the major part of the free arachidonate. Arachidonic acid is metabolized by lipoxygenase in the cytosol to the hydro(peroxy)eicosatetraenoic acids, H(P)ETEs. The reaction depends on reduced glutathion forming a link between the hexosemonophosphate shunt in carbohydrate metabolism and prostanoid metabolism. More important is the oxygenation of arachidonate to the endoperoxides by cyclooxygenase located in the dense tubular system. A minor part is further metabolized to PGD_2, PGE_2, and $PGF_{2\alpha}$, but the major part goes to thromboxane A_2, via catalysis by thromboxane synthetase located in the same membranes. PGG_2, PGH_2, and especially TxA_2 are potent platelet activators, probably acting via receptors of unknown localization. If the formation is abolished, for

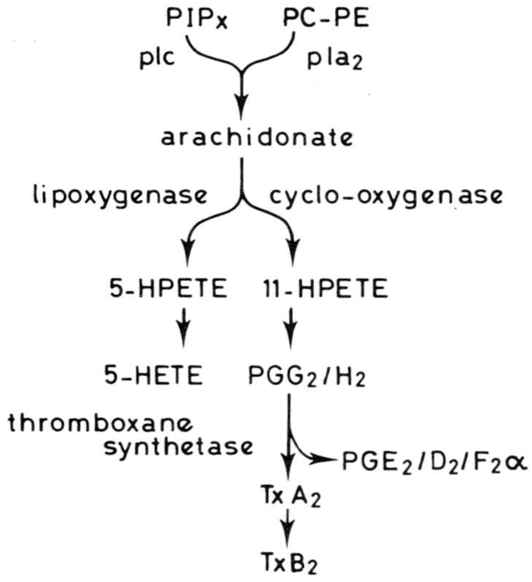

FIGURE 5. Arachidonate metabolism. PIPx — phosphatidylinositol-x-phosphates, PC and PE — phosphatidylcholine and -ethanolamine, H(P)ETE — hydro(peroxy)eicosatetraenoic acids, PG — prostaglandins, and Tx — thromboxanes.

example, by inhibiting cyclooxygenase with aspirin or thromboxane synthetase with imidazole, aggregation and secretion are suppressed and the hemostatic plug formation is retarded.

VI. CYTOSKELETON

The platelet cytoskeleton consists of microtubules and microfilaments. The microtubules appear in resting platelets as a bundle of 8 to 24 circular profiles, each 250 Å in diameter. They consist of polymerized tubulin that is in equilibrium with soluble heterodimers consisting of α and β subunits. The polymerized form is favored by a low cytosolic Ca^{2+} content and GTP, whereas an increase in Ca_i^{2+} shifts the equilibrium to the soluble form. This explains the disappearance of the tubules upon platelet activation. The typical discoid shape of the resting platelet is preserved by the bundle of microtubules. Upon activation the bundle contracts, moves to the center of the cells, and disappears. At the same time pseudopods are formed in which small bundles of polymerized tubulin appear.

The microfilaments are about 50 Å in diameter and form a highly branched network of tiny fibers. Under carefully controlled conditions, they precipitate in a Triton® extract and, depending on the conditions, a membrane skeleton can be discerned from the total cytoskeleton.[104-107] The Triton®-insoluble fraction contains actin, myosin, and the numerous proteins that regulate the different states in which actin is present in the cell (Figure 6A). Actin (mol wt 42,000 daltons) is present in two states, a globular form (G actin) consisting of soluble monomers, each carrying one mole of MgATP, and a fibrillar form (F actin), carrying MgADP.[108,109] The resting platelet continuously converts G to F actin and back, forming a cycle driven by ATP hydrolysis. This so-called "actin treadmilling" consumes as much as 50% of the energy in the resting cells.[110] Part of the G actin is coupled to profilin, forming a storage pool called profilactin. The rise in Ca^{2+} seen upon activation initiates the Ca^{2+}-calmodulin dependent shift of G to F actin, which forms gels, a process enhanced by filamin but retarded by gelsolin. Subsequently, the gels form different types of bundles, a process regulated by α-actinin and vinculin. This facilitates the interaction with myosin,

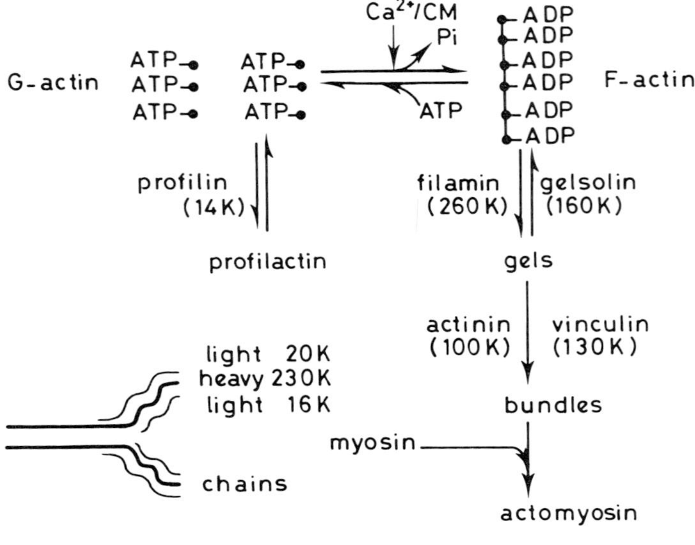

A

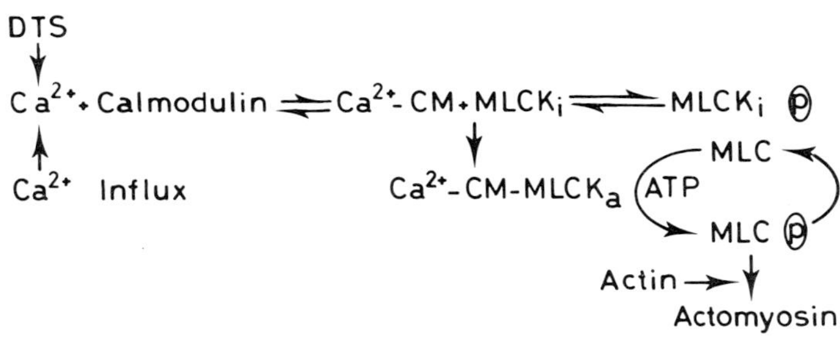

B

FIGURE 6. (A) Actomyosin formation. For details see text. CM — calmodulin. (B) Regulation of myosin light chain phosphorylation. MLCK — myosin light chain kinase, CM — calmodulin, and DTS — dense tubular system.

leading to actomyosin contractile activity and contraction of the platelet plug.[111] A prerequisite for myosin to interact with actin is that one of the constituents, the 20,000-dalton myosin light chain, is phosphorylated (Figure 6B). Also, this process is initiated by Ca^{2+}-calmodulin, which couples to inactive myosin light chain kinase (MLCK), thereby removing it from an extra inactive, phosphorylated storage form. A cAMP-dependent protein kinase catalyzes the rephosphorylation of MLCK. The activated MLCK catalyzes the phosphorylation of the 20,000-dalton light chain enabling the myosin complex (a dimer of one heavy chain and two different light chains) to interact with F actin.[99,112] Phosphorylation of MLC is one of the earliest events during platelet activation and parallels the shift of the discoidal shape to the spherical form.[99]

The composition of the cytoskeleton, as analyzed by the Triton®-insoluble fraction, greatly changes upon platelet activation. Apart from an increase in actin, myosin, actin-binding protein, α-actinin, and tropomyosin, typical membrane constituents appear that are absent in extracts from resting cells, such as glycoproteins Ib[113] and IIb-IIIa.[107] In addition, proteins that become bound to the surface of activated platelets (some secreted products, certain plasma proteins) also appear in the Triton®-insoluble fractions. These findings raise the possibility that, upon activation, the cytoskeleton undergoes a series of alterations that makes it an anchoring network to which specific membrane constituents can attach.[114-116] The role of the glycoprotein IIb-IIIa complex is especially of interest, since in the activated platelet this complex forms the binding site for fibrinogen, which links one platelet to another during the formation of platelet aggregates. A coupling with the cytoskeleton would provide the network that gives strength to an aggregate and through which contraction of the plug can take place.[104]

VII. PLATELET FUNCTIONS

Platelet shape change, aggregation, and secretion of granule components form essential steps in the cessation of bleeding. In a wound the first step in the formation of a platelet plug is probably the contact with collagen fibers that become exposed when the endothelial layer is disrupted. Collagen activates the platelet and induces pseudopod formation, aggregation, secretion, and — especially in combination with thrombin — the generation of procoagulant activity on the platelet surface. Platelet adhesion to the subendothelium at a high shear rate (>800 sec^{-1}) requires vWF, a polymeric glycoprotein (mol wt 2 to 20 $\times$ 10^6 daltons) that circulates in a complex with the antihemophilic factor, factor VIII.[117,118] The vWF binds to the vessel wall, thereby changing in conformation, and interacts with the platelet via binding to glycoprotein Ib.[119,120] A small but significant part of vWF is present in the subendothelial matrix and this also supports the adherence of the platelets.

Following adherence, two processes are initiated that accelerate the formation of the hemostatic plug: (1) prostaglandin-endoperoxides/thromboxane A_2 are formed and (2) the contents of the dense granules are secreted, liberating ADP that triggers other platelets to join the process. Binding sites for fibrinogen are then exposed, enabling fibrinogen to couple the platelets to one another and form aggregates that fill up the wound. Finally, the plug contracts, thereby closing the wound. Simultaneously, the coagulation cascade is initiated, leading to generation of thrombin, which greatly enhances platelet activation and — at later stages — induces formation of fibrin fibers that consolidate the plug.

Platelet aggregation is mediated via exposure of fibrinogen binding sites located on the glycoprotein (GP) IIb-IIIa complex.[121-123] The complex consists of almost equimolar concentrations of GPIIb (IIbα 125,000 and IIbβ 23,000 daltons) and GPIIIa (97,000 daltons) and is stabilized by Ca^{2+} ions. Prolonged incubation with EDTA, high temperature, low pH, or high ionic strength induces dissociation, which is accompanied by loss of fibrinogen binding. The regulation of binding site exposure is poorly understood. Most agonists activate the sites via secretion of ADP,[124] formation of PG-endoperoxides/thromboxane A_2,[125] or both,[126] a process which is inhibited by cAMP.[127] The number of exposed binding sites differs with the type of platelet stimulator, varying from about 40,000 with thrombin to about 80,000 per platelet with ADP.[123] Similarly, the binding properties are different with most agonists inducing only low affinity binding (Kd about 10^{-7} *M*), while PAF[126] and ADP[128] induce two types of binding differing about tenfold in affinity and number. In addition to traditional agonists such as ADP, fibrinogen binding sites can be exposed by treatment with low temperature, chymotrypsin, and dithiothreitol.[123] This type of exposure is not inhibited by cAMP or anticytoskeleton agents and may involve proteolysis of GPIIb-IIIa (chymotrypsin), a reduction of membrane disulfide bonds (dithiothreitol), and a change in membrane fluidity (low temperature). In contrast to the exposure of the sites, which at 22°C and maximal stimulation with PAF is complete within 2 to 5 min, the binding of fibrinogen to the exposed sites is rather slow and requires 30 min or more. In the absence of fibrinogen, exposed sites gradually become inaccessible to fibrinogen.[51]

A second stimulation again exposes binding sites, but whether or not this reflects opening

Table 2
SECRETION GRANULES

Dense granules	Storage ATP-ADP, serotonin, PPi, Pi, Ca^{2+}
α Granules	Proteins, e.g., platelet-specific proteins, coagulation factors, etc.
Lysosomal granules	Lysosomal enzymes, e.g., β-*N*-acetyl-D-glucosaminidase
	α Granules
Homologues of plasma proteins	Fibrinogen, fibronectin, albumin, factor V, plasminogen, HMW-kininogen, vWF, C1-inhibitor, Factor D + β1H globulin of the complement system, PA-inhibitor, α1 antitrypsin, α2-macroglobulin, α2-antiplasmin, antithrombin III, protein S, immunoglobin G
Platelet-specific	Platelet basic protein, β-thromboglobulin, platelet-derived growth factor, platelet factor 4
Others	Thrombospondin, vascular permeability factor, bactericidal factor, chemotactic factor, CFU-M-inhibitor

Note: Abbreviations used: PA — plasminogen activator, CFU-M — colony-forming unit for megakaryocytes.

and closing of a single class of sites is uncertain. Binding studies with fragments of the fibrinogen molecule have revealed which parts are important for aggregation. Platelet recognition sites have been located on the γ chain (397 to 411) and α chains of the fibrinogen molecule.[123]

Aggregation is enhanced by an endogenous lectin that is secreted from the α granules, thrombospondin. This 420,000-dalton protein consists of three identical chains, each containing sites for a variety of different properties, e.g., binding to heparin, fibronectin, fibrinogen, plasminogen, histidine-rich glycoprotein, type V collagen, calcium, and sulfated glycolipids. Apart from the presence in platelets, the protein has been detected in megakaryocytes, aortic smooth muscle cells, fibroblasts, endothelial cells, monocytes, and macrophages. The role in platelet aggregation is thought to be the reinforcement of the macromolecular complex of fibrinogen and GPIIb-IIIa, especially during the second phase of an optical aggregation curve.[129,130]

A great number of other proteins bind to activated platelets. Apart from fibrinogen, vWF[73] and fibronectin[131] bind to exposed GPIIb-IIIa, although the binding properties greatly favor the binding of fibrinogen. The three proteins form a class of adhesive proteins to which different types of binding sites that all recognize an Arg-Gly-Asp sequence can interact.[132]

Activated platelets bind high molecular weight kininogen,[133] plasminogen,[134] coagulation factors XIIIa,[135] XIa,[136] X, II,[137] and protein C.[138] It is uncertain, however, whether in each of these associations specific binding sites are involved or whether binding merely results from the exposure of negatively charged phospholipids.

The exposure of fibrinogen binding sites is, for a major part, mediated via secretion of ADP from the dense granules. Platelets have three types of secretion granules: dense, α, and lysosomal (Table 2). The dense granules are few in number and appear on electron micrographs as black round dots. They are the site of storage of ATP-ADP, in contrast with metabolic ATP-ADP that take part in the various energy-producing and -consuming sequences in the cell. The dense granule membrane is almost completely impermeable to these nucleotides or precursors. A deficiency in storage granules (''storage pool disease'') results in a bleeding tendency (as assessed by the Mielke bleeding time) that is proportional to the amount of dense granule ADP.[139]

The more abundant α granules contain a great variety of proteins, among which are coagulation factors, proteins of the complement and the fibrinolytic systems, and inhibitors of these cascades. A few of the proteins are specific for platelets, such as the heparin-

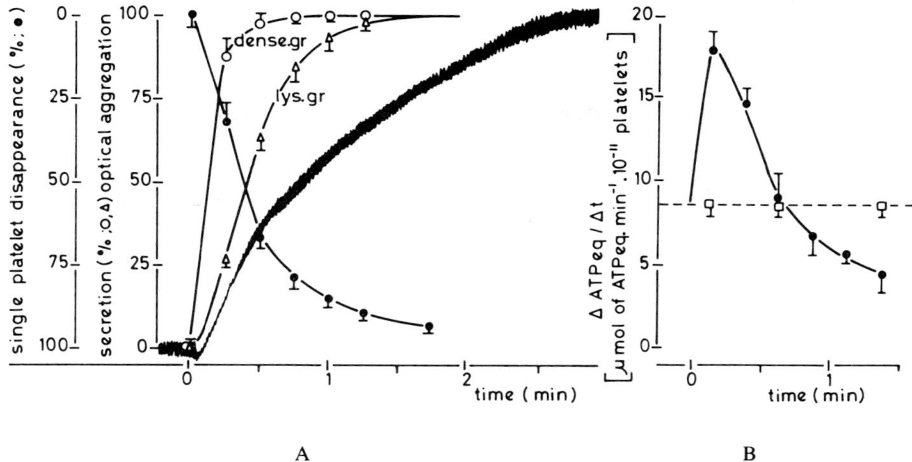

FIGURE 7. Energetics during aggregation and secretion. (A) shows optical aggregation, single platelet disappearance (●), and secretion of dense (○) and lysosomal granule contents (△) by platelets stimulated with 5 U/mℓ thrombin. (B) shows the energy consumption in resting platelets (□) and in platelets stimulated by thrombin (●). (From Verhoeven, A. J. M., Mommersteeg-Leautaud, M. E., and Akkerman, J. W. N., *Biochem. J.*, 221, 777, 1984. With permission.)

neutralizing platelet factor 4 and β thromboglobulin, which make the presence in the extracellular plasma important signs for platelet activation in vivo. Of specific interest is platelet-derived growth factor (PDGF). When PDGF is secreted, it penetrates in the subendothelium and stimulates the smooth muscle cells in the vessel wall to migration and proliferation. This results in thickening of the vessel wall and disturbance of the antihemostatic properties, thereby greatly contributing to formation of an atherosclerotic plaque. A second α-granule protein of interest is plasminogen-activator inhibitor, which retards the activation of the fibrinolytic system by plasminogen activator. Possibly this protein serves in the control of fibrinolysis, giving procoagulant reactions the time to form a plug before degradation can make a beginning.

Platelets contain about 13 different lysosomal enzymes. No patients with severe deficiencies in one or more of these enzymes have been identified so far and the importance of these enzymes is therefore uncertain. Probably, they help to remove the hemostatic plug when damaged tissues are repaired.

The velocity and extent of secretion differ among the three types of secretion granules and greatly depend on the type and dose of the stimulator. When artifacts during isolation of granule markers are prevented, the rate of secretion decreases in the order of dense-, α-, and lysosomal granule secretion with all agonists tested (Figure 7A). Maximal secretion is found with a high dose of thrombin (5 NIHU/mℓ), which liberates all α- and dense-granule contents after about 2 min and about 50% of the lysosomal granules after about 5 min. With lower doses of thrombin or weak activators such as ADP or adrenalin, α and dense granule secretion is incomplete (50 to 70%) and lysosomal secretion becomes almost undetectable (about 10%).

VIII. ENERGY METABOLISM

The maintenance of cell integrity and responsiveness to stimuli, as well as the execution of the different platelet functions, requires a continuous supply of metabolic energy. The energy is made available by the hydrolysis of metabolic ATP, which is rephosphorylated in glycolysis, glycogenolysis, and oxidative phosphorylation. Under aerobic conditions and in the presence of extracellular glucose, glycolytic and mitochondrial ATP resynthesis contribute almost equally to energy generation and produce together 5 to 7 μmol ATP equivalents per minute/10^{11} cells.* Glycolytic ATP regeneration can compensate for impaired mitochondrial energy support and vice versa, since platelets show Pasteur as well as Crabtree effects.[140] At less than 1 m*M* extracellular glucose, glycogen catabolism starts and partly compensates for the impaired glycolytic flux.

In unstimulated platelets, ATP resynthesis and ATP hydrolysis are in equilibrium, as illustrated by the stable levels of metabolic ATP and ADP which are kept at about 4.5 and 0.5 μmol/10^{11} cells, respectively, (equaling a total of 9.5 μmol ATP equivalents per 10^{11} cells). When ATP resynthesis is suddenly blocked, this represents enough energy to support normal aggregation and secretion, indicating that the metabolic price of these functions is below this number.[141] A second and much smaller store of rapidly accessible energy is formed by the glycolytic intermediates, which together represent about 1.5 μmol ATP equivalents per 10^{11} cells. When the metabolic ATP content is low, an excessive decrease in ATP is prevented by first consuming the glycolytic pool.[142] Hence, the phosphorylated carbohydrates "protect" the ATP concentration, a role similar to creatine phosphate in other cells and which is absent in human platelets.

The energy consumption during aggregation and secretion can be assessed quantitatively by inducing rapid blockade of ATP resynthesis with a mixture of inhibitors of glycolytic, glycogenolytic, and oxidative ATP resynthesis. The subsequent fall in metabolic ATP and ADP then reflects the energy consumption of the undisturbed cell and can be compared with the velocities of aggregation and secretion.[144] Following maximal stimulation with thrombin, the energy consumption increases three- to fourfold during the first 20 sec. This is also the time in which most of the aggregation and secretion takes place. When these functions slow down, the energy consumption decreases and even returns to levels below those found in resting platelets (Figure 7). A more detailed comparison between secretion and energy consumption reveals the best correlation when only the increment in energy consumption is considered. This suggests that the various energy-consuming steps in the resting cell continue unchanged during aggregation and secretion. The greatest consumption is found in periods of fast secretion, suggesting that this function requires more energy than shape change or aggregation.

Since the three types of secretion greatly overlap, it is difficult to relate the energy cost to a single type of secretion. However, when ATP hydrolysis is measured in periods of acid hydrolase secretion where dense-granule secretion is completed, the cost of a separate response can be calculated. Thus, complete dense-granule secretion requires 0.5 to 0.8 μmol ATP equivalents per 10^{11} cells, whereas for the combined secretion of α and lysosomal granules (which cannot be sufficiently separated) the price is about 6 μmol (same units). When aggregation is measured as the disappearance of single platelets, the cost for 100% response is about 2.5 μmol (same units). In contrast, shape change is not accompanied by a significant increase in energy consumption, indicating that the energy requirement is small. With a few exceptions, similar numbers are found with other platelet agonists, indicating that most of the energy is consumed in steps that have all agonists in common.[145] An exception is the bivalent cationophore A23187, which induces much more ATP hydrolysis due to a number of aspecific, ATP-dependent effects.

These numbers explain why platelets are capable of normal aggregation and secretion in the absence of ATP regenerating systems. A normal energy content of more than 10 μmol ATP equivalents per 10^{11} cells is more than sufficient to support all platelet functions, as well as the energy demands of the processes already present in the resting cells.

* An ATP equivalent represents the energy liberated in the conversion of 1 ATP to 1 ADP. The energy-rich phosphate in ADP is liberated via the adenylate kinase reaction (2 ADP $\rightleftharpoons$ ATP + AMP) and further hydrolysis of ATP. Hence, ATP and ADP represent 2 and 1 equivalents, respectively.[143,144]

ACKNOWLEDGMENTS

The author gratefully acknowledges the helpful comments of Dr. J. J. Sixma and the excellent secretarial assistance of Maeyken Hoeneveld.

REFERENCES

1. **Beck, W. S., Ed.,** *Hematology,* MIT Press, Cambridge, Mass., 1973, 1.
2. **Levine, R. F., Williams, N., Levin, J., and Evatt, B. L., Eds.,** *Megakaryocyte Development and Function,* Alan R. Liss, New York, 1986.
3. **Kimura, H., Burnstein, S. A., Thorniny, D., Powell, J. S., Harker, L. A., Fialkow, P. J., and Adamson, J. W.,** Human megakaryocytic progenitors (CFU-M) assaying in methylcellulose: physical characteristics and requirements for growth, *J. Cell Physiol.,* 118, 87, 1984.
4. **Williams, N. and Levine, R. F.,** The origin, development and regulation of megakaryocytes, *Br. J. Haematol.,* 52, 173, 1982.
5. **Hoffman, R., Young, H. H., Bruno, E., and Straneva, J. E.,** Purification and partial characterization of a megakaryocyte colony-stimulating factor from human plasma, *J. Clin. Invest.,* 75, 1174, 1985.
6. **Hoffman, R., Mazur, E., Bruno, E., and Floyd, V.,** Assay of an activity in the serum of patients with disorders of thrombopoiesis that stimulates formation of megakaryocyte colonies, *N. Engl. J. Med.,* 305, 533, 1981.
7. **Gewirtz, A. M.,** Human megakaryocytopoiesis, in *Seminars in Hematology 23,* Miescher, P. A. and Jaffe, E. R., Eds., Grune & Stratton, New York, 1986, 27.
8. **Levine, R. F., Hazzard, K. C., and Lamberg, J. D.,** The significance of megakaryocyte size, *Blood,* 60, 1122, 1982.
9. **Breton-Gorius, J. and Vainchenker, W.,** Expression of platelet proteins during the in vitro and in vivo differentiation of megakaryocytes and morphological aspects of their maturation, in *Seminars in Hematology 23,* Miescher, P. A. and Jaffe, E. R., Eds., Grune & Stratton, New York, 1986, 43.
10. **Sporn, L. A., Chavin, S. I., Marder, V. J., and Wagner, D. D.,** Biosynthesis of von Willebrand protein by human megakaryocytes, *J. Clin. Invest.,* 76, 1102, 1985.
11. **Rabellino, E. M., Levene, R. B., Leung, L. K., and Nachman, R. L.,** Human megakaryocytes. Expression of platelet proteins in early marrow megakaryocytes, *J. Exp. Med.,* 154, 88, 1981.
12. **Sporn, L. A., Chavin, S. I., Marder, V. J., and Wagner, D. D.,** Biosynthesis of von Willebrand protein by human megakaryocytes, *J. Clin. Invest.,* 76, 1102, 1985.
13. **Schick, B. P. and Schick, P. K.,** Megakaryocyte biochemistry, in *Seminars in Hematology 23,* Miescher, P. A. and Jaffe, E. R., Eds., Grune & Stratton, New York, 1986, 68.
14. **Schick, P. K., Schick, B. P., Foster, K., and Block, A.,** Arachidonate synthesis and uptake in isolated guinea pig megakaryocytes and platelets, *Biochim. Biophys. Acta,* 795, 341, 1984.
15. **Leven, R. M. and Nachmias, V. T.,** Cultured megakaryocytes: changes in the cytoskeleton after ADP-induced spreading, *J. Cell Biol.,* 92, 313, 1982.
16. **Miller, J. C.,** Characterization of the megakaryocyte secretion response: studies of continuously monitored release of endogenous ATP, *Blood,* 61, 967, 1983.
17. **Leven, R. M., Mulliken, W. H., and Nachmias, V. T.,** Role of sodium in ADP- and thrombin-induced megakaryocyte spreading, *J. Cell Biol.,* 96, 1234, 1983.
18. **Bessman, D.,** Prediction of platelet production during chemotherapy of acute leukemia, *Am. J. Haematol.,* 13, 219, 1982.
19. **White, J. G., Clawson, C. C., and Gerrard, J. M.,** Platelet ultrastructure, in *Haemostasis and Thrombosis,* Bloom, A. L. and Thomas, D. P., Eds., Churchill Livingstone, London, 1981, 22.
20. **White, J. G. and Gerrard, J. M.,** Anatomy and structural organization of the platelet, in *Hemostasis and Thrombosis: Basic Principles and Clinical Practice,* Colman, R. W., Hirsh, J., Marder, V. J., and Salzman, E. W., Eds., Lippincott, Philadelphia, 1982, 343.
21. **Phillips, D. R.,** Receptors for platelet agonists, in *Platelet Membrane Glycoproteins,* George, J. N., Nurden, A. T., and Phillips, D. R., Eds., Plenum Press, New York, 1985, 145.
22. **Haslam, R. J. and Cusack, N. J.,** Blood platelet receptors for ADP and for adenosine, in *Purinergic Receptors,* Burnstock, G., Ed., Chapman and Hall, London, 1981, 223.
23. **Lips, J. P. M., Sixma, J. J., and Schiphorst, M. E.,** Binding of adenosine diphosphate to human blood platelets and to isolated blood platelet membranes, *Biochim. Biophys. Acta,* 628, 451,1980.

24. **Macfarlane, D. E., Mills, D. C. B., and Srivastova, P. C.,** Binding of 2-azidoadenosine[beta-^{32}P]diphosphate to the receptor on intact human blood platelets which inhibits adenylate cyclase, *Biochemistry,* 21, 544, 1982.
25. **Macfarlene, D. E., Srivastava, P. C., and Mills, D. C. B.,** 2-Methylthio adenosine[β-^{32}P]diphosphate. An agonist and radioligand for the receptor that inhibits the accumulation of cyclic AMP in intact blood platelets, *J. Clin. Invest.,* 71, 420, 1983.
26. **Mills, D. C. B., Figures, W. R., Scearce, L. M., Steward, G. J., Colman, R. F., and Colman, R. W.,** Two mechanisms for inhibition of ADP-induced platelet shape change by 5′-p-fluorosulfonylbenzoyladenosine, *J. Biol. Chem.,* 260, 8078, 1985.
27. **Figures, W. R., Scearce, L. M., Wachtfogel, Y., Chen, J., Colman, R. F., and Colman, R. W.,** Platelet ADP receptor and α2-adrenoreceptor interaction, *J. Biol. Chem.,* 261, 5981, 1986.
28. **Hollenberg, M. D.,** Examples of homospecific and heterospecific receptor regulation, *Trends Pharmacol. Sci.,* 6, 242, 1985.
29. **Berndt, M. C. and Phillips, D. R.,** Purification and preliminary physiochemical characterization of human platelet membrane glycoprotein V, *J. Biol. Chem.,* 256, 59, 1981.
30. **Jamieson, G. A. and Okumura, T.,** Reduced thrombin binding and aggregation in Bernard-Soulier platelets, *J. Clin. Invest.,* 61, 861, 1978.
31. **Tam, S. W. and Detwiler, T. C.,** Binding of thrombin to human platelet plasma membranes, *Biochim. Biophys. Acta,* 543, 194, 1978.
32. **Tollefsen, D. M., Faegler, J. R., and Majerus, P. W.,** The binding of thrombin to the surface of human platelets, *J. Biol. Chem.,* 249, 2646, 1974.
33. **Harmon, J. T. and Jamieson, G. A.,** Thrombin binds to a high-affinity ~900,000-dalton site on human platelets, *Biochemistry,* 24,58, 1985.
34. **Tandon, N., Harmon, J. T., Rodbard, D., and Jamieson, G. A.,** Thrombin receptors define responsiveness of cholesterol-modified platelets, *J. Biol. Chem.,* 258, 11840, 1983.
35. **Goldfine, I. D., Gardner, J. D., and Neville, D. M.,** Insulin action in isolated rat thymocytes. I. Binding of ^{125}I-insulin and stimulation of α-aminoisobutyric acid transport, *J. Biol. Chem.,* 247, 6919, 1972.
36. **Holmsen, H., Dangelmaier, C. A., and Holmsen, H. K.,** Thrombin-induced platelet responses differ in requirement for receptor occupancy. Evidence for tight coupling of occupancy and compartmentalized phosphatidic acid formation, *J. Biol. Chem.,* 256, 9393, 1981.
37. **Verhoeven, A. J. M., Gorter, G., Mommersteeg, M. E., and Akkerman, J. W. N.,** The energetics of early platelet responses. Energy consumption during shape change and aggregation with special reference to protein phosphorylation and the polyphosphoinositide cycle, *Biochem. J.,* 228, 451, 1985.
38. **Chiang, T. M., Beachy, E. H., and Kang, A. H.,** Binding of collagen α1 chains to human platelets, *J. Clin. Invest.,* 59, 405, 1977.
39. **Nieuwenhuis, H. K., Akkerman, J. W. N., Houdijk, W. P. M., and Sixma, J. J.,** Human blood platelets showing no response to collagen fail to express surface glycoprotein Ia, *Nature,* 318, 470, 1985.
40. **Regan, J. W., Nakata, H., De Marinis, R. M., Caron, M. G., and Lefkowitz, R. J.,** Purification and characterization of the human platelet α2-adrenergic receptor, *J. Biol. Chem.,* 261, 3894, 1986.
41. **Smith, S. K. and Limbird, L. E.,** Solubilization of human platelet α-adrenergic receptors: evidence that agonist occupancy of the receptor stabilizes receptor-effector interactions, *Proc. Natl. Acad. Sci. U.S.A.,* 78, 4026, 1981.
42. **Sibley, D. R. and Lefkowitz, R. J.,** Molecular mechanisms of receptor desensitization using the β-adrenergic receptor-coupled adenylate cyclase system as a model, *Nature,* 317, 124, 1985.
43. **Cerione, R. A., Regan, J. W., Nakata, H., Codina, J., Benovic, J. L., Gierschik, P., Somers, R. L., Spiegel, A. M., Birnbaumer, L., Lefkowitz, R. J., and Caron, M. G.,** Functional reconstitution of the α2-adrenergic receptor with guanine nucleotide regulatory proteins in phospholipid vesicles, *J. Biol. Chem.,* 261, 3901, 1986.
44. **Alexander, R. W., Cooper, B., and Handlin, R. I.,** Characterization of the human platelet α-adrenergic receptor, *J. Clin. Invest.,* 78, 1146, 1978.
45. **Mukkerjee, A.,** Characterization of α2-adrenergic receptors in human platelets by binding of a radioactive ligand [^{3}H] yohimbine, *Biochim. Biophys. Acta,* 676, 148, 1981.
46. **Kerry, R. and Scrutton, M. C.,** Platelet beta-adreno receptors, *Br. J. Pharmacol.,* 79, 681, 1983.
47. **Winther, K., Klysner, R., Geisler, A., and Andersen, P. H.,** Characterization of human platelet beta-adreno-receptors, *Thromb. Res.,* 40, 757, 1985.
48. **Schick, P. and McKean, M. L.,** Serotonin binding in human platelets, *Biochem. Pharmacol.,* 28, 2667, 1979.
49. **Kloprogge, E., Hasselaar, P., Gorter, G., and Akkerman, J. W. N.,** Stimulus-aggregation coupling in platelets stimulated with PAF-acether, *Biochim. Biophys. Acta,* 883, 127, 1986.
50. **Kloprogge, E. and Akkerman, J. W. N.,** Binding kinetics of PAF-acether (1-O-alkyl-2-acetyl-sn-glycero-3-phosphocholine) to intact human platelets, *Biochem. J.,* 223, 901, 1984.

51. **Kloprogge, E., Mommersteeg, M. E., and Akkerman, J. W. N.,** Kinetics of PAF-acether-induced fibrinogen binding to human blood platelets, *J. Biol. Chem.,* 261, 11071, 1986.
52. **Hwang, S. B., Lee, C. S. C., Cheah, M. J., and Shen, T. Y.,** Specific receptor sites for 1-*O*-alkyl-2-acetyl-sn-glycero-3-phosphocholine (platelet activating factor) on rabbit platelet and guinea pig smooth muscle membranes, *Biochemistry,* 22, 4756, 1983.
53. **Valone, F. H., Coles, E., Reinhold, V. R., and Goetzl, E. J.,** Specific binding of phospholipid platelet-activating factor by human platelets, *J. Immunol.,* 129, 1637, 1982.
54. **Inarrea, P., Gomez-Cambronero, J., Nieto, M., and Sanchez, Crespo M.,** Characteristics of the binding of Platelet-Activating Factor to platelets of different animal species, *Eur. J. Pharmacol.,* 105, 309, 1984.
55. **Wade, P. J., Lunt, D. O., Lad, N., Tuffin, D. P., and McCullagh, K. G.,** Effect of calcium and calcium antagonists on [^{3}H]-PAF-acether binding to washed human platelets, *Thromb. Res.,* 41, 251, 1986.
56. **Valone, F. H.,** Isolation of a platelet membrane protein which binds the platelet-activating factor 1-*O*-hexadecyl-2-acetyl-sn-glycero-3-phosphorylcholine, *Immunology,* 52, 169, 1984.
57. **Thomas, M. E., Osmani, A. H., and Scrutton, M. C.,** Some properties of the human platelet vasopressin receptor, *Thromb. Res.,* 32, 557, 1983.
58. **Vanderwel, M., Lum, D. S., and Haslam, R. J.,** Vasopressin inhibits the adenylate cyclase activity of human platelet particulate fraction through V1-receptor, *FEBS Lett.,* 164, 340, 1983.
59. **Berettini, W. H., Post, R. M., Worthington, E. K., and Casper, J. B.,** Human platelet vasopressin receptors, *Life Sci.,* 30, 425, 1982.
60. **Thibonnier, M. and Roberts, J. M.,** Characterization of human platelet vasopressin receptors, *J. Clin. Invest.,* 76, 1857, 1985.
61. **McDonald, J. W. D. and Stuart, R. K.,** Interaction of prostaglandins E1 and E2 in regulation of cyclic AMP and aggregation in human platelets: evidence for a common prostaglandin receptor, *J. Lab. Clin. Med.,* 84, 111, 1974.
62. **McIntyre, D. E.,** Prostaglandin receptors, in *Platelets in Biology and Pathology,* Gordon, J. L., Ed., Elsevier/North-Holland, Amsterdam, 1981, 211.
63. **Schillinger, E. and Prior, G.,** Prostaglandin I2 receptors in a particulate fraction of various species, *Biochem. Pharmacol.,* 29, 2297, 1980.
64. **Siegl, A. M., Smith, J. B., Silver, M. J., Nicolaou, K. C., and Ahern, D.,** Selective binding site for [^{3}H] prostacyclin on platelets, *J. Clin. Invest.,* 63, 215, 1979.
65. **Cooper, B.,** Agonist regulation of the human platelet PGD2 receptor, *Life Sci.,* 25, 1361, 1979.
66. **Cooper, B. and Ahern, D.,** Characterization of the platelet prostaglandin D2 receptor, *J. Clin. Invest.,* 64, 586, 1979.
67. **Israels, E. D., Nisli, G., Paraskeras, F., and Israels, L. G.,** Platelet Fc receptor as a mechanism for Ag-Ab complex-induced platelet injury, *Thromb. Diath. Haemorrh.,* 29, 434, 1973.
68. **Pfueller, S. and Sosgrove, L. J.,** Activation of human platelets in PRP via their Fc-receptor by antigen-antibody complexes or immunoglobulin G: requirement for particle-bound fibrinogen, *Thromb. Res.,* 20, 97, 1980.
69. **Pfueller, S. L., Kerlero de Rosbo, N., and Bilston, R. A.,** Platelets deficient in glycoprotein I have normal Fc receptor expression, *Br. J. Haematol.,* 56, 607, 1984.
70. **Cheng, C. M. and Hawiger, J.,** Affinity isolation and characterization of immunoglobulin G Fc fragment-binding glycoprotein from human blood platelets, *J. Biol. Chem.,* 254, 2165, 1979.
71. **Karas, S. P., Rosse, W. F., and Kurlander, R. J.,** Characterization of the IgG-Fc receptor on human platelets, *Blood,* 60, 1277, 1982.
72. **Steiner, M. and Luscher, E. F.,** Identification of the immunoglobulin G receptor of human platelets, *J. Biol. Chem.,* 261, 7230, 1986.
73. **De Marco, L., Girolami, A., Zimmerman, T. S., and Ruggeri, Z. M.,** Interaction of purified type IIb von Willebrand factor with the platelet membrane glycoprotein Ib induces fibrinogen binding to the glycoprotein IIb/IIIa complex and initiates aggregation, *Proc. Natl. Acad. Sci. U.S.A.,* 82, 7424, 1985.
74. **Koller, E., Koller, F., and Doleschel, W.,** Specific binding sites on human platelets for plasma lipoproteins, *Hoppe Seyler's Z. Physiol. Chem.,* 363, 395, 1982.
75. **Curtiss, L. K. and Plow, E. F.,** Interaction of plasma lipoproteins with human platelets, *Blood,* 64, 365, 1984.
76. **Bruckendorfer, K. R., Buckley, S., and Hassall, D. G.,** The effect of low-density lipoproteins on the synthesis of cyclic nucleotides induced by prostacyclin in isolated platelets, *Biochem. J.,* 223, 189, 1984.
77. **Hajek, A. S., Joist, J. H., Baker, R. K., Jarett, L., and Daughaday, W. H.,** Demonstration and partial characterization of insulin receptors in human platelets, *J. Clin. Invest.,* 63, 1060, 1979.
78. **Shattil, S. J. and Cooper, R. A.,** Membrane microviscosity and human platelet function, *Biochemistry,* 15, 4832, 1976.
79. **Kramer, R. M., Jakubowski, J. A., Vaillancourt, R., and Deykin, D.,** Effect of membrane cholesterol on phospholipid metabolism in thrombin-stimulated platelets, *J. Biol. Chem.,* 257, 6844, 1982.

80. **Stuart, M. J., Gerrard, J. M., and White, J. C.,** Effect of cholesterol on production of thromboxane B2 by platelets in vitro, *N. Engl. J. Med.*, 302, 6, 1980.
81. **Carvalho, A. C. A., Colman, R. W., and Laes, R. S.,** Platelet function in hyperlipoproteinemia, *N. Engl. J. Med.*, 290, 434, 1974.
82. **Steiner, M. and Luscher, E. F.,** Fluorescence anisotropy changes in platelet membranes during activation, *Biochemistry*, 23, 247, 1984.
83. **Avdonin, P. V., Svitina-Ulitina, I. V., and Kulikov, V. I.,** Stimulation of high-affinity hormone-sensitive GTPase of human platelets by 1-O-alkyl-2-O-acetyl-sn-glyceryl-3-phosphocholine (Platelet Activating Factor), *Biochem. Biophys. Res. Commun.*, 131, 307, 1985.
84. **Billah, M. M. and Lapetina, E. G.,** Platelet-activating factor stimulates metabolism of phosphoinositides in horse platelets: possible relationship to Ca^{2+} mobilization during stimulation, *Proc. Natl. Acad. Sci. U.S.A.*, 80, 965, 1983.
85. **Siess, W., Siegel, F. L., and Lapetina, E. G.,** Arachidonic acid stimulates the formation of 1,2 diacylglycerol and phosphatidic acid in human platelets, *J. Biol. Chem.*, 258, 11236, 1983.
86. **Kaibuchi, K., Takai, Y., Sawamura, M., Hoshijima, M., Fujikura, T., and Nishizuka, Y.,** Synergistic functions of protein phosphorylation and calcium mobilization in platelet activation, *J. Biol. Chem.*, 258, 6701, 1983.
87. **Siess, W., Boehlig, B., Weber, P. C., and Lapetina, E. G.,** Prostaglandin endoperoxide analogues stimulate phospholipase C and protein phosphorylation during platelet shape change, *Blood*, 65, 1141, 1985.
88. **Holmsen, H., Dangelmaier, C. A., and Rongved, S.,** Tight coupling of thrombin-induced acid hydrolase secretion and phosphatidate synthesis to receptor occupancy in human platelets, *Biochem. J.*, 222, 157, 1984.
89. **Leung, N. L., Vickers, J. D., Kinlough-Rathbone, R. L., Reimers, H. J., and Mustard, J. F.,** ADP-induced changes in ^{32}P-phosphate labeling of phosphatidylinositol-4,5-biphosphate in washed rabbit platelets made refractory by prior ADP-stimulation, *Biochem.,Biophys. Res. Commun.*, 113, 483, 1983.
90. **Dean, W. L.,** Purification and reconstitution of a Ca^{2+} pump from human platelets, *J. Biol. Chem.*, 259, 7343, 1984.
91. **Menashi, S., Autki, K. S., Carey, F., and Crawford, N.,** Characterization of the calcium-sequestering process associated with human platelet intracellular membranes, *Biochem. J.*, 222, 413, 1984.
92. **Brass, L. F. and Joseph, S. K.,** A role for IP3 in intracellular Ca^{2+} mobilization and granule secretion in platelets, *J. Biol. Chem.*, 260, 15172, 1985.
93. **O'Rourke, F. A., Halenda, S. P., Zavoico, G. B., and Feinstein, M. B.,** Inositol 1,4,5-triphosphate releases Ca^{2+} from a Ca^{2+} transporting membrane vesicle fraction from human platelets, *J. Biol. Chem.*, 260, 956, 1985.
94. **Watson, S. P., Ruggiero, M. L., Abrahams, S. L., and Lapetina, E. G.,** IP3 induces aggregation and release of serotonin from saponine-permeabilized human platelets, *J. Biol. Chem.*, 261, 5368, 1986.
95. **Massini, P. and Luscher, E. F.,** On the significance of the influx of calcium ions into stimulated human blood platelets, *Biochim. Biophys. Acta*, 436, 652, 1976.
96. **Thompson, N. T. and Scrutton, M. C.,** Intracellular calcium fluxes in human platelets, *Eur. J. Biochem.*, 147, 421, 1985.
97. **Feinstein, M. B., Rodan, G. A., and Cutler, L. S.,** Cyclic AMP and calcium in platelet function, in *Platelets in Biology and Pathology*, Gordon, J. L., Ed., Elsevier/North-Holland, Amsterdam, 1981, 437.
98. **Hallam, T. J., Sandez, A., and Rink, T. J.,** Stimulus-response coupling in human platelets, *Biochem. J.*, 218, 819, 1984.
99. **Daniel, J. L., Molish, I. R., and Holmsen, H.,** Myosin phosphorylation in intact platelets, *J. Biol. Chem.*, 256, 7510, 1981.
100. **Zavoico, G. B. and Feinstein, M. B.,** Cytoplasmic Ca^{2+} in platelets is controlled by cyclic AMP, *Biochem. Biophys. Res. Commun.*, 120, 579, 1984.
101. **Horne, W. C., Norman, N. E., Schwartzs, D. B., and Simons, E. R.,** Changes in cytoplasmic pH and membrane potential in thrombin-stimulated platelets, *Eur. J. Biochem.* 120, 295, 1981.
102. **Siffert, W., Fox, G., Muchenhoff, K., and Scheid, P.,** Thrombin stimulates Na^{+}/H^{+} exchange across the human platelet plasma membrane, *FEBS Lett.*, 172, 272, 1984.
103. **Simon, M. F., Chap, H., and Douste-Blazy, L.,** Activation of phospholipase C in thrombin-stimulated platelets does not depend on cytoplasmic free calcium concentration, *FEBS Lett.*, 170, 43, 1984.
104. **Tuszynski, G. P., Daniel, J. L., and Stewart, G.,** Association of protein with the platelet cytoskeleton, *Semin. Haematol.*, 22, 303, 1985.
105. **Cox, A. C., Caroll, R. C., White, J. G., and Rao, G. H. R.,** Recycling of platelet phosphorylation and cytoskeleton assembly, *J. Cell Biol.*, 98, 8, 1984.
106. **Rotman, A., Heldman, J., and Linder, S.,** Association of membrane and cytoplasmic proteins with the cytoskeleton in blood platelets, *Biochemistry*, 21, 1713, 1982.

107. **Wheeler, M. E., Gerrard, J. M., and Carroll, R. C.,** Reciprocal transmembranous receptor-cytoskeleton interaction in concanavalin A-activated platelets, *J. Cell Biol.,* 101, 993, 1985.
108. **Fox, J. E. B., Boyles, J. K., Reynolds, C. C., and Phillips, D. R.,** Actin filament content and organization in unstimulated platelets, *J. Cell Biol.,* 98, 1985, 1984.
109. **Piazza, G. A. and Wallace, R. W.,** Calmodulin accelerates the rate of polymerization of human platelet actin and alters the structural characteristics of actin filaments, *Proc. Natl. Acad. Sci. U.S.A.,* 82, 1683, 1985.
110. **Daniel, J. L., Molish, I. R., Robkin, L., and Holmsen, N.,** Nucleotide exchange between cytosolic ATP and F-actin-bound ADP may be a major energy-utilizing process in unstimulated platelets, *Eur. J. Biochem.,* 156, 677, 1986.
111. **Caroll, R. C., Butler, R. G., Morris, P. A., and Gerrard, J. M.,** Separable assembly of platelet pseudopodal and contractile cytoskeletons, *Cell,* 30, 385, 1982.
112. **Fox, J. E. B. and Phillips, D. R.,** Role of phosphorylation in mediating the association of myosin with the cytoskeletal structures of human platelets, *J. Biol. Chem.,* 257, 4120, 1982.
113. **Fox, J. E. B.,** Linkage of a membrane skeleton to integral membrane glycoproteins in human platelets. Identification of one of the glycoproteins as glycoprotein Ib, *J. Clin. Invest.,* 76, 1673, 1985.
114. **Fox, J. E. B.,** Identification of actin-binding protein as the protein linking the membrane skeleton to glycoproteins on platelet plasma membranes, *J. Biol. Chem.,* 260, 11970, 1985.
115. **Tuszinski, G. P., Kornecki, R. E., Cierniewski, C., Knight, L. C., Koshy, A., Srivastava, S., Niewiarowsky, S., and Walsh, P. N.,** Association of fibrin with the platelet cytoskeleton, *J. Biol. Chem.,* 259, 5247, 1984.
116. **Carroll, R. G. and Gerrard, J. M.,** Phosphorylation of platelet actin-binding protein during platelet activation, *Blood,* 59, 466, 1982.
117. **Sakariassen, K. S., Bolhuis, P. A., and Sixma, J. J.,** Human blood platelet adhesion to artery subendothelium is mediated by factor VIII-von Willebrand factor bound to the subendothelium, *Nature,* 279, 636, 1979.
118. **Sixma, J. J., Sakariassen, K. S., Stel, H. V., Houdijk, W. P. M., in der Maur, R. J., de Groot, P. H. G., and van Mourik, J. A.,** Functional domains on von Willebrand factor with platelets and with collagen, *J. Clin. Invest.,* 74, 736, 1984.
119. **Ruggeri, Z. M., De Marco, L., Gatti, L., Bader, R., and Montgomery, R. R.,** Platelets have more than one binding site for von Willebrand factor, *J. Clin. Invest.,* 72, 1, 1983.
120. **Fujimoto, T., Ohara, S., and Hawiger, J.,** Thrombin-induced exposure and prostacyclin inhibition of the receptor for factor VIII-von Willebrand factor on human platelets, *J. Clin. Invest.,* 69, 1212, 1982.
121. **Marguerie, G. A., Plow, E. F., and Edginton, T. S.,** Human platelets possess an inducible and saturable receptor specific for fibrinogen, *J. Biol. Chem.,* 254, 5357, 1979.
122. **Bennett, J. S. and Vilaire, G.,** Exposure of platelet fibrinogen receptors by ADP and epinephrine, *J. Clin. Invest.,* 64, 1393, 1979.
123. **Peerschke, E. I. B.,** The platelet fibrinogen receptor, *Semin. Hematol.,* 22, 241, 1985.
124. **Marguerie, G. A. and Plow, E. F.,** The fibrinogen-dependent pathway of platelet aggregation, *Ann. N.Y. Acad. Sci.,* 408, 556, 1983.
125. **Harfenist, E. J., Cuccione, M. A., Packham, M. A., Kinlough-Rathbone, R. L., and Mustard, J. F.,** Arachidonate-induced fibrinogen binding to thrombin-degranulated rabbit platelets is independent of released ADP, *Blood,* 59, 956, 1982.
126. **Kloprogge, E. and Akkerman, J. W. N.,** PAF-acether induces high- and low affinity binding of fibrinogen to human platelets via independent mechanisms, *Biochem. J.,* 240, 403, 1986.
127. **Hawiger, J., Parkinson, S., and Timmons, S.,** Prostacyclin inhibits mobilization of fibrinogen binding sites on human ADP- and thrombin-treated platelets, *Nature,* 285, 195, 1980.
128. **Peerschke, E. I. B., Zucker, M. B., Grant, R. A., Egan, J. J., and Johnson, M. M.,** Correlation between fibrinogen binding to human platelets and platelet aggregability, *Blood,* 55, 841, 1980.
129. **Leung, L. L. K.,** Role of thrombosponding in platelet aggregation, *J. Clin. Invest.,* 74, 1764, 1984.
130. **Lawler, J.,** The structural and functional properties of thrombospondin, *Blood,* 67, 1197, 1986.
131. **Plow, E. F. and Ginsberg, M. H.,** Specific and saturable binding of plasma fibronectin to thrombin-stimulated platelets, *J. Biol. Chem.,* 256, 9477, 1981.
132. **Pytela, P., Pierschbacher, M. D., Ginsberg, M. H., Plow, E. F., and Ruoslahti, E.,** Platelet membrane glycoprotein IIb/IIIa: member of a family of Arg-Gly-Asp-specific adhesion receptors, *Science,* 231, 1559, 1986.
133. **Greengard, J. S. and Griffin, J. H.,** Receptors for HMWK on stimulated washed human platelets, *Biochemistry,* 23, 6863, 1985.
134. **Miles, L. A., Ginsberg, M. H., White, J. C., and Plow, E. F.,** Plasminogen interacts with human platelets through two distinct mechanisms, *J. Clin. Invest.,* 77, 2001, 1986.
135. **Greenberg, C. S. and Shuman, M. A.,** Specific binding of blood coagulation factor VIIIa to thrombin-stimulated platelets, *J. Biol. Chem.,* 259, 14721, 1984.

136. **Sinha, D., Seaman, F. S., Koshy, A., Knight, L. C., and Walsh, P. N.,** Blood coagulation factor XIa binds specifically to a site on activated human platelets distinct from that for factor XI, *J. Clin. Invest.*, 73, 1550, 1984.
137. **Rosing, J., Bevers, E. M., Comfurius, P., Hemker, H. C., van Dieijen, G., Weiss, H. J., and Zwaal, R. F. A.,** Impaired factor X- and prothrombin activation in platelets from a patient with a bleeding disorder, *Blood,* 65, 1557, 1985.
138. **Harris, K. W. and Esmon, C. T.,** Protein S is required for bovine platelets to support activated protein C binding and activity, *J. Biol. Chem.*, 260, 2007, 1985.
139. **Akkerman, J. W. N., Nieuwenhuis, H. K., Mommersteeg-Leautaud, M. E., Gorter, G., and Sixma, J. J.,** ATP-ADP compartmentation in Storage Pool Deficient platelets: correlation between granule-bound ADP and the bleeding time, *Br. J. Haematol.*, 55, 135, 1983.
140. **Akkerman, J. W. N.,** Platelet carbohydrate metabolism, in *Platelet Responses and Metabolism,* Vol. 2, Holmsen, H., Ed., CRC Press, Boca Raton, Fla., 1987, 189.
141. **Akkerman, J. W. N., Holmsen, H., and Driver, H. A.,** Platelet aggregation and Ca^{2+} secretion are independent of simultaneous energy production, *FEBS Lett.*, 100, 286, 1979.
142. **Verhoeven, A. J. M., Mommersteeg, M. E., and Akkerman, J. W. N.,** Balanced contribution of glycolytic and adenylate pool in supply of metabolic energy in platelets, *J. Biol. Chem.*, 260, 2621, 1985.
143. **Atkinson, D. E.,** *Cellular Energy Metabolism and Its Regulation,* Academic Press, New York, 1977, 40.
144. **Verhoeven, A. J. M., Mommersteeg-Leautaud, M. E., and Akkerman, J. W. N.,** Quantification of energy consumption in platelets during thrombin-induced aggregation and secretion, *Biochem. J.*, 221, 777,1984.
145. **Verhoeven, A. J. M., Mommersteeg, M. E., and Akkerman, J. W. N.,** Comparative studies on the energetics of platelet responses induced by different agonists, *Biochem. J.*, 236, 879, 1986.

Chapter 4

ADSORPTION OF COAGULATION FACTORS II, V, AND X AT PHOSPHOLIPID MEMBRANES

Wim Th. Hermens, Jos M. M. Kop, and George M. Willems

TABLE OF CONTENTS

I. INTRODUCTION

The clot-promoting capacity of various nonbiological surfaces, such as glass, was recognized early in the study of blood coagulation. Ever since the famous observation that Hageman's plasma would not coagulate in a glass tube, it was also realized that blood must contain specialized substances needed for surface-mediated coagulation. However, it was not until the 1960s that it was discovered that surface activation of coagulation factors is a normal in vivo phenomenon. In those years several groups of workers concluded that the presence of phospholipids was required for efficient production of thrombin. The concept of the prothrombinase complex of activated factors V and X adsorbed to a phospholipid membrane, as well as the adsorption of factor II to the same membrane as a necessary step to conversion to thrombin, was proposed.[1,2]

The study of the adsorption of coagulation factors, mostly fibrinogen, at artificial surfaces has received new impetus in the development of blood-compatible surfaces. It was realized that almost every protein will adsorb at any surface unless another protein has adsorbed there first.[3] Moreover, the adsorbed amount of protein and specific adsorption of certain plasma proteins to the surface prove to be important determinants of the rate of thrombus formation at such surfaces. Several new techniques for the measurement of protein adsorption have been developed in this field and have recently been reviewed.[4,5]

Progress in the study of adsorption of coagulation factors at phospholipid membranes has been more modest. The preparation of suitable model membranes and the adaptation of existing techniques for the measurement of protein binding at such membranes have posed many difficulties. Reliable values for the binding parameters of factors II, V, and X to membranes of well-defined phospholipid composition have only been obtained in the last decade.

Studies of protein adsorption meet some major obstacles. First, there is still incomplete understanding of the physicochemical principles of protein adsorption. Simple reversible binding to independent binding sites is seldom, if ever, observed. Instead, the binding constants prove to be dependent on the absorbed concentrations of protein, and complicated replacements or sequential adsorptions are observed for mixtures of proteins. There are also strong indications that proteins may initially show reversible adsorption, which then becomes irreversible due to surface-induced transitions in the protein molecule or, in the case of adsorption to phospholipid membranes, due to penetration of protein into the bilayer.

A second major complication is the influence of the hydrodynamic flow conditions on the adsorption process. The rate of surface-mediated activation may easily become transport-limited under the flow conditions prevailing in blood vessels. This implies, for instance, that the concentration of thrombin produced at an endothelial lesion can be orders of magnitude higher closer to the surface than in the plasma. Even in experimental flow systems, one generally uses so-called nonuniformly accessible surfaces with sorption rates dependent on the distance downstream.

A third obstacle is the lack of techniques for routine measurement of protein adsorptions. Until a decade ago, protein adsorptions were mainly measured indirectly, for instance, from activation kinetics, assuming that adsorption is required for activation, or by measurement of protein depletion in suspensions with a large surface-to-volume ratio. Only in the last few years were some techniques introduced allowing direct observation of the adsorption process, such as light scattering in vesicle suspensions, ellipsometry on membranes deposited on solid surfaces, and total internal reflection fluorescence (TIRF).[5] These techniques were often already known in other areas of research, but had to be adapted for the study of protein-lipid interactions. They are still subject to experimental limitations, and a number of assumptions is required to allow the calculation of binding parameters from experimentally measured variables.

Due to the complications just mentioned, there are still few generally accepted data on the adsorption of coagulation factors to phospholipid membranes. Different techniques have produced different results, and results obtained for vesicle suspensions have also differed from those obtained with planar model membranes or biological membranes, such as platelets. Some of these discrepancies can be explained, however, and Section V shows that for the coagulation factors II, V, and X, which are the only factors that have presently been studied by a variety of techniques, a more or less consistent picture is emerging. In order to do so, the three complicating aspects just mentioned must be shortly discussed.

II. PRINCIPLES OF PROTEIN ADSORPTION

A. Introduction

Protein adsorption can be described in two complementary ways. First, there is the thermodynamic description, based on general physicochemical principles such as the conservation of energy. In this approach one is not interested in the specific mechanisms of adsorption. It is irrelevant, for instance, whether the binding occurs due to electrostatic attraction or hydrophobic bonding. The essential point is that the free energy of the system can be defined and is decreased by the binding process. Adsorption will then occur spontaneously. The thermodynamic approach is useful for the acquisition of a general picture of the adsorption process. It is of limited value, however, in the description of actual protein binding experiments. This is mainly due to the fact that most protein adsorptions are, at least partly, irreversible, and this interferes with the calculation of the free energy change during binding.

Consequently, another approach is more often used in the analysis of protein binding data. This second approach starts by proposing a specific mechanism for the adsorption process. Using such a model, the observed variables such as the adsorbed concentration of protein or the rate of adsorption can be "translated" in the model parameters. This translation is usually performed by statistically averaging, and this approach is, therefore, often called the statistical method. It has the advantage of allowing the incorporation of detailed information on the mechanism of adsorption in the proposed model, but the results will obviously not be of general validity and will often produce discussions about the correctness of the proposed model. As it turns out, the same phenomena can often be explained by completely different models. In this section we will briefly discuss these two complementary approaches, focusing on a few special features of protein adsorption that are still partly unexplained.

B. Thermodynamic Description of Protein Adsorption

Within the framework of thermodynamics, one first proceeds by defining a set of measurable variables, such as temperature (T), pressure (P), volume (V), or surface area (A), which together completely specify the physicochemical state of the system. If such a set is found, the variables included are called the state variables of the system. The next step consists of defining a few thermodynamic functions, the so-called state functions, such as the enthalpy H and the entropy S, which are also completely determined by the state variables P, T, V, or A, but in addition show a behavior determined by a number of general physical laws. One of these laws states that the energy (U) of the system is always conserved (first law of thermodynamics). This law implies that if one performs external work on a system, this system can only return to the initial state if it performs the same amount of work on the external world or releases an equivalent quantity of heat. Another general law states that in an isolated system any spontaneously occurring process will lead to an increase of the entropy S (second law of thermodynamics).

A state function of particular importance for the prediction of spontaneously occurring processes and for the formulation of equilibrium conditions is the free energy, or Gibbs energy (G). Using the first and second laws of thermodynamics, one can prove that in systems with constant temperature and pressure any spontaneous process will proceed such that the value of G will be lowered. This implies that ΔG, i.e., the change in G, will always be negative. As G will always keep a positive value, a state of equilibrium is reached at which G will assume the minimal value. Such a state of equilibrium will be stable because a change in this state would imply $\Delta G > 0$, and such a change could never occur spontaneously. If the process considered is the spontaneous adsorption of protein to a surface, the value of ΔG is expressed per mole of adsorbed protein and called the binding affinity.

The change in G is often divided into two separate parts according to the relation:

$$(\Delta G)_{T,P} = (\Delta H)_{T,P} - T(\Delta S)_{T,P} < 0 \quad (1)$$

where the indices T and P, added to the parenthesis, indicate that temperature and pressure are kept constant.

Equation 1 shows that a process will occur spontaneously if by proceeding the enthalpy H of the system is lowered (enthalpy-driven or enthalpic process) or the entropy S is increased (entropy-driven or entropic process). The lowering of enthalpy can often be measured independently; it corresponds to the quantity of heat liberated in a closed calorimeter kept at constant temperature and pressure. Equation 1 thus implies that exothermic reactions will tend to proceed spontaneously. Calorimetric experiments have, however, often shown endothermic protein adsorptions, i.e., adsorptions that take up heat instead of liberating it ($\Delta H > 0$). Such adsorptions can only be entropy driven, and the entropic contribution must more then balance the enthalpic one.

An enthalpy-driven process can be easily grasped intuitively. A state of higher energy is spontaneously changing to a state of lower energy, and the energy difference is released as heat. It is more difficult to acquire a feeling for an entropy-driven process. The physical picture of increasing entropy is a growing degree of randomization or chaos in the system. The unfolding of a tightly coiled polypeptide chain presents an example of such an increase in degrees of freedom. Liberation of a structured layer of counterions by an adsorbing protein molecule is another example. The second law of thermodynamics states that physical systems have a general tendency towards such randomizations, and Equation 1 shows that this tendency can be the driving force of physical processes.

A useful thermodynamic concept in interfacial systems is the existence of a surface tension σ in the interface between two nonmixing phases. A simple example is a droplet of water in air. The adhesive interactions between water molecules will not be balanced for the molecules in the outer water layer, and such molecules will be subject to a net inward force. As a result, the droplet will tend to minimize the surface area, and one may often fruitfully assume that the droplet is covered by a contractile skin. The surface tension σ is defined such that the work needed to increase the surface area A by an amount ΔA is equal to $\sigma\Delta A$. This implies that σ has the dimension of a force per unit length (N/m). For the water-air interface, one may measure the magnitude of σ by determination of the weight and the circumference of water drops falling from a dripping tab; just before falling, the weight of the drop equals the product of σ and the circumference. At room temperature a value of approximately 72×10^{-3} N/m (= 72 dyne/cm) is thus found. Knowing this value, one may, for instance, determine the value of σ as a function of the area per molecule of phospholipid monolayers at the air-water interface. This is done by spreading the phospholipids on the aqueous subphase of a Langmuir film balance as shown in Figure 1. If the barrier is exerting a force of, for instance, 30 mN/m, it must be remembered that the water-air surface exerts a counter force on the barrier of 72 mN/m. Accordingly, the phospholipid monolayer is contracting with a force of 42 mN/m.

The interface between two nonmixing phases has a positive free energy. This is a consequence of the fact that a negative contribution to the free energy of the system would

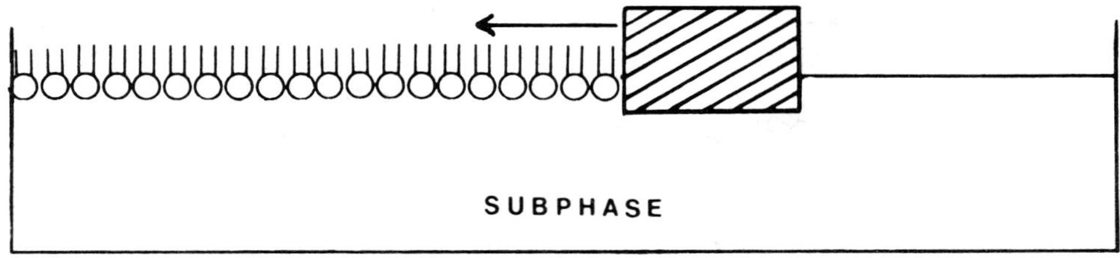

FIGURE 1. A Langmuir film balance with a monolayer phospholipid compressed by a movable barrier.

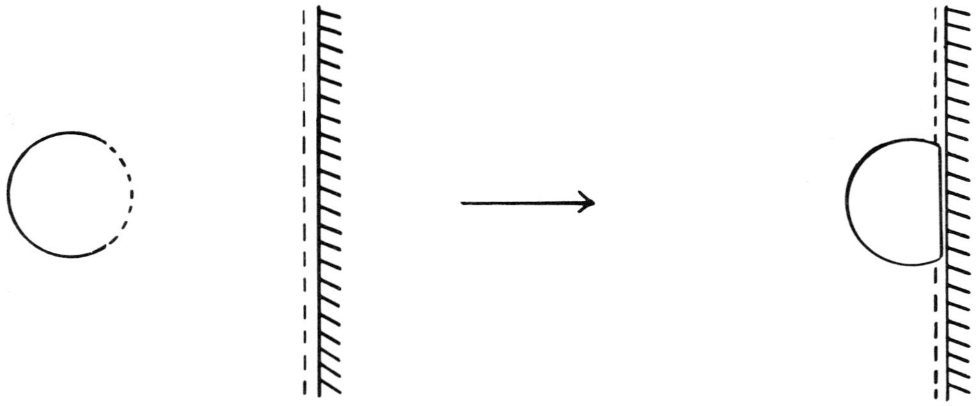

FIGURE 2. Decrease of surface areas with positive free energy as a mechanism of protein adsorption.

result in spontaneous enlargement of the interfacial area until complete mixing would be obtained. A hydrophobic surface in water or a hydrophobic part of a protein molecule will thus increase the free energy of the system. A decrease of the surface area can in that case be the driving force of adsorption with a contribution $\sigma\Delta A < 0$ to the decrease of free energy. This is shown schematically in Figure 2. Such a phenomenon can be interpreted as the thermodynamic description of protein adsorption by hydrophobic bonding.

C. Model-Dependent Description of Protein Adsorption

In the simplest model for the adsorption of proteins, the process of binding is pictured analogous to a reversible chemical reaction between protein molecules in solution and independent binding sites at the surface. Statistical averaging then results in the equivalent of the law of mass action:

$$\frac{d}{dt}\Gamma = k_{on}(\Gamma_{max} - \Gamma)\,C_b - k_{off}\,\Gamma \tag{2}$$

where Γ is the surface concentration, i.e., the adsorbed mass of protein per unit surface area, C_b is the concentration of protein in the solution, Γ_{max} is the maximal value of Γ and equal to the number of binding sites per unit surface area multiplied by the mass per protein molecule, and k_{on} and k_{off} are the sorption rate constants which are assumed to be independent of Γ and C_b.

If equilibrium is established, i.e., $d\Gamma/dt = 0$ and $\Gamma = \Gamma_{eq}$, Equation 2 is reduced to the classical Langmuir adsorption isotherm:

$$\Gamma_{eq} = \Gamma_{max}[C_b/(K_d + C_b)], \quad \text{with} \quad K_d = k_{off}/k_{on} \tag{3}$$

However, such simple reversible binding to independent binding sites is seldom observed. In contrast, one finds phenomena such as Γ-dependent values of k_{on} and k_{off}, incomplete desorption after removal of protein from the solution, different values of Γ_{eq} if the protein is added in steps instead of as a single dose to the solution, adsorptions showing an overshoot before the plateau value of Γ_{eq} is reached, etc. A host of models has been proposed to account for these observations (see References 4 and 5 for a review). These models involve specific assumptions, such as the presence of different sets of binding sites, lateral interactions between adsorbed molecules, inhomogeneous adsorption in patches of adsorbed protein, surface-induced changes in adsorbed molecules leading to altered binding affinity, or loss of binding capacity of desorbed molecules. Although these proposed models allow accurate description of sorption data in specific cases, little evidence has been presented for the physical reality of the proposed mechanisms, and it must be concluded that the modelling of protein adsorption is still in its infancy.

Much more detailed work, experimentally as well as theoretically, has been done with respect to the adsorption of flexible polymers. The structure of such chain molecules can often be rigidly controlled during synthesis, allowing a more precise description of the conformation of adsorbed molecules, as shown in Figure 3. The probability of different chain conformations can be calculated by various statistical methods.[6,7] In this approach the chain molecule is divided into segments placed in a lattice. The conformation of the molecules may change by a random walk of the segments through the lattice. By assuming different energies for a segment adsorbed to the surface or a segment surrounded by solvent, one may then calculate the density distribution of segments in a direction perpendicular to the surface and the adsorbed quantity of polymer. Such calculations for well-characterized chain molecules have shown good agreement between experimental results and theoretical predictions in bulk systems. Verification of calculated adsorptions is, however, still hampered by the lack of techniques for the measurement of actual segment distributions close to the adsorbing surface.

Modeling of the adsorption of flexible polymers has produced some features that are also observed in protein adsorption. The most important similarity is a tendency to irreversible adsorption. Even for relatively weak interactions between single segments and the surface, the large number of segments that may eventually become attached to the surface may result in a large overall binding affinity, and the probability that all segments are desorbed at the same moment — a condition required for the desorption of the complete chain molecule — may become very small. The validity of such comparisons between adsorbed polymers and proteins is not self-evident. Some experimental findings indicate essential differences. The maximal quantities of polymer adsorbed, for instance, generally exceed full monolayer coverage, and the large number of loops could never be accommodated so that all segments are in contact with the surface. In contrast, protein adsorption generally shows less than full monolayer coverage. In this respect, protein molecules seem to behave more like compact structures that may prevent the adsorption of additional molecules even before the surface is fully covered. A number of proteins also have high packing densities in solution, close to the value in crystallized preparations,[5] and this also favors a picture of the protein molecule as a tightly coiled structure, quite unlike the expanded chain molecules of flexible polymers. As a rule, polymers also show a decrease of entropy upon adsorption, corresponding to a loss of degrees of freedom in the adsorbed molecule. This implies that polymer adsorptions are enthalpy driven. In contrast, protein adsorptions may be entropy driven,[5] suggesting that at least some peripheral domains are unfolding upon adsorption.

III. THE INFLUENCE OF FLOW CONDITIONS ON PROTEIN ADSORPTION

A. Introduction

The in vivo production of thrombin will often occur at the vessel wall, e.g., at activated

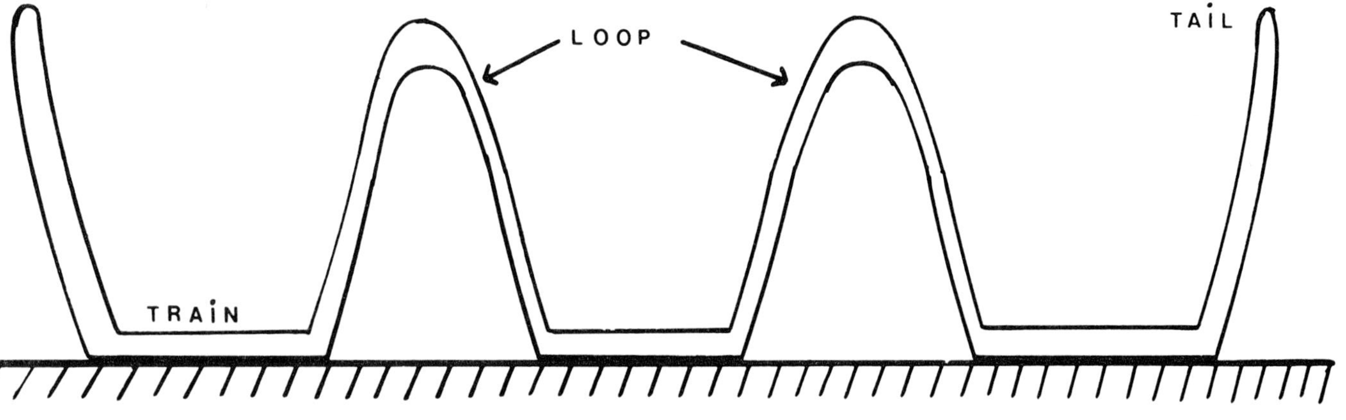

FIGURE 3. Model for an adsorbed chain molecule. Regions adsorbed to the surface (trains) are alternating with extensions in the solution (loops and tails).

platelets adhering to an endothelial lesion. Due to the laminar flow conditions prevailing in blood vessels, there is a region of sluggish flow close to the endothelial surface. Traditionally, this region has been called the "unstirred layer", and has often been modeled as a stagnant layer of 5- to 150-μm thickness directly adjacent to the surface. It has the effect of imposing a limit value on the rate of protein adsorption to the surface. It can be intuitively understood that a rapid blood flow close to the surface will diminish the influence of this transport barrier, because such rapid flow will provide a fresh supply of protein and thereby prevent protein depletion of the boundary layer. As the flow velocity approaches zero at the surface, a rapid flow close to the surface can only be obtained for a large gradient in the flow velocities, i.e., a large shear rate, close to the surface.

With respect to the influence of flow conditions on the rate of protein adsorption, three different situations may occur. For proteins with very low intrinsic adsorption rates, i.e., low values of k_{on}, the transport capacity of diffusion is sufficient to keep the protein concentration close to the surface approximately equal to the bulk concentration, and there is no transport barrier. The sorption rate constants thus measured are the true intrinsic rate constants. For proteins with very high values of k_{on}, there is almost complete depletion of the boundary layer. This is the so-called transport-limited case with sorption rates that are completely determined by diffusion and convection. Such transport-limited adsorption also implies transport-limited desorption, because a high value of k_{on} has the effect that desorbing molecules have a high chance of adsorbing again unless they are rapidly transported from the surface to the bulk. The third situation is the intermediate case, with sorption rates determined by both the intrinsic sorption rates and by flow conditions. As will be discussed in Section V, the initial phase of the adsorption of factors II, X, and V is completely transport limited. Higher surface concentrations of these coagulation factors have the effect of decreasing the values of k_{on}, and this brings the sorption kinetics in the intermediate case.

A useful concept in the study of transport limitations in protein adsorption is the so-called uniformly accessible surface. This is a surface for which the combined effects of diffusion and convection result in a transport of protein with a uniform velocity towards the surface; that is, the velocity component perpendicular to the surface is independent of the position on the surface. Such a uniformly accessible surface can be described by an equivalent unstirred layer model with uniform layer thickness. As shown below, this allows a simple interpretation of actually measured "apparent" adsorption rates in terms of the true intrinsic rate constants and the model parameters. As shown in Section III.C, however, a surface in a laminar flow field is far from uniformly accessible. This implies, for instance, that the rate of adsorption of coagulation factors on activated platelets adhering to the vessel wall will be site dependent. A numerical example of this situation will be given in Section III.D.

B. Apparent and Intrinsic Sorption Rates in the Unstirred Layer Model

Figure 4 shows the classical unstirred layer model. A protein-adsorbing surface, situated at $x = 0$, is separated from a perfectly mixed bulk solution by an unstirred layer of thickness d. Protein molecules can only pass through the unstirred layer by diffusion. It is assumed that there is initially no protein present in the solution, and that at time $t = 0$ the protein concentration in the solution is changed abruptly to a fixed bulk value C_b. For reversible binding to independent binding sites one then obtains (see Equation 2):

$$\frac{d}{dt}\Gamma(t) = k_{on}[\Gamma_{max} - \Gamma(t)]\, C(0, t) - k_{off}\,\Gamma(t) \qquad (4)$$

where $\Gamma(t)$ is the surface concentration of protein at time t, k_{on} and k_{off} are the intrinsic adsorption and desorption rate constants, and $C(0,t)$ is the protein concentration in the solution at $x = 0$, i.e., directly adjacent to the surface, at time t. By solving the diffusion equation

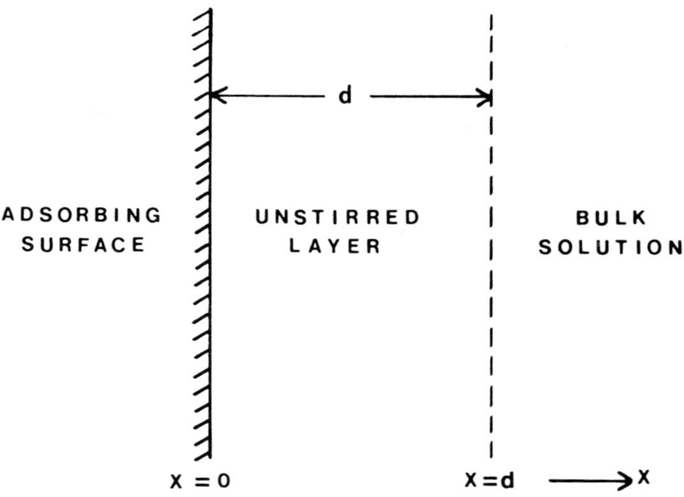

FIGURE 4. The unstirred layer model.

for C(x,t), it can be shown[8] that within a second after addition of protein to the bulk solution, a linear concentration gradient of protein will be established in the unstirred layer. After some time the concentration C(0,t) will start to increase, and the concentration gradient will become less steep, but it will remain linear for practically the whole period of adsorption. This behavior can also be understood from general considerations. The transport capacity of diffusion and the capacity for adsorption of the surface are both large, compared to the quantity of protein in the unstirred layer. Under these circumstances a steady-state concentration profile will be rapidly established in the unstirred layer, and a linear gradient is the only possible steady state. This latter fact follows from the circumstance that the diffusional flux of protein is proportional to the concentration gradient, and a local change in the flux, i.e., a departure from a linear gradient, would cause a change in the local protein concentration or a disturbance of the steady state.

Due to this linearity, one may also write $d\Gamma/dt = D[C_b - C(0,t)]/d$, with D the diffusion constant of the protein. Eliminating C(0,t) from Equation 4 by use of this expression, one obtains after rearrangement of terms:

$$\frac{d}{dt}\Gamma(t) = k_{on}^{app}[\Gamma_{max} - \Gamma(t)]\, C_b - k_{off}^{app}\,\Gamma(t) \qquad (5)$$

with

$$k_{on}^{app} = k_{on}/[1 + k_{on}(\Gamma_{max} - \Gamma)d/D]$$

$$k_{off}^{app} = k_{off}/[1 + k_{on}(\Gamma_{max} - \Gamma)d/D] \qquad (6)$$

Some interesting conclusions follow from these expressions. For small values of k_{on}, i.e., for $k_{on}\Gamma_{max}\, d/D << 1$, there is no influence of diffusion on sorption kinetics, and the intrinsic sorption rate constants k_{on} and k_{off} are equal to the apparent constants k_{on}^{app} and k_{off}^{app} obtained from sorption experiments. In practical applications one first measures $d\Gamma/dt$ as a function of time after addition of protein to the solution at $t = 0$. After adsorption of a sufficient quantity of protein, the rate of desorption is measured after suddenly changing the buffer concentration of protein to zero by rapidly flushing the cuvette with fresh buffer. Flushing

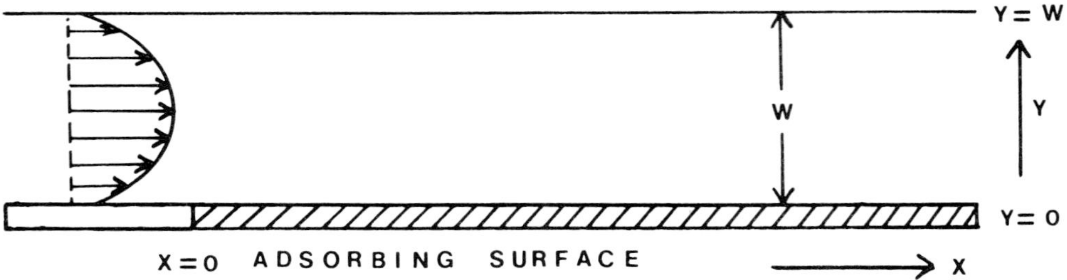

FIGURE 5. Laminar flow in a narrow slit.

is continued, at a slower rate, during desorption in order to prevent accumulation of desorbed protein. For $C_b = 0$ Equation 5 reduces to $d\Gamma/dt = -k_{off}^{app}\,\Gamma(t)$ and k_{off}^{app} can thus be obtained by measurement of the rate of desorption as a function of the surface concentration. Knowing k_{off}^{app}, the value of k_{on}^{app} can be obtained from the earlier measured adsorption phase, because Equation 5 can be written as $k_{on}^{app} = (d\Gamma/dt + k_{off}^{app}\Gamma)/[(\Gamma_{max} - \Gamma)C_b]$.

Equation 6 shows that for large values of k_{on}, the intrinsic rate constants will be grossly underestimated if they are equated to k_{on}^{app} and k_{off}^{app}. As explained before, this is also true for the desorption rate constant because of the high chance of readsorption. Even for high value of k_{on}, however, the differences between intrinsic and apparent rate constants will vanish if $\Gamma(t)$ approaches Γ_{max}, i.e., close to maximal surface coverage (see Equation 6). Theoretically, one could thus estimate the intrinsic values k_{on} and k_{off} by measuring the sorption rates close to Γ_{max}. In practice, however, high values of k_{on} may already result in large differences between apparent and intrinsic sorption constants for values for Γ close to Γ_{max}. Accurate assessment of $d\Gamma/dt$ requires some range of values for Γ and such a range close to Γ_{max} will often be too small for accurate measurements. As a result, one can only obtain lower limits for k_{on} of the order of $10^6\ M^{-1}\ sec^{-1}$,[8] whereas the values of k_{on} for factors II, X, and V are about one to two orders of magnitude higher (see Section V). It is important to note from Equation 6 that the value of the dissociation constant $K_d = k_{off}/k_{on}$ equals the ratio $k_{off}^{app}/k_{on}^{app}$, and may thus be determined from sorption kinetics, even for transport-limited sorption.

C. Uniformly Accessible Surfaces

Figure 5 shows a narrow slit of width w. An adsorbing surface is situated at $x > 0$. A buffer solution containing protein at a concentration C_b starts flowing into the slit at a time $t = 0$. The protein concentration at a site x,y in the slit, and at time t is indicated by $C(x,y,t)$, and the flow of protein through this site is indicated by the two components, J_x and J_y. The value of $C(x,y,t)$ can only change in time if at least one of the flows J_x or J_y changes the value at the site x,y (conservation of protein mass) and accordingly we have:

$$\frac{\partial}{\partial t} C(x, y, t) = -\frac{\partial}{\partial x} J_x - \frac{\partial}{\partial y} J_y \tag{7}$$

The minus signs in the right-hand side of this equation express the fact that the local protein concentration will be decreased if the local flux is increasing and vice versa.

If the inner surface of the slit has a sufficiently large capacity for protein adsorption, i.e., large compared to the protein content of thin boundary layer with $y/w << 1$, a steady state $C_s(x,y)$ will be rapidly established as explained in the preceding section. In that case, the left-hand side of Equation 7 will vanish. The quantity of interest in this equation is J_y, the

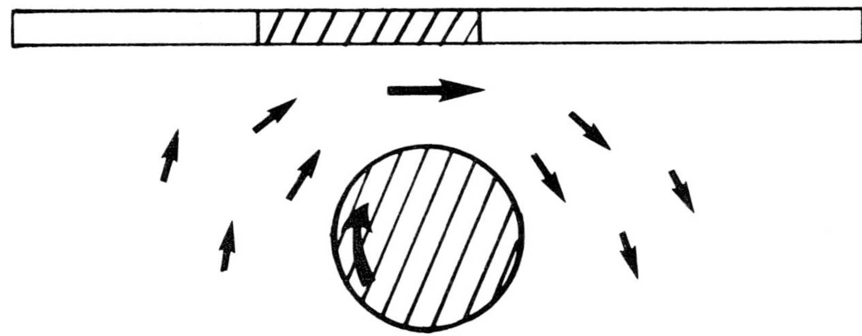

FIGURE 6. A rotating cylinder close to the adsorbing surface.

flow of protein directed to the surface, because in the steady state it must equal the rate of protein adsorption and the diffusional transport to the surface:

$$J_y = -\frac{d}{dt}\Gamma = -D\left(\frac{\partial C_s}{\partial y}\right)_{y=0} \tag{8}$$

The latter equality in this equation is a consequence from the fact that the buffer flow is strictly parallel to the surface, and transport in the y direction can only be effected by diffusion.

If a stable laminar flow is established in the slit, the corresponding parabolic flow profile can be written as $v(y) = \gamma y(1 - y/w)$, where $v(y)$ is the flow velocity at a distance y from the surface. One may check that this expression satisfies the conditions $v(y) = 0$ for $y = 0$ and $y = w$ and that $\gamma = (\partial v/\partial y)_{y=0}$ is the shear rate at the surface. In the steady state and close to the surface ($y/w << 1$) one thus obtains: $J_x = v(y)C_s(x,y) = \gamma y C_s(x,y)$. Inserting this expression for J_x and Equation 8 for J_y into Equation 7, one obtains an equation that can be solved[9] with the following result:

$$\frac{d}{dt}\Gamma = 0.54(\gamma D^2/x)^{1/3}\, C_b \tag{9}$$

This expression implies that the adsorbing surface in Figure 5 is not uniformly accessible, because the rate of adsorption or the flow of protein towards the surface will decrease for increasing x. An equivalent, unstirred layer model would need an unstirred layer of increasing thickness in the x direction.

Equation 9 shows that for increasing values of the shear rate γ at the surface, the rate of protein adsorption will also increase. This circumstance offers opportunities of devising uniformly accessible surfaces. Figure 6 shows one of these systems.[8] A rotating cylinder produces a vortex flow close to the protein-adsorbing surface. The shear rate increases in the narrow space between the surface and the cylinder. Somewhat more to the left, the lower shear rate is compensated by a flow component in the direction of the surface. Due to this compensation, the shaded area in the adsorbing surface will be approximately uniformly accessible.

A more fundamental solution is obtained by considering the adsorption of proteins on a rotating disc, as shown in Figure 7. Again, a compensation mechanism occurs with high shear rates at the edges and a flow parallel to the surface, in contrast to low shear rates and a flow directed towards the surface in the middle. This setup was originally introduced in the design of electrodes in electrochemistry[10] and has recently also been applied to the study of the adsorption of Factor II.[11]

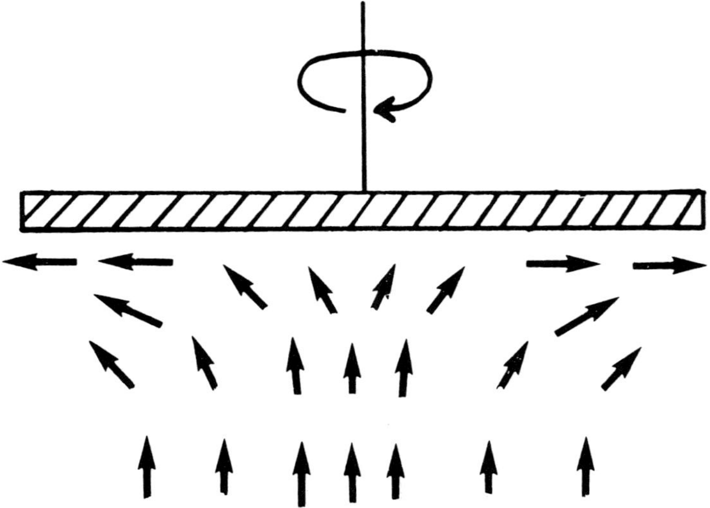

FIGURE 7. Flow pattern at a rotating disc.

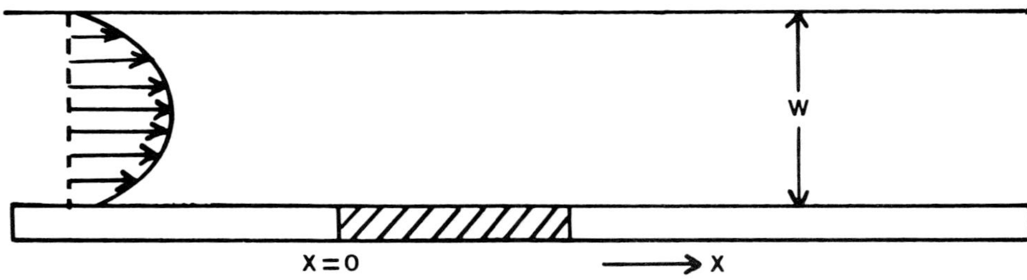

FIGURE 8. A small arteriole with a lesion starting at x = 0.

D. A Numerical Example: Adsorption of Prothrombin at an Endothelial Lesion

As will be discussed in Section V, the value of k_{on} for the adsorption of factor II on phospholipid model membranes and the value of Γ_{max} for such membranes are such that the initial phase of adsorption is, indeed, completely transport limited. For biological membranes, however, values of Γ_{max} are difficult to estimate, because the capacity for adsorption of coagulation factors may be largely diminished by the adsorption of plasma proteins such as albumin and fibrinogen, which are present in large excess. A more reasonable estimate for the rate of factor II adsorption occurring in vivo can be obtained from measurements of the thrombin-generating capacity of activated platelets in buffer solutions containing excess ovalbumin.[12] For platelets activated by thrombin and collagen, it was found that a single platelet can produce about 10^{-6} pmol factor II_a per second. This value can be used to estimate the thrombin-generating capacity of an endothelial lesion covered with activated platelets.

Figure 8 shows a small arteriole of about 30-μm diameter with an endothelial lesion covered with activated platelets. Assuming a surface density of 10^7 platelets per square centimeter, i.e., about 50% of complete coverage,[13] the maximal production of thrombin by a single layer of adhering platelets would be about 10 pmol of factor IIa per square centimeter per second. The question to be answered is whether this rate of thrombin production can be realized or is restricted by limitation of transport of factor II to the surface.

The midstream blood velocity in an arteriole of this diameter is about 3 mm/sec.[14] For a parabolic flow velocity profile, $v(y) = \gamma y(1 - y/w)$ (see the preceding section) one has a midstream velocity $v(w/2) = \gamma w/4$. Inserting the values $v(w/2) = 3$ mm/sec and $w = 30$ μm, one obtains the value of $\gamma = 400\ sec^{-1}$ for the shear rate at the surface. The diffusion constant for factor II is $6.2 \times 10^{-7}\ cm^2/sec$,[15] and the concentration of factor II in plasma is about 1.5 nmol/mℓ. Inserting these values into Equation 9 one obtains:

$$\begin{aligned} x &= 10^{-4}\ cm \quad & d\Gamma/dt &= 20\ pmol/cm^2/sec \\ x &= 10^{-3}\ cm \quad & d\Gamma/dt &= 4.4\ pmol/cm^2/sec \\ x &= 10^{-2}\ cm \quad & d\Gamma/dt &= 2.0\ pmol/cm^2/sec \\ x &= 10^{-1}\ cm \quad & d\Gamma/dt &= 0.9\ pmol/cm^2/sec \end{aligned} \tag{10}$$

These values imply that only for a lesion as small as a single platelet the rate of thrombin production will not be hampered. In contrast, a lesion of about 1 mm in diameter will show a strong transport limitation with respect to thrombin generation. It is interesting to note from this example that platelets are just small enough to allow unrestricted production of thrombin by an activated platelet adhering to the vessel wall. Any plug of platelets, however, will show transport limitations. This conclusion remains essentially unaltered for larger blood vessels, because the simultaneous increase of vessel diameter and blood velocity leaves the value of γ in the range of 200 to 1000 sec^{-1}. For larger vessels Equation 9 will be approximately valid because it was derived for a flat surface situated in a narrow slit. For small vessels — in fact, also for the example just presented — the effect of transport limitation will be even more severe, because curvature will cause an additional protein depletion of the central bulk solution.

The plasma concentration of factor II is about 1.5 μ*M* and high, if compared to the Michaelis constant for factor II activation which is of the order of $K_m = 0.1\ \mu M$.[16] It follows from this example, however, that such a high plasma concentration is needed to overcome transport limitations. During steady-state production of thrombin, the factor II concentration close to the vessel wall will be lowered to a value close to K_m, and the large gradient thus created will ensure a rapid transport of factor II from the bulk to the surface.

Another effect of transport limitation will be that during steady-state production of thrombin there is a large accumulation of thrombin at the vessel wall. In fact, the situation is complementary and the thrombin concentration at the vessel wall will approximately equal the factor II concentration in the bulk. Apart from the low flow velocities at the wall, this high thrombin concentration will promote platelet activation, thus contributing to the efficiency of platelet adherence to endothelial lesions.

IV. METHODS FOR THE DETERMINATION OF BINDING PARAMETERS

A. Introduction

As mentioned in Section I, the concept of the prothrombinase complex of activated factors Xa and Va situated on a phospholipid surface was developed about 20 years ago. Evidence for this model came mainly from the measurement of the kinetics of thrombin production as a function of the concentrations of factors Xa, Va, and phospholipid. It was found, for instance, that excess phospholipid inhibits the production of thrombin, and this suggests a "surface dilution" effect. In such kinetic experiments one does not directly observe the adsorption of coagulation factors on the phospholipid membrane, and the binding constants obtained are thus apparent constants, depending on the specific assumptions about the mechanism of factor II activation. Although this lack of direct verification of the binding process is a definite disadvantage, the kinetic method for the estimation of binding parameters still has superior sensitivity compared to the direct methods that have since been developed.

At the time when the concept of the prothrombinase complex was established, the first direct ellipsometric measurements of the adsorption of proteins from buffer solutions to various solid substrates had already been performed.[17-19] The preparation of phospholipid model membranes and the techniques for purification of coagulation factors were, however, insufficiently developed to allow an ellipsometric study of the prothrombinase complex. It took another decade before the first direct observations of the association of factor II with phospholipid vesicles were made by means of light scattering.[20] Since then a variety of techniques has been applied that will be shortly discussed below.

B. Binding Parameters Obtained from the Kinetics of Thrombin Production

In a solution containing factors II, Xa, and Va it is assumed that factor II is activated by a stoichiometric complex of factors Xa and Va: $Xa + Va \rightleftarrows XaVa$ with a dissociation constant $K_d = [Xa][Va]/[XaVa]$. This assumption implies that noncomplexed factor Xa may also activate factor II, but at a rate that can be neglected compared to the rate of activation by the XaVa complex.[16]

For a low initial concentration of $[Xa]_o$, i.e., $[Xa]_o << K_d$, one may choose a series of initial concentration $[Va]_o$ such that $[Va]_o$ is much larger than $[Xa]_o$, but different values of $[Va]_o$ will still result in different values of [XaVa]. In that case, one may write $[Va] \cong [Va]_o$ and $[Xa] = [Xa]_o - [XaVa]$. The rate of thrombin production v will be proportional to the concentration [XaVa] and one has $v/v_{max} = [XaVa]/[Xa]_o$. Inserting these relations into the expression for K_d one obtains:

$$1/v = (K_d/v_{max})(1/[Va]_o) + 1/v_{max} \qquad (11)$$

A plot of $1/v$ vs. $1/[Va]_o$ will thus produce a straight line with an intercept at the ordinate of $1/v_{max}$ and an intercept $1/K_d$ at the abcissa. A similar equation may be obtained if a fixed low concentration [Va] of factor Va is titrated with factor Xa. By preincubation of either factor Va or Xa with a phospholipid suspension, one may thus obtain the binding parameters of the various factors in the complete prothrombinase complex.[21]

C. Determination of the Protein Depletion of Solutions

One of the simplest methods for the determination of binding parameters is based on phospholipid preparations that can be separated from the bulk solution. If the adsorbed amount of protein forms an appreciable part of the total quantity of protein in the system, one may simply calculate the bound fraction. This method has been applied for the binding of factors II, X, and V to large unilamellar vesicles[22] and to platelets.[23,24] In both cases the phospholipids can be separated from the bulk solution by means of centrifugation.

In practical applications of this depletion technique, one is often hampered by the fact that for the measurement of K_d values of the order of 10^{-9} *M* or below, the protein concentrations in the solution become too low for accurate measurement. This limitation can be overcome by the use of radiolabeled protein preparations, but the purification and labeling procedures involved may introduce artefacts due to different parameters for labeled and native molecules.[25]

D. Binding to Phospholipid Monolayers at the Air/Water Interface

The adsorption of coagulation factors to phospholipid monolayers spread on the aqueous subphase of a Langmuir trough has been studied by some authors (see Figure 1). The surface concentration of adsorbed protein was measured either by direct detection of surface radioactivity after addition of radiolabeled proteins to the subphase,[26,27] or by registration of the changes in surface pressure due to adsorption.[27] The latter measurements have shown a strong dependence of obtained results on the initial surface pressure. This is a complicating factor because it is not a priori apparent which surface pressure should be chosen. Ill-defined flow conditions and large surface/volume ratios may also complicate the interpretation of these data, especially of measured sorption rates.

E. Measurement of the Electrical Resistance and Capacitance of Phospholipid Monolayers

The change in the electrical capacitance of a phospholipid monolayer due to the adsorption of proteins has been used for the measurement of the adsorption kinetics of factor II.[28,29] An important feature of this technique is that it may allow differentiation between adsorption and penetration in the phospholipid monolayer. Both phenomena have different effects on the capacitance, and penetration may also be detected by the contact of protein with the electrode, because several amino acids can be recognized by the specific voltage-dependent conductivity.[30] Although this technique is especially suited for the measurement of adsorption rates, it does not allow the determination of the intrinsic value of k_{on} for factor II because of the transport limitations discussed in Section III.

F. Protein-Lipid Binding Measured by Gel Filtration

This technique was introduced as a general method for the measurement of binding of various substances to proteins.[31] A column of cross-linked dextran is incubated with a buffer solution containing radiolabeled protein. The phospholipid preparation is applied to the column as a small volume of uniformly sized vesicles, and the column is eluted with the incubation medium. The protein-vesicle complexes have a larger size than the protein molecules. As a result, these complexes have a smaller distribution volume in the column and will travel down the column more rapidly than the uncomplexed protein molecules in the initial phospholipid-protein mixture. A peak of increased radioactivity is eluted from the column, corresponding to the bound quantity of protein. This peak is followed by a pit of decreased radioactivity due to protein depletion of the buffer. If the peak and the pit are completely separated, as can be checked from the equality of excess counts and missing counts, one can be sure that the phospholipid vesicles were exposed to the initial protein concentration in the buffer. By varying this concentration, one obtains the dissociation constant K_d.

G. Light Scattering in Phospholipid Suspensions

A macromolecular solution will scatter a fraction of the light intensity traveling through the solution. The light intensity i_θ, in a direction at an angle θ to the incoming lightbeam, is given by[6]

$$i_\theta = F.I_o\, c\, n^2(\partial n/\partial c)^2(1 + \cos^2\theta)/(1/M + 2Bc + 3Cc^2 + \ldots) \qquad (12)$$

with I_o as the total intensity of the incoming lightbeam, c the concentration of macromolecules in the solution, n the refractive index of the solution, M the molecular mass of the scattering macromolecules, and B and C the second and third virial coefficient that correct for the nonideality of the solution due to particle interactions. The factor F is a system-dependent constant given by $F = 2\pi^2/N\lambda^4r^2$ with N the number of Avogadro, λ the wavelength of light, and r the distance between the scattering sample and the light detector. The important parameter $\partial n/\partial c$ can be determined on a differential refractometer at the same wavelength as used for the scattering experiments. For dilute solutions the terms 2Bc and $3Cc^2$ can be neglected, while n^2 can be replaced by n_o^2 with n_o as the refractive index of the buffer.

In 1977, Nelsestuen and Lim[20] introduced light scattering as a method for the measurement of the adsorption of factor II to phospholipid vesicles. The small (16 to 20 nm diameter) unilamellar vesicles, with a molecular weight of approximately $M = 10^7$, are effective light-scattering "macromolecules" and this scattering is much enhanced if they become coated with protein. The scattering of unbound protein molecules may be neglected in first approximation. Experiments are usually performed at an angle $\theta = 90°$. In that case it follows from Equation 12 that the ratio of the scattering intensities for the protein-vesicle complex (I_2) to that of the vesicles without protein (I_1) is equal to $I_2/I_1 = (\partial n_2/\partial c_2)^2 M_2c_2/[(\partial n_1/\partial c_1)^2M_1c_1)]$. As the number of light-scattering particles is not changed by the adsorption, i.e., $c_1/M_1 = c_2/M_2$, one obtains:

$$I_2/I_1 = (\partial n_2/\partial c_2)^2 M_2^2/[(\partial n_1/\partial c_1)^2M_1^2] \quad (13)$$

In practical applications Equation 13 is solved by an iterative procedure. As a first approximation one assumes that $(\partial n_2/\partial c_2)/(\partial n_1/\partial c_1) = 1$ and estimates M_2/M_1 from the measured intensities I_2 and I_1. The ratio of protein to phospholipid in the complex, as calculated from M_2/M_1, is then used to calculate $\partial n_2/\partial c_2$ by interpolation between the values for pure lipid, i.e., $\partial n_1/\partial c_1$, and the corresponding value for pure protein. This calculated value is then inserted into Equation 13 and M_2/M_1 is again estimated. This process is repeated until M_2/M_1 becomes constant.

An important advantage of this technique is that it allows determination of intrinsic adsorption and desorption rate constants. Due to the reduction of the size of the adsorbing phospholipid membranes to macromolecular dimensions, there is no buildup of boundary layers, as discussed in the preceding section. The upper limit of the measurable rate of adsorption thus equals the maximal rate of a bimolecular chemical conversion that is of the order of 10^9 M^{-1} sec^{-1}. This advantage was used in a stopped-flow version of the light-scattering system.[32]

A drawback of this method is the relatively high phospholipid concentration, of the order of 0.1 m*M*, required for sufficient scattering intensities. Any appreciable binding of protein to this quantity of lipid will rapidly deplete the pool of unbound protein if the concentration of protein is low. Such protein depletion cannot be checked because the vesicles cannot be separated from the solution, and this puts a lower limit of 10^{-7} to 10^{-8} *M* to the values of K_d that can be measured.

H. Ellipsometry

Ellipsometry is an optical technique for the measurement of the refractive index (n) and the thickness (d) of thin layers (0.1 to 100 nm) deposited on reflecting surfaces. The reflecting surface can be a chromium slide covered with a monolayer[33] or double layer[8] of phospholipid by means of the Langmuir-Blodgett technique for the stacking of fatty acid multilayers.[34] The adsorption of proteins to such a phospholipid-covered slide can be measured in buffer solutions and the surface concentration of adsorbed protein can be calculated from the measured values of n and d by using the following relation:

$$\Gamma = 3d(n^2 - n_b^2)/\{(n^2 + 2)[r(n_b^2 + 2) - v(n_b^2 - 1)]\} \quad (14)$$

This relation is a consequence of the classical Lorentz-Lorenz relation[35] and contains the specific refractivity (r) and the partial specific volume (v) of the adsorbed protein, as well as the refractive index n_b of the buffer solution. Equation 14 is used if the adsorbed layer consists of a mixture of protein and buffer. If, in contrast, the adsorbed layer consists of pure protein, this equation is reduced to:

$$\Gamma = d(n^2 - 1)/[r(n^2 + 2)] \quad (15)$$

Ellipsometry allows simultaneous measurement of the surface concentration Γ and buffer concentration of protein C_b. Depletion of the buffer solution can be avoided, even for very low protein concentrations, by using a continuous flow of solution through the cuvette

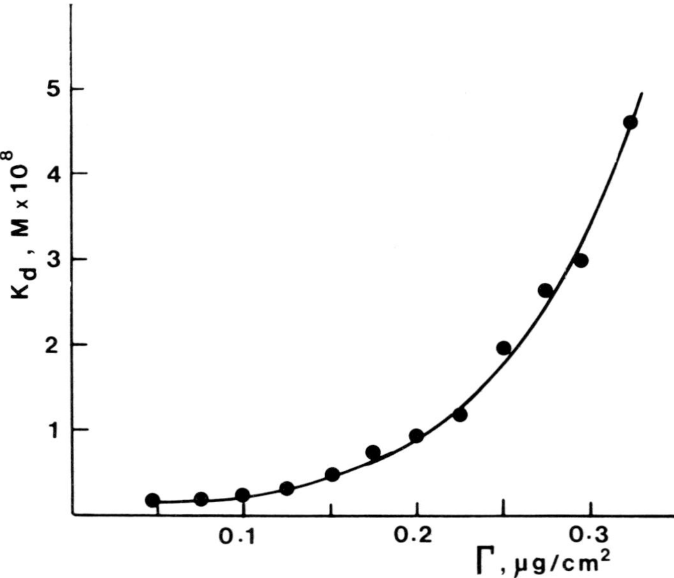

FIGURE 9. The dissociation constant K_d as a function of the surface concentration Γ for the adsorption of factor II on a di 18:1 PS double layer.

containing the adsorbing slide. This allows determination of K_d values as low as 10^{-10} to 10^{-11} *M*.[33,35] However, such experiments are time consuming because the adsorption is usually transport limited, and the diffusional flux of protein to the surface becomes very slow for such low protein concentrations in the buffer.

V. BINDING PARAMETERS FOR THE ADSORPTION OF COAGULATION FACTORS II, V, AND X ON PHOSPHOLIPID MEMBRANES

A. Introduction

In Section II some complicating features of protein adsorption were discussed. Two of these aspects are particularly relevant in a review of binding parameters. First, it is often found that the value of the dissociation constant K_d only remains constant in a domain of low surface concentration. Beyond this range K_d will increase by further adsorption. Figure 9 shows this phenomenon for the adsorption of factor II on a di C 18:1 PS double layer. Up to a value of about $\Gamma = 0.20$ μg/cm² the value of K_d is of the order of 10^{-9} *M*, but for higher values of Γ the value of K_d increases by several orders of magnitude. As it is difficult to imagine the presence of different binding sites on a homogeneous membrane consisting of a single phospholipid, it is tempting to explain this behavior by assuming that for a surface concentration of about 0.20 μg/cm² the adsorbed protein molecules become subject to lateral interactions hampering further adsorption. In order to avoid ambiguity, the values of K_d quoted in the tables below are initial values measured for low surface coverage.

A second complicating factor is the apparently reversible behavior during protein adsorption, which sometimes proves irreversible if desorption is attempted. Higher protein concentrations in the buffer solution result in higher surface concentrations, but only limited desorption occurs if the solution is replaced by pure buffer. An example of such behavior is the adsorption of fibrinogen on di C 18:1 PS double layers[8] and the adsorption of factor V on phospholipid membranes of various composition (unpublished results). Until now this phenomenon has not been explained satisfactorily, and it should be kept in mind, considering the values of K_d for factor V in the tables below. Such values were measured by adsorption experiments, and desorption would indicate much lower, or even zero, values for K_d.

Binding of the γ-carboxyglutamic acid containing factors II and X to phospholipid membranes requires the presence of Ca^{2+} or other divalent metal ions. As the descarboxy factors, induced by therapy with vitamin K antagonists, do not bind to such membranes, it has been generally assumed that the binding mechanism consists of the formation of a calcium-mediated complex between the carboxyglutamic acid residues and the phospholipids. A chelation type of binding has been proposed[36,37] in order to account for the limited influence of ionic strength on the binding process. It has also been suggested that the carboxyglutamic acid residues are only involved in a calcium-dependent transition in the factor II molecule that unmasks the binding site for phospholipids.[38]

The effect of calcium on the values of K_d for factor II is mainly restricted to the range of 0 to 2 m*M* Ca^{2+}. A further increase of the calcium concentration, for instance, to 10 m*M* Ca^{2+}, will only slightly lower the value of K_d. Similar results have been shown for prothrombin fragment 1[39] and factor X.[40] The compilation in the tables was therefore restricted to values measured at calcium concentrations in the range of 2 to 10 m*M*.

Apart from the presence of Ca^{2+}, the binding of factors II and X also requires the presence of negatively charged (acidic) phospholipids in the adsorbing membrane. For percentages between 0 to 20% of acidic phospholipids, values of Γ_{max} for factor II increase approximately linearly from 0 to 0.20 μg/cm², while a further increase of this percentage has a progressively less effect.[26,33] In order to explain this observation, it was suggested that the binding of factors II and X to mixtures of neutral and charged phospholipids is effected by clustering of acidic phospholipids. This would create domains to which the protein molecules can bind. Some studies, using fluorescent lipid-soluble probes, have produced evidence supporting this hypothesis.[41,42] However, more recent studies, using similar methods, indicate that clustering of acidic phospholipids is absent or very limited during binding of factor II to such mixed membranes.[43,44]

The percentage of acidic phospholipids not only determines the value of Γ_{max}, but also has a large effect on the value of K_d, as shown in Figure 10. Between 20 and 100% of phosphatidylserine (PS) the affinity of the membrane for factors II and X is much increased, and the values of K_d are decreased by two orders of magnitude.[33] The effect of surface concentration on the values of K_d vanishes for lower percentages of acidic phospholipids. This implies that for membranes containing less than 20% of acidic phospholipids, the effect of Γ on the value of K_d has disappeared and the adsorption can be described as reversible binding to independent binding sites. Again, this suggests that the value of Γ_{max} for 20% acidic phospholipids, i.e., about 0.20 μg/cm² (see Table 1), is the limit value for the surface concentration at which steric hindrance of adsorbed factor II molecules starts. Efficient adsorption of factor V also requires the presence of acidic phospholipids in the membrane. In contrast, however, calcium is not required and high calcium concentrations even inhibit adsorption.

Because most experiments have been done for phosphatidylserine/phosphatidylcholine mixtures, the tables have been restricted to such membranes. Substitution of PG for PS results in somewhat lower binding affinities.[39] The effect of temperature on the values of the dissociation constants is limited in the range 10 to 37°C,[36] and values measured at different temperatures were pooled.

B. Parameters Obtained from Binding Isotherms

Values of K_d and the maximal surface concentration Γ_{max} are usually obtained from the so-called binding isotherm, i.e., the surface concentration Γ measured as a function of the buffer concentration of protein C_b. In such experiments a set of values for C_b is chosen and the corresponding equilibrium values of Γ are determined. In equilibrium one has k_{on} C_b

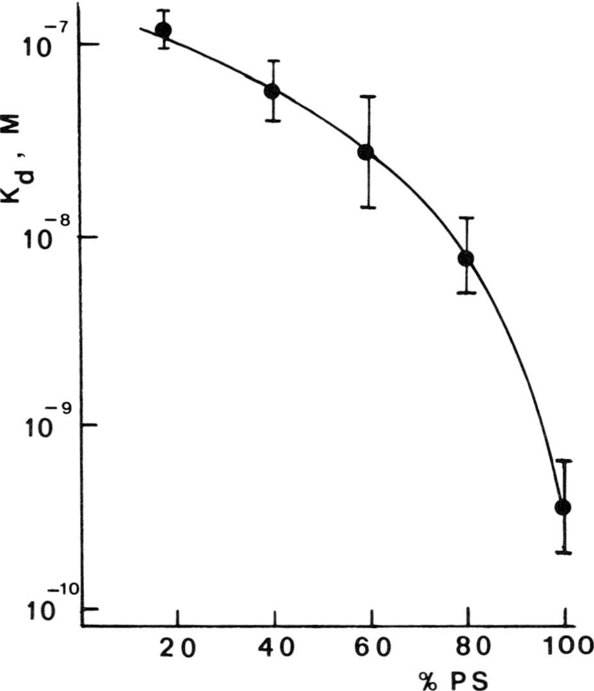

FIGURE 10. The dissociation constant K_d as a function of the percentage of PS for the adsorption of factor II on phospholipid monolayers consisting of di 18:1 PC/di 18:1 PS mixtures.

$(\Gamma_{max} - \Gamma) = k_{off}\Gamma$ or $K_d = k_{off}/k_{on} = C_b(\Gamma_{max} - \Gamma)/\Gamma$. This relation is usually written as:

$$1/\Gamma = (K_d/\Gamma_{max})(1/C_b) + 1/\Gamma_{max} \tag{16}$$

and a double-reciprocal plot, i.e., $1/\Gamma$ as a function of $1/C_b$, will thus yield a straight line, allowing determination of K_d and Γ_{max} from the intercepts $-1/K_d$ and $1/\Gamma_{max}$ with the horizontal and vertical axis. Transport limitations do not occur in this approach, because only equilibrium states are observed and all gradients in the solution will have vanished. As discussed in the preceding section, deviations from linearity will often occur due to nonreversible or interacting binding sites. Values of K_d and Γ_{max} are then extrapolated from the initial part of the curve, i.e., for low values of C_b, with inherent risks for biased values of Γ_{max} and K_d.

Table 1 shows selected data from the literature obtained with a variety of techniques. The binding parameters were obtained essentially by application of Equation 16 or from related expressions. For factors II and X, a rather uniform picture is apparent, with only a somewhat higher value for Γ_{max} as determined by light scattering. These latter values can only be calculated by using specific assumptions on protein orientation, vesicle size, and distribution of phospholipids over outer and inner membranes, while the other techniques considered in Table 1 allow more direct determination of surface concentrations. Accordingly, it seems safe to assume that the maximal surface concentrations of factors II and X on membranes containing 20% PS will be of the order of 0.20 $\mu g/cm^2$. A considerable higher value of about 0.50 $\mu g/cm^2$ is found for factor V. Calculations of the quantity of protein in a closely packed monolayer suffer from incertainties with respect to molecular dimensions and ori-

Table 1
PARAMETERS OBTAINED FROM BINDING ISOTHERMS FOR THE ADSORPTION OF FACTORS II, X, AND V ON MODEL MEMBRANES

Protein (phospholipid preparation)	Method	K_d (*M*)	Γ_{max} ($\mu g/cm^2$)	Ref.
	Factor II			
Brain PS/egg PC SUV	Light scattering	3×10^{-7}	± 0.50	40
di 18:1 PS/di 18:1 PC LUV	Protein depletion	2×10^{-7}	0.14	22
di 18:1 PS/di 18:1 PC monolayer	Ellipsometry	1.6×10^{-7}	0.22	33
	Prothrombin Fragment 1			
Brain PS/egg PC monolayer	Film balance	3×10^{-7}	0.12	26
	Factor X			
Brain PS/egg PC SUV	Light scattering	2×10^{-7}	± 0.50	40
di 18:1 PS/di 18:1 PC SUV	Thrombin generation	1×10^{-7}	0.14	45
di 18:1 PS/di 18:1 PC LUV	Protein depletion	1.6×10^{-7}	0.10	46
	Factor V			
di 18:1 PS/di 18:1 PC LUV	Protein depletion	3×10^{-7}	0.55	46
di 18:1 PS/di 18:1 PC monolayer	Film balance	10^{-11}	0.45	27
di 18:1 PS/di 18:1 PC double-layer	Ellipsometry	2×10^{-9}	0.30	58

Note: Membranes contained 20—25% of PS and 80—75% of phosphatidylcholine (PC). All values were measured in Tris buffer, pH = 7.0—7.5, containing 2—10 m*M* $CaCl_2$ and 0.1 *M* NaCl. Temperatures ranged from 10—37°C. SUV = small unilamellar vesicles and LUV = large unilamellar vesicles.

entations. However, it seems safe to say that the values of Γ_{max} in Table 1 correspond to less than 50% of full surface coverage. In this respect, it is interesting to note that the value of Γ_{max} for factor II is almost doubled on 100% PS membranes.[8,33] Table 1 shows rather ambiguous values for the dissociation constant of factor V. Values of $K_d = 10^{-7}$ to 10^{-8} *M* have also been reported for factor V under identical conditions.[49] As further discussed below, these discrepancies reflect conflicting results with respect to the reversibility of factor V binding.

C. Measurement of Sorption Rate Constants

Table 2 shows values of the intrinsic sorption rate constants k_{on} and k_{off}, measured by stopped-flow light scattering. The reversibility of factor II binding is apparent from the fact that the value of K_d in Table 2, calculated from $K_d = k_{off}/k_{on}$, equals the equilibrium value presented in Table 1. The value of $k_{on} = 10^7\ M^{-1}\ sec^{-1}$ shown in Table 2 corresponds to a collisional efficiency of about 15%, that is, 15% of the number of collisions between protein molecules and vesicles, as calculated from Smoluchowski's theory,[32] results in binding.

The data in Table 2 suggest reversibility of factor V binding, although desorption is very slow. The calculated value of $K_d = 10^{-11}$ *M* was in agreement with experiments on the binding of ^{125}I-factor V to monolayers at the air/water interface[27] (see Table 1). In these experiments, factor V adsorbed to the monolayer could be displaced by a large excess of phospholipid vesicles added to the subphase. However, factor V or Va adsorbed to di C

Table 2
PARAMETERS OBTAINED FROM THE SORPTION KINETICS OF FACTORS II AND V ON MODEL MEMBRANES

Protein (phospholipid preparation)	k_{on} (M^{-1} sec^{-1})	k_{off} (sec^{-1})	K_d (M)
	Factor II		
Brain PS/egg PC SUV	1.5×10^7	4	3×10^{-7}
Brain PG/egg PC SUV	6×10^6	25	4×10^{-6}
	Factor V		
Brain PS/egg PC SUV	10^8	5×10^{-3}	5×10^{-11}

Note: Conditions were as described in Table 1. All values were measured by stopped-flow light scattering.[32,47]

18:1 PS/di C 18:1 PC double layers does not desorb if the protein solution is replaced by buffer.[58] This discrepancy resembles the observation that radiolabeled albumin adsorbed irreversibly in pure buffer may readily desorb if an excess of unlabeled albumin is added to the buffer.[48] Apparently, net desorption may be impossible, while exchange between adsorbed molecules and molecules in the solution can occur. Freshly added phospholipid vesicles could have some ''scavenger activity'' which enables them to displace factor V from the membrane. The value of k_{on} for factor V in Table 2 is very high and corresponds to a collisional efficiency of about 30%.[47]

D. Interactions Between Adsorbed Factors II, Xa, and Va

Protein adsorption from a solution containing a binary mixture of proteins may show sequential adsorptions. If one component is present in large excess, but the other component has a higher binding affinity, the surface will first be covered with the abundant protein, which will then be gradually replaced by the scarce component. Plasma contains many proteins with binding affinities and concentrations that may differ by orders of magnitude. Accordingly, such sequential adsorptions will often occur, but they are not commonly observed because most techniques only measure the total concentration of adsorbed protein and cannot differentiate between the components in an adsorbed mixture. Vroman et al.[3,50] have elegantly demonstrated such sequential adsorption by studying the adsorption from thin films of plasma that become depleted of the scarce components. This will stop the sequence at various stages, depending on the thickness of the plasma layer.

Dilution of protein solutions may also change the ratio of adsorbed proteins. More puzzling, however, is the observation that this ratio may pass through a maximal value for increasing dilution.[50-52] This phenomenon cannot be explained by the classical binding model based on the law of mass action. A tentative explanation is that the adsorption of the proteins is inhibited to a different degree by increasing surface concentrations.[53]

Similar phenomena are observed in studies on the adsorption of mixtures of factors II, Xa, and Va to model membranes. For instance, preadsorption of factor Va will strongly inhibit the rate of adsorption of factor II, which may even drop below the rate of thrombin production as measured after addition of factor Xa.[58] This indicates that the production of thrombin cannot be described by the binding of factor II molecules to the membrane, which then travel along the surface until they meet a Xa-Va complex and are converted. For such a mechanism, the rate of thrombin production could never exceed the rate of factor II adsorption. Instead, it seems as if factor II molecules in the solution react directly with the

Table 3
EFFECT OF PREADSORPTION OF FACTOR Va ON THE ADSORPTION OF FACTORS II AND Xa

Protein (phospholipid preparation)	Method	K_d (*M*)	Γ_{max}/Γ_{Va} (mol/mol)	Ref.
	Factor II			
di 18:1 PS/di 18:1 PC LUV	Protein depletion	4×10^{-9}	1.20	22
	Factor Xa			
di 18:1 PS/di 18:1 PC LUV	Protein depletion	1×10^{-9}	0.96	22
Brain PS/egg PC SUV	Thrombin generation	5×10^{-10}	0.85	55
Unstimulated platelets	^{125}I-Xa Depletion	6×10^{-10}	0.91	56
Lymphocytes	Thrombin generation	1.3×10^{-10}	—	24

Note: Conditions were as described in Table 1.

prothrombinase complex on the surface in a simple bimolecular reaction with a high reaction rate. A similar conclusion was drawn from the observation that vesicles containing progressively less acidic phospholipids (20 to 2%) are also binding less factor II, but without impairment of the thrombin-producing capacity.[54]

In spite of the inhibition of the rate of adsorption, Table 3 shows that preadsorption of factor Va stimulates the binding affinity for factors II and Xa. This means that the rates of desorption are inhibited even more than the rates of adsorption. The overall effect is a lowering of the dissociation constants K_d with two to three orders of magnitude (see Tables 1 and 3).

Addition of factor Xa to phospholipid membranes preincubated with factors Va and II results in the production of thrombin, but only after some time lag that can be influenced by the ''fluidity'' of the phospholipids in the membrane.[57] This finding was interpreted as indicating that the assembly of Xa-Va complexes, from factor Xa and Va molecules adsorbed to the surface, forms a rate-limiting step.[57] This suggestion is difficult to reconcile, however, with the data presented in Tables 1 and 3. If factor Xa is added in concentrations below 10^{-9} *M*, factor Xa can only bind directly to the Va-membrane complex, but the time lag is still observed.[58] An alternative hypothesis could, therefore, be that the Xa-Va complex undergoes an intramolecular transition before it acquires prothrombinase activity. The last column in Table 3 shows that the quantities of factors II and X that bind with high affinity after preadsorption of factor Va equal the quantity of adsorbed factor Va in moles per unit surface area. This implies that the factor Va molecules adsorbed at the membrane act as receptor molecules with a binding affinity of $K_d \cong 10^{-9}$ *M*. For factors II or Xa concentrations exceeding about 10^{-8} *M*, additional binding sites become available with an affinity $K_d \cong 10^{-7}$ *M*. Because the Xa-Va complex in solution has a dissociation constant of about 10^{-9} *M*,[21] adsorption of factor Xa will often occur in coadsorption with factor Va.

The data given in this section on mutual stimulation and inhibition of adsorbing proteins may also be strongly influenced by the presence of a large excess of plasma proteins such as albumin and fibrinogen. Taken together, all these aspects picture a complex situation and this probably explains why studies directly relating the production of thrombin to data on the surface concentrations of factors II, Xa, and Va are scarce.

REFERENCES

1. **Hemker, H. C., Esnouf, M. P., Hemker, P. W., Swart, A. C. W., and Macfarlane, R. G.,** Formation of prothrombin converting activitiy, *Nature,* 214, 248, 1967.
2. **Jobin, F. and Esnouf, M. P.,** Studies on the formation of the prothrombin converting complex, *Biochem. J.,* 102, 666, 1967.
3. **Vroman, L. and Adams, A. L.,** Identification of rapid changes at plasma-solid interfaces, *J. Biomed. Mater. Res.,* 3, 43, 1969.
4. **Ivarsson, B. and Lundström, J.,** Physical characterization of protein adsorption on metal and metaloxide surfaces, *Crit. Rev. Biocompatibility,* 2(1), 1, 1986.
5. **Andrade, J. D. and Hlady, V.,** Protein adsorption and materials biocompatibility: a tutorial review and suggested hypotheses, *Adv. Pol. Sci.,* 79, 1, 1986.
6. **Tanford, C.,** *Physical Chemistry of Macromolecules,* John Wiley & Sons, New York, 1967.
7. **Andrade, J. D.,** Introduction to surface chemistry and physics of polymers, in *Surface and Interfacial Aspects of Biomedical Polymers,* Vol. 1, 1985, 1.
8. **Corsel, J. W., Willems, G. M., Kop, J. M. M., Cuypers, P. A., and Hermens, W. T.,** The role of intrinsic binding rate and transport rate in the adsorption of prothrombin, albumin and fibrinogen to phospholipid bilayers, *J. Colloid Interface Sci.,* 111, 544, 1986.
9. **Bird, R. B., Stewart, W. E., and Lightfoot, E. N.,** *Transport Phenomena,* John Wiley & Sons, New York, 1960, 363.
10. **Levich, V. G.,** *Physicochemical Hydrodynamics,* Prentice-Hall, Englewood Cliffs, N.J., 1962.
11. **Willems, G. M., van der Voort, J. M. Q., and Hermens, W. Th.,** Ellipsometric determination of protein sorption kinetics at a rotating disc surface, in *Proc. 7th Int. Symp. Affinity Chromatography,* Oberammergau, in press.
12. **Rosing, J., van Rijn, J. L. M. L., Bever, E. M., van Dieijen, G., Comfurius, F., and Zwaal, R. F. A.,** The role of activated human platelets in prothrombin and factor X activation, *Blood,* 65, 319, 1985.
13. **Williams, W. J., Bentler, E., Erslev, A. J., and Wayne, R. R.,** *Hematology,* McGraw-Hill, New York, 1972, 999.
14. **Guyton, A. C.,** *Textbook of Medical Physiology,* W. B. Saunders, Philadelphia, 1976, 238.
15. **Lim, T. K., Bloomfield, V. A., and Nelsestuen, G. L.,** Structure of the prothrombin — and blood clotting factor X — membrane complexes, *Biochemistry,* 16, 4177, 1977.
16. **Rosing, J., Tans, G., Govers-Riemslag, J. W. P., Zwaal, R. F. A., and Hemker, C.,** The role of phospholipids and factor Va in the prothrombinase complex, *J. Biol. Chem.,* 255, 274, 1980.
17. **Rothen, A.,** The ellipsometer, an apparatus to measure thickness of thin surface films, *Rev. Sci. Instrum.,* 16, 26, 1945.
18. **Trurnit, H. J.,** Studies of enzyme systems at a solid-liquid interface. I. The system chymotrypsin-serum albumin, *Arch. Biochem. Biophys.,* 47, 251, 1953.
19. **Vroman, L. and Lukosevicius, A.,** Ellipsometer recordings of changes in optical thickness of adsorbed films associated with surface activation of blood clotting, *Nature,* 204, 701, 1964.
20. **Nelsestuen, G. L. and Lim, T. K.,** Equilibria involved in prothrombin — and blood clotting factor X — membrane binding, *Biochemistry,* 16, 4164, 1977.
21. **Lindhout, T., Govers-Riemslag, J. W. P., Van de Waart, P., Hemker, H. C., and Rosing, J.,** Factor Va-factor Xa interaction. Effects of phospholipid vesicles of varying composition, *Biochemistry,* 21, 5494, 1982.
22. **Van de Waart, P., Hemker, H. C., and Lindhout, T.,** Interaction of prothrombin with factor Va-phospholipid complexes, *Biochemistry,* 23, 2838, 1984.
23. **Kane, W. H., Lindhout, M. J., Jackson, C. M., and Majerus, P. W.,** Factor Va-dependent binding of factor Xa to human platelets, *J. Biol. Chem.,* 255, 1170, 1980.
24. **Tracy, P. B., Eide, L. L., and Mann, K. G.,** Human prothrombinase complex assembly and function on isolated peripheral blood cell populations, *J. Biol. Chem.,* 260, 2119, 1985.
25. **Van der Scheer, A., Feyen, J., Klein Elhorst, J., Krugers Dagneaux, P. G. L. C., and Smolders, C. A.,** The feasibility of radiolabeling for human serum albumin (HSA) adsorption studies, *J. Colloid Interface Sci.,* 66, 136, 1978.
26. **Lecompte, M. F., Miller, J. R., Elion, J., and Benarous, R.,** Interaction of prothrombin and its fragments with monolayers containing phosphatidylserine. I. Binding of prothrombin and its fragment I to phosphatidylserine-containing monolayers, *Biochemistry,* 19, 3434, 1980.
27. **Mayer, L. D., Pusey, M. L., Griep, M. A., and Nelsestuen, G. L.,** Association of blood coagulation factors V and X with phospholipid monolayers, *Biochemistry,* 22, 6226, 1983.
28. **Lecompte, M. F. and Miller, J. R.,** Interaction of prothrombin and its fragments with monolayers containing phosphatidylserine. II. Electrochemical determination of lipid layer perturbation by interacting prothrombin and its fragments, *Biochemistry,* 19, 3439, 1980.

29. **Lecompte, M. F., Rubinstein, J., and Miller, J. R.,** Adsorption kinetics of prothrombin, *J. Colloid Interface Sci.*, 91, 12, 1983.
30. **Miller, J. R. and Rishpon, Y.,** Structure and permeability of lipid monolayers interacting with proteins and polypeptides, in *Electrical Phenomena at the Biological Membrane Level*, Roux, E., Ed., Elsevier, Amsterdam, 1977, 93.
31. **Hummel, J. P. and Dreyer, W. J.,** Measurement of protein-binding phenomena by gel filtration, *Biochim. Biophys. Acta*, 63, 530, 1962.
32. **Wei, G. J., Bloomfield, V. A., Resnick, R. M., and Nelsestuen, G. L.,** Kinetic and mechanistic analysis of prothrombin-membrane binding by stopped-flow light scattering, *Biochemistry*, 21, 1949, 1982.
33. **Kop, J. M. M., Cuypers, P. A., Lindhout, T., Hemker, H. C., and Hermens, W. T.,** The adsorption of prothrombin to phospholipid monolayers quantitated by ellipsometry, *J. Biol. Chem.*, 259, 13993, 1984.
34. **Blodgett, K. B.,** Films built by depositing successive monomolecular layers on a solid surface, *J. Am. Chem. Soc.*, 57, 1007, 1935.
35. **Cuypers, P. A., Corsel, J. W., Janssen, M. P., Kop, J. M. M., Hermens, W. T., and Hemker, H. C.,** The adsorption of prothrombin to phosphatidylserine multi-layers quantitated by ellipsometry, *J. Biol. Chem.*, 258, 2426, 1983.
36. **Resnick, R. M. and Nelsestuen, G. L.,** Prothrombin-membrane interaction. Effects of ionic strength, pH and temperature, *Biochemistry*, 19, 3028, 1980.
37. **Zell, A., Enspahr, H., and Bugg, C. E.,** Model for calcium binding to γ-carboxyglutamic acid residues of proteins: crystal structure of calcium α-ethylmalonate, *Biochemistry*, 24, 533, 1985.
38. **Borowski, M., Furie, B. C., Bauminger, S., and Furie, B.,** Prothrombin requires two sequential metal-dependent conformational transitions to bind phospholipid, *J. Biol. Chem.*, 261, 14969, 1986.
39. **Dombrose, F. A., Gitel, S. N., Zawalich, K., and Jackson, C. M.,** The association of bovine prothrombin fragment I with phospholipid, *J. Biol. Chem.*, 254, 5027, 1979.
40. **Nelsestuen, G. L. and Broderius, M.,** Interaction of prothrombin and blood-clotting factor X with membranes of varying composition, *Biochemistry*, 16, 4172, 1977.
41. **Mayer, L. D. and Nelsestuen, G. L.,** Calcium- and prothrombin-induced lateral phase separation in membranes, *Biochemistry*, 20, 2457, 1981.
42. **Mayer, L. D. and Nelsestuen, G. L.,** Membrane lateral phase separation induced by proteins of the prothrombinase complex, *Biochim. Biophys. Acta*, 734, 48, 1983.
43. **Jones, M. E. and Lentz, B. R.,** Phospholipid lateral organization in synthetic membranes as monitored by pyrene-labeled phospholipids: effect of temperature and prothrombin fragment l binding, *Biochemistry*, 25, 567, 1986.
44. **Prigent-Dachary, J., Faucon, J.-F., Boisseau, M.-R., and Dufourcq, J.,** Topology of the binding site of blood-clotting factors in model membranes, a fluorescence study, *Eur. J. Biochem.*, 155, 133, 1986.
45. **Van Dieijen, G., Tans, G., Van Rijn, J., Zwaal, R. F. A., and Rosing, J.,** Simple and rapid method to determine the binding of blood clotting factor X to phospholipid vesicles, *Biochemistry*, 20, 7096, 1981.
46. **Van de Waart, P., Bruls, H., Hemker, H. C., and Lindhout, T.,** Interaction of bovine blood clotting factor Va and its subunits with phospholipid vesicles, *Biochemistry*, 22, 2427, 1983.
47. **Pusey, M. L., Mayer, L. D., Wei, G. J., Bloomfield, V. A., and Nelsestuen, G. L.,** Kinetic and hydrodynamic analysis of blood clotting factor V-membrane binding, *Biochemistry*, 21, 5262, 1982.
48. **Brash, J. L., Uniyal, S., and Samak, Q.,** Exchange of albumin adsorbed on polymer surfaces, *Trans. Am. Soc. Artif. Int. Organs*, 20, 69, 1974.
49. **Bloom, J. W., Nesheim, M. E., and Mann, K. G.,** Phospholipid binding properties of bovine factor V and factor Va, *Biochemistry*, 18, 4419, 1979.
50. **Vroman, L., Adams, A. L., Fischer, G. C., Munoz, P. C., and Stanford, M.,** Proteins, plasma, and blood in narrow spaces of clot-promoting surfaces, in *Advances in Chemistry*, Ser. 199, Cooper, S. L. and Peppas, N. A., Eds., American Chemical Society, Washington, D.C., 1982, 264.
51. **Horbett, T. A.,** Mass action effects on competitive adsorption of fibrinogen from hemoglobin solutions and from plasma, *Thromb. Haemostas. Stuttg.*, 51, 174, 1984.
52. **Brash, J. L. and Ten Hove, P.,** Effect of plasma dilution on adsorption of fibrinogen to solid surfaces, *Thromb. Haemostas. Stuttg.*, 51, 326, 1984.
53. **Cuypers, P. A., Willems, G. M., Hemker, H. C., and Hermens, W. T.,** Adsorption kinetics of protein mixtures. A tentative explanation of "the Vroman effect", *Ann. N.Y. Acad. Sci.*, 516, 244, 1987.
54. **Pusey, M. L. and Nelsestuen, G. L.,** The physical significance of K_m in the prothrombinase reaction, *Biochem. Biophys. Res. Commun.*, 114, 526, 1983.
55. **Nesheim, M. E., Eid, S., and Mann, K. G.,** Assembly of the prothrombinase complex in the absence of prothrombin, *J. Biol. Chem.*, 256, 9874, 1981.
56. **Tracy, P. B., Nesheim, M. E., and Mann, K. G.,** Coordinate binding of factor Va and factor Xa to the unstimulated platelet, *J. Biol. Chem.*, 256, 743, 1981.

57. **Higgins, D. L., Callahan, P. J., Prendergast, F. G., Nesheim, M. E., and Mann, K. G.,** Lipid mobility in the assembly and expression of the activity of the prothrombinase complex, *J. Biol. Chem.*, 260, 3604, 1985.
58. **Kop, J. M. M.,** unpublished results.

Chapter 5

LIPID INVOLVEMENT IN CONTACT ACTIVATION

Guido Tans and Jan Rosing

TABLE OF CONTENTS

I. INTRODUCTION

When human blood comes into contact with negatively charged surfaces such as glass, kaolin, dextran sulfate, or sulfatides, contact activation occurs. In vitro studies have shown that contact activation can initiate major pathways involved in the defense of the human body against injury, i.e., blood coagulation and the fibrinolytic system, the complement system, the kinin forming pathways, and the renin-angiotensin system. Although it is as yet not clear whether contact activation actually plays a role in the in vivo initiation of these pathways, the in vitro studies suggest that the contact system may have a regulatory function in maintaining the balance between these pathways.

Four proteins that circulate freely in the blood are involved in contact activation — Factor XII, Factor XI, prekallikrein, and high molecular weight kininogen (high M_r kininogen). Factors XII and XI and prekallikrein are the zymogen forms of active serine proteases (Factor XII_a, Factor XI_a, and kallikrein). These zymogens become activated during contact activation. The fourth contact factor, high M_r kininogen, is thought to function as a cofactor in these activations.

Contact activation requires the presence of a suitable negatively charged surface. Since the early discovery that the glass tube was an absolute requirement for in vitro intrinsic coagulation, a wide variety of negatively charged surfaces has been shown to be also capable of initiating the contact system. Most of these substances cannot serve as a physiological model for contact activation, since they are not present in the human body. However, in recent years physiological substances such as lipopolysaccharides, heparin, and membrane lipids (sulfatides and phospholipids) have also been shown to stimulate in vitro contact activation. This chapter contains a review of our current knowledge on the mode of action of these lipid components in the mediation of contact activation. For more detailed information about the physiology and biochemistry of contact activation reactions, the reader is referred to other reviews.[1-3]

II. THE PROTEINS OF CONTACT ACTIVATION

Four proteins appear to be involved in contact activation of human plasma — the zymogens Factor XII, Factor XI, prekallikrein, and the protein cofactor high M_r kininogen. In this paragraph we will briefly summarize the structural and functional properties of these proteins as far as these are pertinent to understand the function of procoagulant surfaces in contact activation.

A. Factor XII

Factor XII, which is also known as Hageman factor, is the zymogen form of the serine protease, Factor XII_a. Factor XII is a glycoprotein with a molecular weight of 80,000 daltons,[4,5] which is present in human plasma at a concentration of approximately 30 $\mu g/m\ell$.[4,6] Recently, the amino acid sequence of the human molecule was reported and a two-dimensional folding model, schematically shown in Figure 1, was proposed.[7-9] It was found that the aminoterminal region of Factor XII (approximately 40,000 daltons) consists of domains homologous with the type II and I regions of fibronectin,[10] epidermal growth factor,[11,12] and with the kringle structures that have also been found in prothrombin,[13] plasminogen,[14] tissue type plasminogen activator,[15,16] and urokinase.[17-19] The precise functions of these domains in the Factor XII molecule are as yet undefined, but since the amino terminal region of the molecule is required for binding to negatively charged surfaces,[20] it may be that one or more of these domains is involved in the binding of Factor XII to the surface. The 40,000-dalton region is followed by a connecting region of 12,000 daltons, which is unusually rich in proline. This region does not share homology with any other

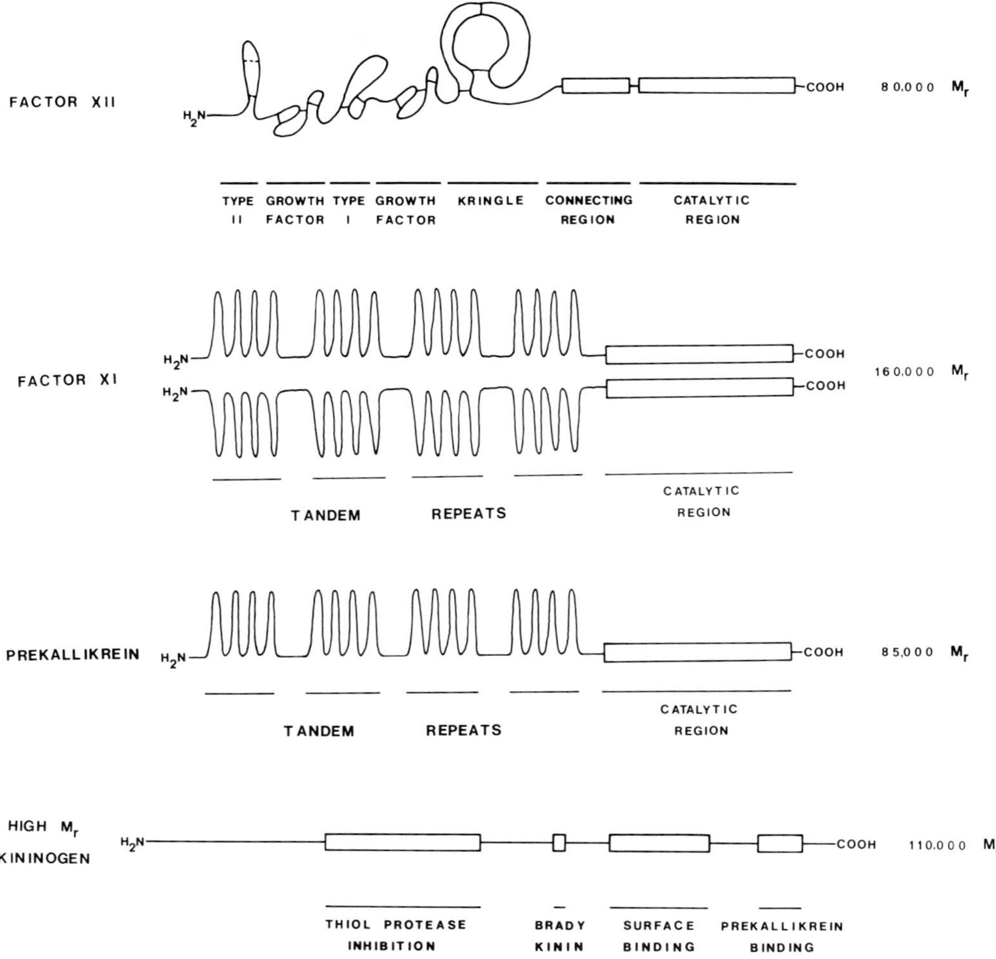

FIGURE 1. Schematic models for contact activation proteins. The models shown in this figure are based on the primary amino acid sequences reported in literature. Factor XII from References 7 to 9, prekallikrein from Reference 28, Factor XI from Reference 35, high M_r kininogen from References 49 to 51 and 66.

known protein, and the biological function is not known. The connecting region links the amino terminal region to the catalytic domain of 28,000 daltons, which shows extensive homology with trypsin and contains the amino acids (Ser, His, Asp) of the catalytic triad of serine proteases.[7]

Activation of Factor XII is brought about by cleavage of a single peptide bond (Arg_{353}-Val_{354}). The resulting two-chain enzyme, α-Factor XII_a, consists of a heavy chain (52,000 daltons), which is linked via a disulfide bridge to a light chain (28,000 daltons) that contains the active site. α-Factor XII_a can undergo further proteolysis in the heavy chain just outside the disulfide bridge that links the heavy and light chain together.[21-23] The enzyme thus remaining is called β-Factor XII_a (also known as Hageman factor fragment) and has a molecular weight of 30,000 daltons.[7,22,23] Since β-Factor XII_a lacks the amino terminal region of Factor XII, it does not bind to negatively charged surfaces and, consequently, has negligible clotting activity.

B. Prekallikrein

Prekallikrein, like Factor XII, is a single-chain zymogen of a serine protease which can be activated by cleavage of a single peptide bond. Prekallikrein is a glycoprotein with a molecular weight of approximately 85,000 daltons[24,25] and is present in plasma at a concentration of some 50 μg/mℓ.[26,27] The molecular model for prekallikrein is shown in Figure 1. It is based on the primary structure recently reported by Chung et al.[28] The amino terminal part of the molecule was found to contain four tandem repeats of 90 or 91 amino acid residues in length. This region of prekallikrein is highly homologous with the amino terminal part of the Factor XI monomer (see also Figure 1). The tandem repeats appear unique for prekallikrein and Factor XI, since thus far no other proteins have been reported to contain such a structure. The precise function of this region in prekallikrein and Factor XI is not known, but since this part of the molecule is essential for the binding to high M_r kininogen[29-31] (see also Section IV), these regions may function as the high affinity binding site. Prekallikrein occurs in plasma in two forms with a small difference in molecular weight, and SDS-gels of prekallikrein show a closely spaced doublet at approximately 85,000 daltons.[25] Activation of prekallikrein occurs upon cleavage of Arg_{371}-Ile_{372} within a disulfide bridge.[28] The resulting two-chain enzyme consists of a heavy chain of approximately 50,000 daltons and a light chain of 33,000 or 36,000 daltons, which contains the active site.[29] Thus, the difference in the two forms of prekallikrein appears to be located in the catalytic region of the molecule. It has not yet been solved whether this difference in molecular weight is caused by different degrees of glycosylation or by a difference in peptide chain length.

The heavy and light chains of kallikrein have been separated and isolated.[29] After this procedure the light chains of kallikrein retained full catalytic capacity. These fragments have proven to be very useful tools in unraveling some of the functions of these domains in contact activation interactions (see also Sections IV and V).

C. Factor XI

The Factor XI molecule takes up a rather unique place among the plasma zymogens identified thus far. It appears to be built up of two identical single-chain subunits of 80,000 daltons that are held together by one or more disulfide bonds.[32,33] Like the other zymogens of contact activation, Factor XI is a glycoprotein. The concentration of Factor XI in human plasma is approximately 6 μg/mℓ.[34] The amino acid sequence of Factor XI has been reported,[35] and a schematic model of the molecule is shown in Figure 1. The amino terminal region of each Factor XI subunit was found to contain the same four tandem repeats that are also present in prekallikrein. As already mentioned, these regions may function in the high affinity binding of Factor XI to high M_r kininogen. The carboxy-terminal part of each subunit was found to be highly homologous to trypsin and contains the amino acids of the catalytic triad.[35] Thus, each subunit contains a potential catalytic region, the active site of which becomes exposed upon cleavage of Arg_{369}-Ile_{370} within a disulfide bridge. Factor XI_a, therefore, is an enzyme with two active sites, one at each subunit. Each subunit consists of a heavy chain of 50,000 that is linked via a disulfide bridge to a light chain of 30,000 daltons, which contains the active site.[31]

D. High M_r Kininogen

High M_r kininogen is thought to act as a cofactor in the contact activation reactions.[36-40] It is a single chain glycoprotein of 110,000 daltons,[41] and the concentration of high M_r kininogen in plasma is 70 to 90 μg/mℓ.[27,42,43] A model for high M_r kininogen with structural and functional domains is shown in Figure 1. High M_r kininogen is one of the major sources of the vasoactive peptide bradykinin, which is liberated from the molecule by plasma kallikrein to give two-chain kininogen of which one chain is further cleaved to result in a stable

Table 1
SURFACES THAT PROMOTE CONTACT ACTIVATION

Nonlipid	Ref.	Lipid or lipid-like	Ref.
Glass, kaolin, celite	67	Bacterial lipopolysaccharides	75
Diatomaceous earth	68	Glycolipids (sulfatides, gangliosides)	76
Ellagic acid	69	Cholesterol sulfate	77
Dextran sulfate	70	Long-chain saturated fatty acids	76, 78—80
Amylose sulfate	71	Platelets	81
Heparin, chondroitin sulfate	72	Endothelial cells	82
L-Homocystine	73	Acidic phospholipids	83
Sodium urate crystals	74		

light chain.[44,45] The molecular weights of the heavy and light chains are approximately 64,000 and 54,000 daltons as judged by SDS-gelelectrophoresis.[44-46] However, more careful determination by gel filtration in 6 *M* guanidine-HCl and by equilibrium sedimentation showed the molecular weights of the heavy and light chains of high M_r kininogen to be 50,000 and 30,000 daltons, respectively.[46] It has been suggested that cleavage of the molecule is necessary to express activity in contact activation.[47,48]

The amino acid sequence of high M_r kininogen has been reported[49-51] and, from comparison with the sequence of other proteins, it was found that the heavy chain of high M_r kininogen is highly homologous to cysteine (thiol) protease inhibitors.[52-54] However, it is not likely that this region of the molecule has a function in contact activation, since the isolated light chain of high M_r kininogen retains full ability to promote in vitro contact activation in.[41,44,46,55,56] A region in the molecule of some 40 amino acid residues which contains 27% histidine, 27% glycine, and 17% lysine[57,58] appears to be essential for the procoagulant activity of high M_r kininogen. In bovine high M_r kininogen, this region can be split off, resulting in a loss of contact activation-promoting activity.[56,59-61] It is thought that this positively charged region plays a function in the binding to negatively charged surface.

High M_r kininogen has a high affinity for plasma prekallikrein and Factor XI (see also Section IV). This explains why prekallikrein and Factor XI circulate in plasma in a 1:1 stoichiometric complex with high M_r kininogen.[62,63] The high affinity binding site for plasma prekallikrein and Factor XI, which is also present on the light chain of high M_r kininogen,[46,64,65] has recently been located within a region comprising 40 amino acids (residues 185 to 224) near the carboxy terminus of the kininogen light chain.[66]

III. SURFACES THAT STIMULATE CONTACT ACTIVATION

Contact activation shows an absolute requirement for negatively charged surfaces. In the absence of a proper surface the reactions are far too slow for significant activation to occur. Over the past 25 years a wide variety of substances has been shown to stimulate in vitro contact activation. Table 1 shows a selection of these. The list is certainly far from complete, but it illustrates the general sort of substances which have been found thus far to be capable of propagating contact activation reactions. What these materials appear to have in common is the fact that they all contain a net negative charge and provide a surface onto which the contact activation proteins can bind and at which they can interact with each other. Strictly speaking, not all substances mentioned in Table 1 will actually provide a real surface. Some compounds (dextran sulfate, heparin, amylose sulfate, and chondroitin sulfate) are large macromolecules (polymers) with high charge density, which apparently provide ample binding sites to promote the interactions and reactions of the proteins involved in contact activation. For the sake of simplicity we will, however, also classify these compounds as ''surface''. Not much more is known concerning the structural and chemical requirements for a surface to be active. Most of the substances listed in Table 1 are rather ill defined both chemically and/or physically, and this has seriously hampered progress in understanding the mode of action of the surface in contact activation. Only recently more detailed information about the structure-function relationship of procoagulant surfaces has become available.

Although the division into nonlipid and lipids or lipid-like substances in Table 1 is rather arbitrary on a functional basis, it will, however, facilitate a discussion concerning the physical nature of the various contact-activating surfaces.

A. Nonlipid Surfaces

A large amount of inorganic materials (of which only a small selection is shown in Table 1) has been shown to promote contact activation. The best known and most widely used is kaolin, a sort of clay with a net negative charge. The disadvantage of materials such as kaolin is that they are rather ill defined. Kaolin, apart from sites with which the contact proteins can favorably interact, also appears to have inhibitory binding sites which will irreversibly bind and inhibit the proteins involved in contact activation.[84] Ellagic acid has long been thought to be the exception to the rule that contact activation requires a surface for the proteins to bind to. It was thought that soluble ellagic acid interacted with the proteins and stimulated the contact activation reactions. Since ellagic acid is a chemically well-defined substance with known charge, it has gained widespread attention. However, later it was shown that contact activation by ellagic acid did not occur by the action of the soluble monomeric molecules, but was actually promoted by larger (centrifugable) ellagic acid-metal ion aggregates present in the ellagic acid preparations.[85]

Sulfated polysaccharides such as amylose sulfate, amylopectin sulfate, and dextran sulfate appear to be very strong contact activators.[70,71] Other well-known polysaccharides, such as chondroitin sulfate and heparin, can also initiate contact activation,[71,72,86,87] though less efficiently.[71] The contact activation-promoting activity appears to be dependent upon the size and the charge density of the polysaccharide. Thus the most active amylose sulfates are those with highest molecular weight which contain the most sulfate groups.[71] Likewise, dextran sulfate molecules of lower molecular weight show diminished activity.[87] Heparin, which is usually much smaller (15,000 to 20,000 average M_r), is, therefore, also less active and small molecular weight heparin fragments hardly show any activity at all.[168]

L-Homocystine and sodium urate crystals are contact activators that may have potential physiological significance. Homocystinuria is a rare metabolic disorder that is associated with the deficiency of an enzyme required to convert homocysteine to cysthathione (see Reference 73). As a result, homocysteine cannot be metabolized and is excreted in the urine in the form of homocystine, and high levels of L-homocystine occur in the blood of patients with homocystinuria. Crystals of L-homocystine have been shown to stimulate contact activation, and this may provide a rationale for understanding the often fatal thrombotic problems occurring in patients with this disease.[73] Urate crystals play a primary role in the clinical syndrome of acute gouty arthritis.[74] Moreover, since synovial fluid contains Factor XII,[88] and mixtures of joint fluid and sodium urate crystals have been shown to promote Factor XII activation,[89] it has been proposed that the contact activation system plays a role in the initiation of the inflammatory process occurring in the joints of patients suffering from an attack of acute gouty arthritis.[74,89]

B. Lipid or Lipid-Like Surfaces

From the early days a number of lipids or lipid-containing materials have been recognized as a potential model for contact activation in vivo. Early literature contains reports that suggest contact activation to occur with long-chain saturated fatty acids.[76,78-80] Endothelial

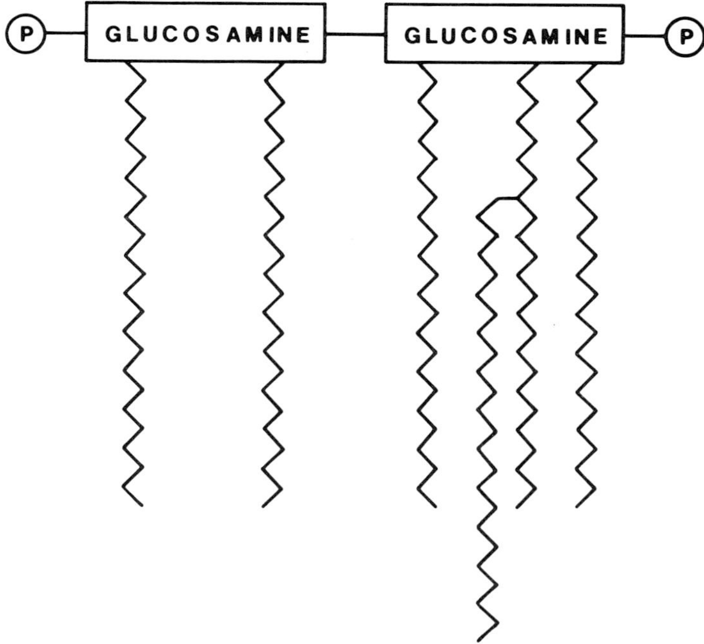

FIGURE 2. Schematic structure of the lipid A backbone of lipopolysaccharides from Gram-negative bacteria.

cells[82] and activated human platelets[81,90] have also been reported to promote activation of Factor XII. Which components of these activators (membrane lipid or protein) are responsible for these activities is as yet not known. Over the past years, however, a variety of artificial membranes of known lipid composition have been defined to stimulate contact activation.

1. Bacterial Lipopolysaccharides

It has been recognized that episodes of bacterial shock result in contact activation and kinin formation[75,91,92] and are accompanied by a significant decrease in the plasma levels of contact activation proteins.[91] The bacterial component for this is most likely endotoxin, i.e., bacterial lipopolysaccharide (LPS). The LPS structure of Gram-negative bacteria shares a common core glycolipid structure which contains a polysaccharide linked by a 2-keto-3-deoxyoctonate-trisaccharide to lipid A. The structural components of LPS responsible for contact activation appears to be the lipid A part,[75] the chemical structure of which is shown in Figure 2. Lipid A consists of six fatty acid chains linked to two glucosamines, to which two phosphate groups are attached.[93] Presumably, the phosphate groups provide the surface with the negative charge required for the stimulation of contact activation.

2. Cholesterol Sulfate

Recently, Shimada et al.[77] tested a number of steroids and steroid sulfates for the capacity to stimulate contact activation. Of the substances tested, cholesterol sulfate proved to be a very potent stimulator of contact activation. Cholesterol acetate and sulfodeoxycholic acid showed some activity, whereas other steroid sulfates tested were not active. The procoagulant effect is dependent upon the sulfate group, since cholesterol had no or little activity by itself. The fact that cholesterol sulfate was the only steroid sulfate that had a high activity suggests that the hydrophobic chain is essential for micelle formation,[77] thereby providing a negatively charged surface at which the proteins can interact.

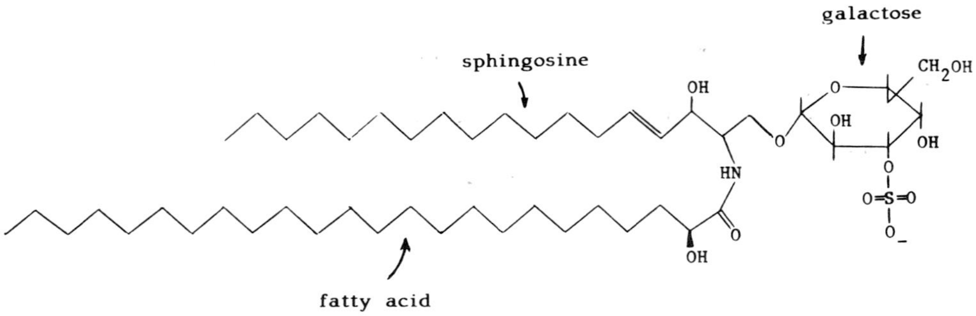

galactose
sphingosine
CH_2OH
OH
OH
OH
HN
O
O=S=O
O
O
OH
fatty acid

FIGURE 3. Chemical structure of cerebroside sulfates (sulfatides).

3. Sulfatides

The most promising compounds in providing a well-defined model system for in vivo contact activation are cerebroside sulfates (sulfatides). Fujikawa et al.[76] reported that sulfatides are strong stimulators of the activation of purified bovine contact factors. They also appear to be very potent in propagating contact activation in human plasma[94] and in promoting reactions between purified human contact factors.[71,95-99] Sulfatides have been found in many mammalian tissues (for a review see Reference 100), e.g., in brain, nerve,[100-102] and kidney tissue.[100,103] Small quantities of sulfatides have also been demonstrated in red blood cells.[104] The function of sulfatides in these tissues is not yet understood, but it has been suggested that they may play a role in the Na^+/K^+-ATPase[100,103] and in opiate as well as β-endorphin receptors[100,105,106] at the cell surface.

Figure 3 shows the chemical structure of sulfatides. It is a glycosphingolipid built up of a long chain base (sphingosine) to which a fatty acid is attached via an amide bond. The hydroxyl group at the first carbon is linked to a galactose head group which is sulfated at the 3 position. The composition of the long chain base in human brain sulfatides is almost exclusively (94%) dihydroxy 18:1 (sphingosine, the structure used in the figure) with very small amounts of dihydroxy 18:0 (4%) and dihydroxy 18:2 (2%).[107] There is more variation in the fatty acid part of sulfatides. About two thirds of the fatty acids in sulfatides from brain tissue are 2-hydroxy fatty acids (mostly 24:0 and 24:1) and one third are normal fatty acids (mostly 24:1, see References 101 and 108). Thus, although many fatty acids with different chain lengths are found, the most abundant are those that contain 24 carbon atoms (Figure 3). Sulfatides are recognized to contain a hydrophobic part (built up by the long chain base and the fatty acid) and a hydrophylic head group with a net negative charge due to the sulfate group. Such a structure makes it suitable to become embedded in a membrane. Indeed, in well-defined model systems sulfatides have been shown to be incorporated in phosphatidylcholine bilayers.[109,110]

Some ambiguity appears to exist in literature concerning the physical form of pure sulfatides in an aqueous environment. It appears that sulfatides show a polymorphism analogous to that displayed by phospholipids (see Chapters 2 and 7). Sulfatides have been reported to form micelles[109,111,112] the size of which is 180 sulfatide molecules per micelle, as determined by ultracentrifugation.[111,112] However, considerably larger structures have been observed in the ultracentrifuge as well.[112] In 1972, Abrahamsson et al.,[108] using X-ray diffraction, observed that depending on the temperature and water content both the micellar and the lamellar forms can exist.

Recently, we have shown that when sulfatides are dispersed at high temperature (above the 55°C phase transition, see below) by means of vortexing, very large particles are obtained that elute in the void volume of a Sepharose® 2B column (Figure 4A).[169] Freeze-fracture electron microscopy revealed that such preparations contain very large spherical liposomes with extended fracture faces as expected for lamellar structures. The size distribution ranged from 2 to 5 μm in diameter. Figure 4B shows a typical fracture face obtained with such a large spherical liposome. The fracture faces of the bilayers display ordered corrugations similar to those observed on fracture faces of synthetic lipids in the $P_{\alpha\beta}$ or $P_{\beta'}$ phase.[113-115] Since these phases are typical for a lipid bilayer in the solid gel state, this indicates that at the temperature from which the sulfatides were quenched (room temperature) the lipid is in the solid gel state. This is supported by recent differential scanning calorimetric data for sulfatides from bovine brain[116] which report a phase transition temperature of approximately 55°C for the transition from the solid gel to the liquid crystalline phase.

Upon mild sonication (again above 55°C), small single-shelled vesicles are obtained ranging in size from 400 to 2000 Å diameter. From such a preparation it is possible to obtain vesicles with well-defined diameters by gel filtration on Sepharose® 2B (Figure 4C). Figure 4D shows the fracture face of gel-filtered sonicated sulfatides, displaying spherical and flattened vesicles with a diameter around 500 Å. The finding that sulfatides are present as bilayers appears in contrast with earlier literature reporting that sulfatides form micelles upon sonication.[109,111,112] It is possible that differences in the sonication procedure (e.g., sonication time, intensity of sonication, and temperature at which the sonication is performed) may account for the different forms. Even after mild sonication, sulfatides did not form a homogeneous membrane preparation. We observed that after sonication above the phase transition, approximately 20 to 30% of the sulfatides may be present in the micellar form, since this percentage of the sulfatides did not sediment after centrifugation and eluted at the end of the Sepharose® 2B column. It is likely, however, that micelles are less potent in promoting contact activation, since the activation of purified human Factor XII is strongly diminished with these particles.[170] This indicates that the sulfatide bilayer is the biologically most active form, which strongly promotes contact activation in human plasma.

4. Phospholipids

Only recently it was reported that negatively charged phospholipids such as phosphatidylserine (PS), phosphatidyglycerol (PG), and phosphatidylinositol (PI) were capable of stimulating kallikrein-dependent activation of Factor XII in a purified system.[83] It appears, however, that Factor XII activation on acidic phospholipids only occurs at very low salt concentration.[83] Therefore, the physiologic importance of the finding that acidic phospholipids can stimulate Factor XII activation remains as yet unclear. Negatively charged phospholipids only stimulated Factor XII activation when the lipid bilayer was in the solid gel state. Since at 37°C sulfatides are also in the solid gel state (see above), this may be an important parameter for a membrane to be active in contact activation.

IV. EQUILIBRIUM BINDING STUDIES

The reactions of contact activation require the presence of a negatively charged surface and the protein cofactor high M_r kininogen. The stimulation by the surface is thought to result from the binding of the various contact factors, which enables effective interaction at the surface.

Early studies have shown that Factor XII readily binds to kaolin,[5,20,21,38,39,117-120] and that binding of Factor XII is essential for activation of this zymogen, probably as the result of a conformational change in the molecule which renders it more susceptible to proteolytic activation.[120] Purified Factor XI will adsorb to a variety of materials, such as polystyrene, polyethylene, glass, and kaolin.[121,122] Prekallikrein also binds to kaolin, but in that case the bound prekallikrein is no longer available for activation.[84] In a plasmatic environment, however, Factor XI and prekallikrein do not bind effectively to kaolin unless high M_r kininogen is present.[123] This protein cofactor stimulates the binding of Factor XI and prek-

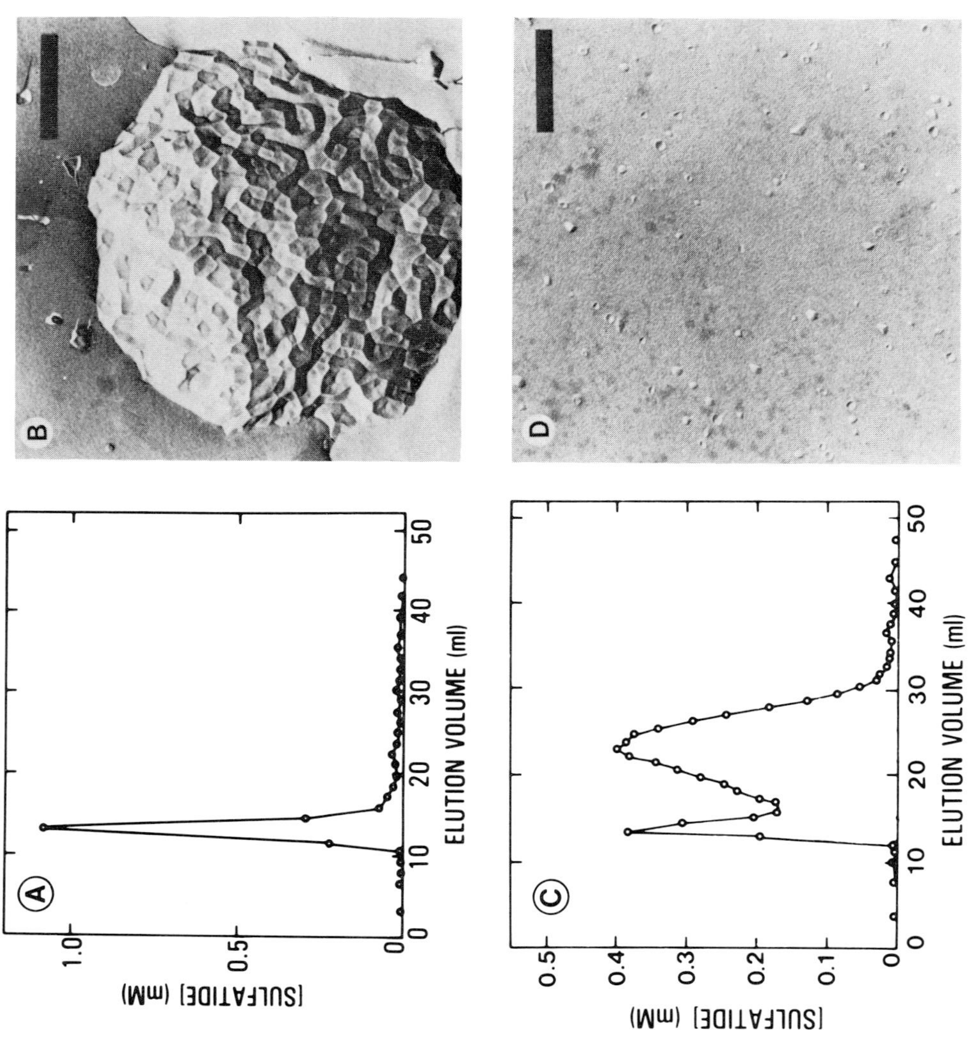
A
B
C
D
[SULFATIDE] (mM)
ELUTION VOLUME (ml)
[SULFATIDE] (mM)
ELUTION VOLUME (ml)

FIGURE 4. Gel permeation chromatography on Sepharose® 2B and freeze fracture electron microscopy of sulfatides. A and B: 5 mℓ of a 2-m*M* solution of bovine brain sulfatides in chloroform/methanol (1/1; v/v) was dried under a stream of nitrogen, and the lipid was subsequently resuspended in 2 mℓ 50 m*M* Hepes (pH 7.4), 75 m*M* NaCl by vigorous vortexing at 70°C for 2 min. Of this solution, 0.75 mℓ was passed over Sepharose® 2B (0.9 × 30 cm) at a flow rate of 5 mℓ/hr at room temperature, and 1-mℓ fractions were collected (panel A). The material eluting in the void volume was concentrated by centrifugation at 100,000 × *g* in a Beckman® TL 100 ultracentrifuge and subjected to freeze-fracture electron microscopy. Panel B shows a typical example of a particle found in the freeze-fracture replicas of vortexed sulfatides at 30,000 × magnification. C and D: A 2-mℓ suspension of vortexed sulfatides (5 m*M*) was sonicated at 70°C for 5 min, using a model W-375 sonicator from Heat Systems Inc. at a 60% pulse at setting 2. After sonication the preparation was centrifuged for 5 min in an Eppendorf microfuge to remove possible contaminating pieces originating from the sonicator probe. 1.5 mℓ was subsequently passed over Sepharose® 2B (0.9 × 30 cm) at a flow rate of 5 mℓ/hr at room temperature and 1-mℓ fractions were collected (panel C). Panel D shows a freeze-fracture replica obtained from this material at × 43,000 magnification. Horizontal bars in panels B and D represent 3 cm in length. (From Tans, G., Verkley, A. J., Yu, J., and Griffin, J. W., *Biochem. Biophys. Res. Commun.*, 149, 1002, 1987. With permission.)

allikrein to kaolin,[84,123] and it is thought that it localizes these zymogens at the surface in a favorable way for interaction with surface-bound Factor XII.[63,84]

Thus, it can be seen that the individual dissociation constants of the protein-protein and protein-surface complexes are important parameters that need careful evaluation in order to appreciate the mode of action by which surface and protein cofactors stimulate the contact activation reactions. Unfortunately, most of the surface materials that have been studied are rather ill defined. Thus, for example, kaolin will not only bind contact factors favorably, but also exposes binding sites that will irreversibly bind contact factors. It is, however, to be expected that with the availability of better-defined surface components such as sulfatides, equilibrium binding studies can be more successfully performed. In this paragraph we will review the current data available concerning the protein- and lipid-protein interactions of contact activation.

A. Protein-Protein Interactions

Shortly after the discovery of high M_r kininogen as a cofactor of contact activation, it was found that plasma prekallikrein and Factor XI circulate in plasma complexed with high M_r kininogen.[62,63] This indicates that these proteins must have a high affinity for each other. Thus far, no direct high affinity interaction has been reported for Factor XII with high M_r kininogen. Table 2 summarizes the binding data thus far available in literature for the binding of high M_r kininogen to prekallikrein (kallikrein) and Factor XI (Factor XI_a). These data have all been obtained using fluorescent-labeled proteins.[30,46,66,124,125]

As can be seen, the binding of these proteins to each other appears to be very strong and is characterized by dissociation constants in the nanomolar range. The binding site of high M_r kininogen for prekallikrein and Factor XI is exclusively located within the light chain region of the kininogen molecule,[46,64,65] and the site for prekallikrein binding has been narrowed to a stretch of 40 amino acid residues near the carboxy-terminal end of the light chain.[66] The structural information in prekallikrein for binding to high M_r kininogen is exclusively located in the heavy chain region of this molecule,[29,30] and the same appears to hold for Factor XI.[31]

B. Lipid-Protein Interactions

Only recently the first data concerning binding of contact activation proteins to lipids have become available. With the exception of one study,[83,126] all binding experiments have been carried out with sulfatides (liposomes or vesicles). It appears that Factor XII binds with high affinity to sulfatides.[83,98,124,126] The dissociation constant for the human protein was estimated to be less than 7 n*M*,[126] whereas the bovine protein binds with a K_d of some 20 n*M*.[124] High M_r kininogen purified from bovine plasma also displays high affinity for sulfatides and forms a complex with a dissociation constant of 38 n*M*.[124] It appears that high M_r kininogen and Factor XII compete for the same binding sites on sulfatides.[97,124]

Some disagreement exists in literature as to whether prekallikrein and kallikrein bind to sulfatides. Griep et al.[83] and Shimada et al.[124] failed to detect significant binding of prekallikrein to sulfatides. However, Rosing et al.[98] showed that kallikrein can bind to sulfatides and that it is actually the heavy chain region of the molecule that is responsible for binding. In this latter study it was shown that the binding of kallikrein was strongly dependent on the salt concentration and on the pH of the buffer (increased binding at decreasing pH and salt concentrations), which may explain why this binding was not observed in the other studies. In any case, it will be clear that the affinity of prekallikrein or kallikrein for sulfatides is much weaker than that of Factor XII and high M_r kininogen. Finally, Factor XI and Factor XI_a have also been shown to bind to sulfatides.[127]

Griep et al.[126] reported that Factor XII also binds to phospholipid vesicles composed of pure phosphatidylethanolamine or pure PS. It appears, however, that binding of Factor XII

Table 2
EQUILIBRIUM BINDING DATA FOR THE INTERACTION OF HIGH M_r KININOGEN OR THE LIGHT CHAIN OF HIGH M_r KININOGEN WITH PREKALLIKREIN, KALLIKREIN, AND DERIVED PEPTIDES, AND WITH FACTORS XI AND XI_a

	High M_r kininogen		High M_r kininogen light chain		
Ligand	K_d (n*M*)	Stoichiometry (mol/mol)	K_d (n*M*)	Stoichiometry (mol/mol)	Refs.
Prekallikrein	12[a]	1.2[a]	14[a]	1.1[a]	30
			16[b]	1.0[b]	46
			18[c]		66
			38[d]	1.2[d]	124
Kallikrein	15[a]	1.3[a]	17[a]	0.9[a]	30
Kallikrein heavy chain	14[a]	1.4[a]	14[a]	1.2[a]	30
Kallikrein light chain	Not detectable		Not detectable		
Factor XI	32[e]	2[e]			125
Factor XI_a	32[e]	2[e]			125

[a] Human proteins.
[b] Human proteins.
[c] Human proteins.
[d] Bovine proteins.
[e] Human proteins.

per se is not sufficient to explain the surface stimulation of Factor XII activation. Thus, it was shown that Factor XII binds equally well to phospholipid surfaces either in the fluid or in the solid gel state, but Factor XII activation only occurred on surfaces that were in the solid gel state. It was, therefore, concluded that lipid surfaces only function efficiently when they are in the solid gel state[126] (see also Section III), presumably because such surfaces allow Factor XII to obtain a favorable conformation after binding the surface.

V. KINETICS AND MECHANISM OF CONTACT ACTIVATION REACTIONS

Progress in understanding the molecular mechanisms involved in contact activation reactions and insight in the mode of action of the negatively charged surfaces and the protein cofactor high M_r kininogen has been seriously hampered by the fact that many feedback reactions occur during the activations of the contact activation zymogens. Moreover, the fact that the binding of contact factors to surfaces is frequently accompanied by a loss of protein available for activation (References 84 and 128) increases the difficulties of interpreting kinetics of contact activation. Therefore, most information concerning the various zymogen activations has been obtained by studying the separate contact activation reactions using purified proteins. Figure 5 schematically summarizes the interactions and reactions that have been defined thus far.

During contact activation the zymogens prekallikrein and Factor XII are thought to be involved in a so-called reciprocal activation mechanism in which Factor XII_a activates prekallikrein to kallikrein, which in turn converts Factor XII into Factor XII_a. Factor XII_a appears to be the central enzyme in contact activation since it can:

1. Activate prekallikrein to kallikrein, thereby contributing to the rate of activation

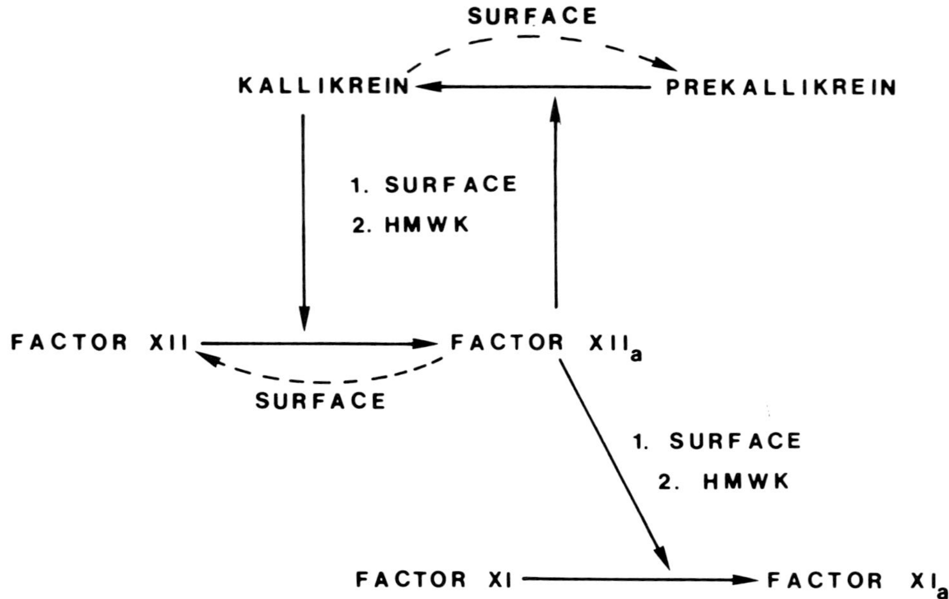

FIGURE 5. Zymogen activations occurring during contact activation.

2. Activate its own zymogen Factor XII in a surface-dependent autoactivation, thereby contributing even more to the rate of activation
3. Activate Factor XI to Factor XI_a, which propagates the initial trigger into the intrinsic coagulation cascade, since Factor XI_a subsequently activates coagulation Factor IX

Recently, we have observed that under certain experimental conditions prekallikrein can also be activated by the enzymatically active form, kallikrein. Like Factor XII autoactivation, the autoactivation of prekallikrein is a surface-dependent reaction[99] (see below). A possible negative feedback mechanism, not indicated in the figure, is the conversion of α-Factor XII_a into β-Factor XII_a by kallikrein. Since the surface binding site of α-Factor XII_a is lost after this reaction, this results in a loss of the procoagulant activity of the Factor XII_a molecule. The appearance of β-Factor XII_a is, however, slow as compared to the appearance of α-Factor XII_a during contact activation.

A. Factor XII Activation

The conversion of Factor XII into Factor XII_a is by far the best-studied reaction occurring during contact activation, and we will, therefore, treat this reaction in detail. Moreover, the mechanism by which the negatively charged surface acts in this reaction may be an example for the function of the surface in the other contact activation reactions. Activation of the zymogen Factor XII is accompanied by the cleavage of Arg_{353}-Val_{354}, producing so-called α-Factor XII_a,[7,8,129] a two-chain serine protease consisting of a heavy chain (52,000 M_r) and a light chain (28,000 M_r) held together by a disulfide bridge. Although other plasma enzymes may activate Factor XII, kallikrein is the major enzyme responsible for the activation of Factor XII in plasma.[21,39,130-134] One other reaction may contribute to Factor XII_a formation and that is autoactivation of the zymogen Factor XII by the active form α-Factor XII_a.[22,95,96,135-138]

1. Autoactivation of Factor XII

As first demonstrated in 1979 by Wiggins and Cochrane[135] for rabbit Factor XII and subsequently for the human protein,[136] the zymogen Factor XII will undergo spontaneous activation upon incubation with a suitable negatively charged surface. Due to the fact that bovine Factor XII does not autoactivate,[139] this reaction has long been controversial. By means of rigorous kinetic analysis, it was established that autoactivation of human Factor XII resulted from a so-called intermolecular process in which Factor XII is cleaved and activated by the enzymatically active form, α-Factor XII_a.[96] Autoactivation requires the presence of a procoagulant surface such as sulfatides or dextran sulfate, and for optimal activation both the enzyme (α-Factor XII_a) and the substrate (Factor XII) need to be bound to the negatively charged surface. This is suggested by the fact that:

1. Autoactivation is not detectable in the absence of surface.
2. β-Factor XII_a, the 30,000 M_r form of Factor XII_a, that lacks the ability to bind to negatively charged surfaces, is not capable of activating Factor XII.[96,136]
3. Excess surface diminishes the rate of autoactivation.[95,96,126]

The observed rate constants of autoactivation are in the order of magnitude of 10^4 to 10^5 M^{-1} sec^{-1}.[83,96,126,137] Such numbers should, however, be treated with some caution, since autoactivation is a surface-bound process, the rate of which depends on the amount of negatively charged surface present. Therefore, the rate constant must be regarded as an apparent rate constant. From our own experience the k_2^{app} of autoactivation with sulfatides or dextran sulfate under optimal conditions will yield values around 10^5 M^{-1} sec^{-1}, which likely represent the maximal attainable rates for autoactivation of Factor XII.

2. Activation of Factor XII by Plasma Kallikrein

Although autoactivation may contribute to the activation of Factor XII, the finding that Factor XII_a formation is greatly retarded in prekallikrein-deficient plasmas[21,39,130-134] is indicative for a major role of plasma kallikrein in the activation of Factor XII during contact activation. Due to the fact that inhibitors of kallikrein are present in plasma (e.g., Cl inhibitor), the only quantitative information on the efficiency of kallikrein-dependent Factor XII activation has been obtained from studies with the purified proteins.

Activation of Factor XII by kallikrein is greatly stimulated by negatively charged surfaces[76,98,120,126,137] and to a lesser extent by high M_r kininogen.[38-40,76,120,140,141] Part of this stimulation is likely due to the binding of Factor XII to the surface per se. Griffin[120] reported that ^{125}I-Factor XII bound to kaolin was much more susceptible to proteolytic activation by fluid-phase enzymes. The increase in ^{125}I-Factor XII cleavage after binding of Factor XII to the surface varied from some 4-fold with trypsin to some 300-fold with kallikrein. Based on this observation, Griffin[120] proposed that binding of Factor XII to the surface is followed by a conformational change of the molecule, which renders it much more susceptible to proteolytic cleavage.

More recently, kinetic data have become available concerning kallikrein-dependent Factor XII activation in the presence of dextran sulfate,[137] kaolin,[140] or sulfatides.[83,98,126] Table 3 summarizes the kinetic parameters of Factor XII activation by kallikrein thus far reported in literature. Using human proteins, Tankersley and Finlayson[137] found that dextran sulfate stimulated the catalytic efficiency (k_{cat}/K_m) of kallikrein-dependent Factor XII activation some 11,000-fold.[137] This increase was due to a 500-fold increase in k_{cat} and a 20-fold decrease in K_m. Sugo et al.[140] determined the kinetic parameters of bovine Factor XII activation at optimal concentrations of kaolin and high M_r kininogen and found a catalytic efficiency similar to that observed for human Factor XII activation (Table 3).

It will be clear that due to the process of autoactivation it is difficult to obtain the rates of kallikrein-dependent Factor XII activation in those cases where autoactivation contributes to the reaction rates. Tankersley and Finlayson[137] solved this problem by approximating the contributions of autoactivation and kallikrein using an iterative computer program to fit the

Table 3
KINETIC PARAMETERS OF KALLIKREIN-DEPENDENT FACTOR XII ACTIVATION

Activator	k_{cat} (sec^{-1})	K_m (μM)	k_{cat}/K_m ($M^{-1}\ sec^{-1}$)	Ref.
Kallikrein[a]	0.01	11	0.96×10^3	137
Kallikrein + dextran sulfate[a]	5.7	0.51	11.2×10^6	137
Kallikrein + kaolin + high M_r kininogen[b]	0.21	0.004	5.2×10^7	140

[a] Human proteins, pH 8.0, 37°C, with and without 25 μg/mℓ dextran sulfate.
[b] Bovine proteins, pH 8.0, 37°C, 33 μg/mℓ kaolin, 11 n*M* high M_r kininogen.

experimental data. This procedure was also adopted by Griep et al.[83,126] Rosing et al.[98] presented an analytical solution to the rate equations that can be used at substrate concentrations where the reactions are still second order (i.e., below K_m). In that case the experimental data can be fitted to a mathematical equation in order to obtain the rate constant of kallikrein-dependent activation. Figure 6 shows a representative experiment illustrating this.[98] At Factor XII concentrations below K_m the reactions contributing to Factor XII activation can be written as:

$$XII \xrightarrow{k_1'} XII_a \qquad (1)$$

$$XII + XII_a \xrightarrow{k_2} 2 \times XII_a \qquad (2)$$

Reaction 1 is the formation of Factor XII_a by kallikrein, which is characterized by a pseudo first-order rate constant, k_1', which equals the second-order rate constant k_1 times the kallikrein concentration. Reaction 2 represents Factor XII autoactivation which is described by the second-order rate constant k_2. The rate equations can be solved[98] to result in an expression for the formation of Factor XII_a with time, which contains only two unknown variables (k_1' and k_2). One of these, k_2, can be determined independently, since in the absence of kallikrein only autoactivation occurs. In that case a plot of $\ln(XII/XII_a)$ vs. time should give a straight line from which k_2 is determined (Figure 6, closed circles; see also References 96 and 98). Thus, in the presence of kallikrein the expression for Factor XII_a formation then contains only one unknown variable, k_1', which can be determined by curve fitting of the experimental points as illustrated in Figure 6.

Rosing et al.[98] and Griep et al.[126] attempted to correlate the stimulating effect of negatively charged surfaces with the binding of the reactants involved (i.e., Factor XII/XII_a and kallikrein/prekallikrein). Although in both studies sulfatides were used as a model surface, they reached opposite conclusions for the mode of action of sulfatides in the activation of Factor XII. Both groups showed that Factor XII readily and quantitatively binds to sulfatides, which is to be expected with a K_d of less than 7 n*M*.[126] Griep et al.[126] did not observe significant binding of prekallikrein and they proposed that: (1) the stimulation of kallikrein-dependent Factor XII activation by sulfatides is solely due to the fact that Factor XII upon binding becomes a better substrate for kallikrein and (2) that kallikrein acts out of solution on surface-bound Factor XII. In such a model maximum stimulation is achieved once all Factor XII is bound, and a further increase of the amount of surface will not further influence the rate of activation. This is in contrast to a process in which both enzyme and substrate must be bound to the surface in order to obtain optimal reaction rates. In such a case, once all reactants are bound, an increase in surface will result in a decreased density of reactants at

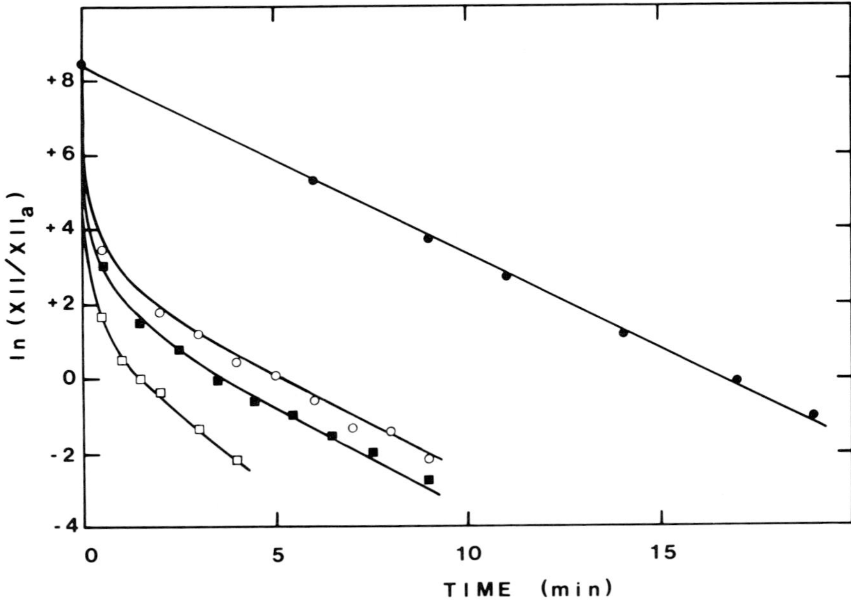

FIGURE 6. Determination of kallikrein-dependent activation of Factor XII in the presence of sulfatides. 0.1 μM Factor XII was allowed to activate at 37°C in 70 mM Hepes (pH 7.2), 80 mM NaCl, 1 mg/mℓ ovalbumin, and 100 μM sulfatides in the absence (●) and in the presence of 0.08 nM kallikrein (○), 0.16 nM kallikrein (■), or 0.64 nM kallikrein (□). At the time intervals indicated, samples were withdrawn from the reaction mixture to determine the amounts of Factor XII_a formed (see Reference 98) and the ratio of ln (Factor XII/Factor XII_a) was calculated and plotted vs. time. The drawn lines represent a computer fit of the experimental data using k_1 of $8.5 \times 10^6 M^{-1} sec^{-1}$ and a k_2 of $4.4 \times 10_4 M^{-1} sec^{-1}$. (From Rosing, J., Tans, G., and Griffin, J. H., *Eur. J. Biochem.*, 151, 531, 1985. With permission.)

the surface and, hence, in a decreased reaction rate. Griep et al.[126] observed that autoactivation difference was observed between the ability of kallikrein or the light chain to activate Factor XII. Both the rates of kallikrein- and light chain-dependent activation of Factor XII were stimulated in the presence of sulfatides. However, the light chain-dependent reaction was stimulated some 30-fold, as compared to a 3400-fold stimulation of kallikrein-dependent Factor XII activation. Rosing et al.[98] also showed that in the presence of sulfatides the pH of Factor XII was much more sensitive to an increase of the sulfatide concentration than kallikrein-dependent Factor XII activation. Although in the latter case reaction rates did diminish somewhat at higher sulfatide concentrations, these data were interpreted to support their proposal that surface-bound Factor XII is activated by fluid-phase kallikrein.[126]

Rosing et al.,[98] however, made a number of observations which do not fit in such a model. They compared the kinetics of Factor XII activation by, respectively, kallikrein and the isolated light chain of kallikrein. Kallikrein is a two-chain enzyme, the light chain of which contains the active site.[29] A fully enzymatically active light chain can be obtained by mild reduction and alkylation of kallikrein, followed by affinity chromatography over Sepharose® to which high M_r kininogen is coupled.[29] It has been shown that both kallikrein and the isolated light chain have approximately the same enzymatic activities towards the natural substrates of kallikrein, i.e., Factor XII, Cl inhibitor, α_2-macroglobulin, and high M_r kininogen.[29,142,143] In a clotting assay the light chain of kallikrein is, however, much less procoagulant than the parent molecule, kallikrein.[29] The likely explanation for this can be found in Table 4, in which it is shown that kallikrein and the light chain were virtually indistinguishable in the ability to convert the small oligopeptide substrate H-D-pro-phe-arg-p-NA (S2302) and fluid-phase Factor XII. However, in the presence of sulfatides a large

Table 4
COMPARISON OF THE CATALYTIC PROPERTIES OF KALLIKREIN AND LIGHT CHAIN[a]

	k (M^{-1} sec^{-1})	
Substrate	**Kallikrein**	**Light chain**
H-D-pro-phe-arg-pNA (S2302)	1.45×10^6	1.34×10^6
Factor XII	1.57×10^3	1.51×10^3
Factor XII + sulfatides	5.34×10^6	4.17×10^4

[a] Human proteins, pH 7.0, 37°C.

From Rosing, J., Tans, G., and Griffin, J. H., *Eur. J. Biochem.*, 151, 531, 1985. With permission.

dependency of Factor XII activation was different for both enzymes, whereas in the absence of surface this was not the case. Finally, in the absence of surface, Factor XII activation was insensitive to variations in the NaCl concentration, whereas in the presence of sulfatides, kallikrein-dependent Factor XII activation became highly sensitive to changes in the NaCl concentration, in contrast to the light chain-dependent reaction which remained insensitive.[98] In all these experiments Factor XII was found to be quantitatively bound to sulfatides. Kallikrein did also bind, albeit with a much weaker affinity than Factor XII_a. The light chain of kallikrein did not show any affinity for the negatively charged surface. Since the observed effects of pH and NaCl on the rate of Factor XII activation correlated well with their effects on the surface binding of kallikrein, Rosing et al.[98] concluded that this indicates that in experiments with kallikrein, surface-bound Factor XII was activated by surface-bound kallikrein, and that in the case of the light chain, surface-bound Factor XII was activated by soluble light chain acting out of solution.

This proposal is in disagreement with the proposal of Griep et al.[126] As already mentioned, these authors compared the effect of the concentration of sulfatides on the rate of Factor XII activation by autocatalysis and by kallikrein. They found that at higher sulfatide concentration the rate of kallikrein-dependent activation was relatively independent of the sulfatide concentration, as compared to a large decrease in the rate of autoactivation.[126] These data may, however, also be explained in terms of a model in which kallikrein must be bound to the surface in order to attain maximal reaction rates. In the case of autoactivation both Factors XII and XII_a have a very high affinity for sulfatides, and at relatively low sulfatide concentrations they will be quantitatively bound. Increasing the sulfatide concentration will then decrease the concentrations of reactants at the surface and, hence, the rate of the reaction will decrease (e.g., see Reference 96). Considering the weak affinity of kallikrein for sulfatides, an increase of the sulfatide concentration will result in an increased binding of kallikrein, which may counteract the decrease in the reaction rate due to a decrease of the concentration of Factor XII at the surface. Thus, it is likely that the differences in the dependency of autoactivation and of kallikrein-dependent Factor XII activation on the sulfatide concentration are merely a reflection of the much weaker affinity of kallikrein for sulfatides.

We feel that the currently available data concerning the mode of action of the negatively charged surface in the activation of Factor XII by kallikrein are best explained in a model in which the stimulatory effect of the surface is the result of two distinct additive effects (Figure 7):

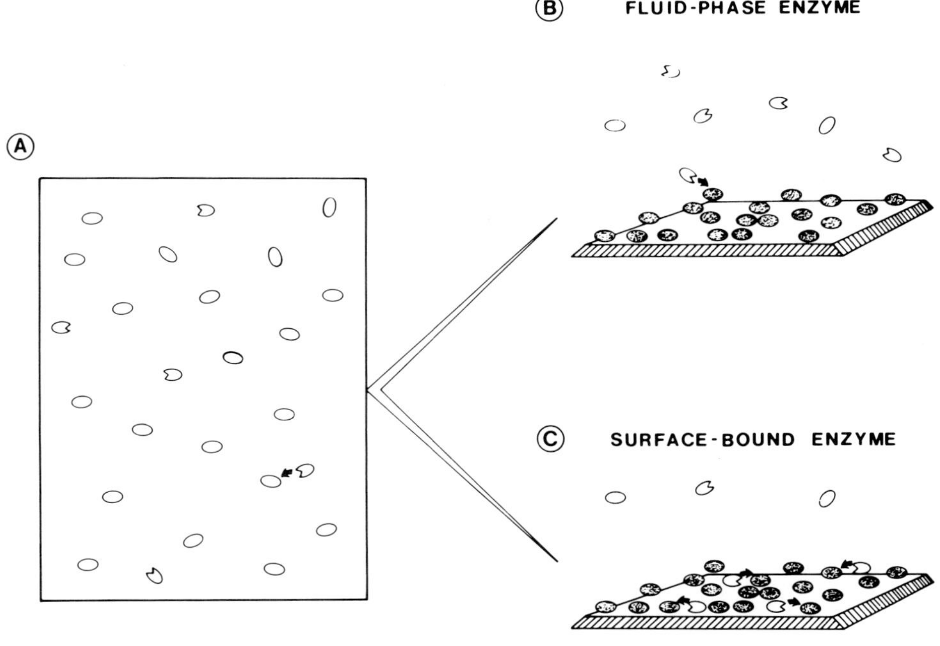

FLUID-PHASE REACTION SURFACE-DEPENDENT REACTION

NEGATIVELY CHARGED SURFACE

FACTOR XII; CONFORMATIONALLY CHANGED FACTOR XII; ENZYME

FIGURE 7. Model for the effect of negatively charged surfaces on the activation of Factor XII. Panel A represents the reaction in the fluid phase in the absence of a negatively charged surface. When a procoagulant surface is introduced, Factor XII will bind and undergo a conformational change, which renders it more susceptible to proteolytic activation. This explains the stimulation of Factor XII activation observed with fluid phase enzymes, e.g., trypsin, plasmin (see Reference 120) or the light chains of kallikrein (see Reference 98). This situation is shown in panel B. Panel C shows the situation when the enzyme also binds to the negatively charged surface, e.g., kallikrein (see Reference 98). In that case, the rate of Factor XII activation increases because: (1) bound Factor XII is a better substrate than fluid phase Factor XII and (2) both enzyme and substrate become localized at the negatively charged surface, a situation which greatly facilitates the formation of productive enzyme-substrate complexes. This will result in an additional increase of the reaction rates.

1. Binding of Factor XII to the negatively charged surface renders the molecule more susceptible to proteolytic activation.[120] This explains the observed stimulation of Factor XII activation by fluid-phase enzymes, such as the light chain of kallikrein,[98] trypsin, or plasmin,[120] and part of the stimulation of kallikrein-dependent Factor XII activation.
2. Binding of kallikrein to the surface further facilitates the interaction with surface-bound Factor XII, since it promotes the formation of productive enzyme-substrate complexes, which causes an additional increase in the rate of Factor XII activation when kallikrein is used as the enzyme.

3. Relative Importance of Autoactivation and Kallikrein-Dependent Factor XII Activation

When the rate constants for autoactivation (10^5 M^{-1} sec^{-1}) are compared with the catalytic efficiencies (k_{cat}/K_m) reported for kallikrein-dependent Factor XII activation (10^7 to 10^8 M^{-1} sec^{-1}), it will be evident that the kallikrein-dependent reaction is much more efficient. Tankersley and Finlayson[137] estimated that at the prekallikrein and Factor XII concentrations present in plasma the reciprocal activation of Factor XII will be some 2000-fold more rapid than autoactivation. Thus, certainly in the initial stages of contact activation kallikrein-dependent activation of Factor XII will be much more important than autoactivation.

B. Prekallikrein Activation

Activation of prekallikrein in human plasma is completely dependent on the presence of Factor XII.[70] Although this would suggest that no other enzymes contribute to prekallikrein activation, we have recently observed that under certain experimental conditions purified prekallikrein will undergo autoactivation in the presence of a suitable negatively charged surface.[99] Thus, two reactions may contribute to the activation of prekallikrein, i.e., autocatalytic and Factor XII_a-dependent prekallikrein activation.

1. Autoactivation of Human Plasma Prekallikrein

When purified human plasma prekallikrein is incubated with sulfatides or dextran sulfate, spontaneous activation occurs, as judged by the appearance of amidolytic activity towards the chromogenic substrate S2302.[99] Using various inhibitors, it was shown that the enzyme kallikrein and the process of prekallikrein autoactivation exhibited exactly the same sensitivity and selectivity for inhibitors, indicating that under these circumstances prekallikrein is indeed activated by kallikrein. This new observation is illustrated by the experiment shown in Figure 8. The time course of appearance of amidolytic activity shows a typical sigmoidal behavior in which an apparent lag phase is followed by a relatively rapid activation, after which a plateau is reached. Analysis of the time course of activation in terms of a second-order mechanism of autoactivation, as shown before to occur for Factor XII,[96] showed that a straight line was obtained when ln (prekallikrein/kallikrein) was plotted vs. time (Figure 8; see also Figure 6). This indicates that the reaction can be described as:

$$\text{prekallikrein} + \text{kallikrein} \xrightarrow{k_2} 2.\ \text{kallikrein}$$

in which k_2 is the rate constant of the reaction. Prekallikrein autoactivation shows an absolute requirement for surface, since in the absence of sulfatides no activation was observed. In view of the low affinity of prekallikrein and kallikrein for sulfatides (see also Section V.A.2) and the ionic strength dependence of these binding interactions, it will not be surprising that prekallikrein autoactivation is extremely sensitive to variations in the NaCl concentration, and that there is a considerable decrease in the rate of the reaction at increasing NaCl concentrations. Although the rate constant of activation must be interpreted as an apparent rate constant because of the multiple binding equilibria involved, rough estimates of k_2 at optimal conditions yield values of approximately 10^5 M^{-1} sec^{-1}, which are comparable to the catalytic efficiencies observed for Factor XII autoactivation.[96]

2. Prekallikrein Activation by Factor XII_a

Human plasma prekallikrein is readily activated by β-Factor XII_a.[24,144] The activation follows Michaelis-Menten kinetics with a k_{cat} of 3 sec^{-1} and a K_m that is strongly influenced by ionic strength (K_m = 2 μM at I = 0.12).[144] In the absence of a procoagulant, surface α-Factor XII_a and β-Factor XII_a have the same activity towards prekallikrein.[137] Prekallikrein activation by α-Factor XII_a is enhanced by negatively charged surfaces[123,137,140] and by high

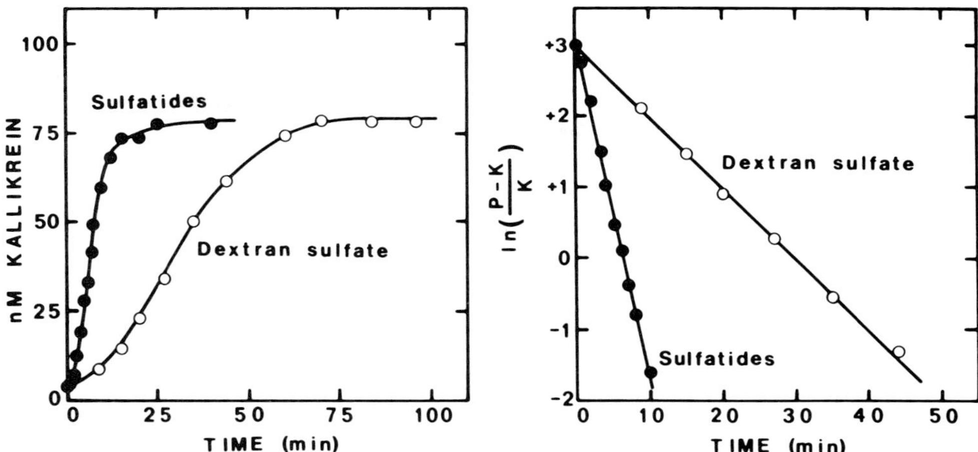

FIGURE 8. Autoactivation of human prekallikrein in the presence of sulfatides or dextran sulfate. Purified human plasma prekallikrein (290 n*M*) was allowed to activate at 37°C in 50 m*M* Hepes (pH 7.2), 32.5 m*M* NaCl, 0.5 mg/mℓ ovalbumin, and 50 μ*M* sulfatides (●) or 0.5 μg/mℓ dextran sulfate (○). At the time intervals indicated, the kallikrein formed in the reaction mixture was determined using the oligopeptide H-D-pro-phe-arg-p-nitroanilide (S2302) as a substrate for kallikrein. The second-order logarithmic plots shown in panel B were constructed using the amounts of kallikrein (K) determined and the plateau value of kallikrein reached (P) to calculate ln[(P − K)/(K)]. (From Tans, G., Rosing, J., Berrettini, M., Lämnole, B., and Griffin, J. H., *J. Biol. Chem.*, 262, 11308, 1987. With permission.)

M_r kininogen.[123,140] No data are available on the effect of these accessory components on β-Factor XII_a-dependent prekallikrein activation. Table 5 summarizes the kinetic parameters of prekallikrein activation by α-Factor XII_a reported thus far for the human and bovine proteins. As can be seen, the rate enhancement brought about by the accessory components are much less than those observed in the case of Factor XII activation (Tables 4 and 5; see also Section V.A). The rate enhancement induced by the surface appears mainly due to a decrease in K_m. The effect of high M_r kininogen on prekallikrein activation will be discussed in Section V.D.

Thus far there are no further data available on the kinetics and mechanism of surface-dependent prekallikrein activation. In analogy with the role of the negatively charged surface in Factor XII activation discussed above, it is likely that the stimulation of the negatively charged surface on the rate of prekallikrein activation is due to the fact that enzyme (α-Factor XII_a) and substrate (prekallikrein) have affinity both for each other and for the surface, and that the surface will, therefore, promote the formation of productive enzyme-substrate complexes which will result in increased activation rates.

3. Relative Importance of Autoactivation and of Factor XII_a-Catalyzed Prekallikrein Activation

The rate constant of prekallikrein autoactivation ($10^5\ M^{-1}\ sec^{-1}$) determined under optimal conditions is an order of magnitude less than the rate constant observed for prekallikrein activation by α-Factor XII_a in the presence of dextran sulfate ($4 \times 10^7\ M^{-1}\ sec^{-1}$).[137] Thus, even under favorable conditions prekallikrein autoactivation is less efficient than Factor XII_a-dependent kallikrein formation. Moreover, since both prekallikrein and kallikrein have weak affinity for the surface, autoactivation rates will be much more sensitive to an increase of the NaCl concentration. It is, therefore, plausible that autoactivation of prekallikrein will not significantly contribute to prekallikrein activation in plasma.

Table 5
KINETIC PARAMETERS OF PREKALLIKREIN ACTIVATION BY α-FACTOR XII_a

Activator	k_{cat} (sec^{-1})	K_m (μM)	k_{cat}/K_m (M^{-1} sec^{-1})
α-Factor XII_a[a]	1.03	1.8	5.7×10^5
α-Factor XII_a + dextran sulfate[a]	3.6	0.091	390×10^5
α-Factor XII_a[b]	0.05	1.0	0.5×10^5
α-Factor XII_a + kaolin[b]	0.056	0.8	0.7×10^5
α-Factor XII_a + high M_r kininogen[b]	0.05	0.26	1.9×10^5
α-Factor XII_a + kaolin + high M_r kininogen[b]	0.04	0.04	10.0×10^5

[a] From Reference 137, human proteins, pH 8.0, 37°C, 5 μg/mℓ dextran sulfate.
[b] Calculated from Reference 140, bovine proteins, pH 8.0, 37°C, 8.3 μg/mℓ kaolin, 0.42 μg/mℓ high M_r kininogen.

C. Factor XI Activation

The enzyme responsible for the activation of Factor XI in plasma is α-Factor XII_a.[32] In the absence of surface, the activation of Factor XI by α-Factor XII_a and β-Factor XII_a is very slow, and large amounts of enzyme and substrate are required in order to attain appreciable rates of Factor XI activation.[32,33,145] The presence of a suitable negatively charged surface and high M_r kininogen greatly enhances the rate of Factor XI activation.[32,123,145] The magnitude of the rate enhancements vary between 2- and 30-fold for surface stimulation[145] and from 10-[145] to 60-fold[123] for high M_r kininogen. Since no further kinetic data are available, the precise mode of action of the negatively-charged surface and the protein cofactor in Factor XIIa-catalyzed Factor XI activation is not yet known.

D. The Effect of High M_r Kininogen

With the exception of the autoactivation reactions, high M_r kininogen has been reported to act as a rate-enhancing cofactor in all contact activation reactions. This protein cofactor appears to be subject to regulation of activity during contact activation, since it has been reported that it needs to be cleaved in order to exert a stimulatory effect.[47,48] The major enzyme responsible for this activation is plasma kallikrein, although it has been reported that Factors XII_a[146] and XI_a[147] are also capable of converting high M_r kininogen into an active form. Factor XI_a will eventually destroy the cofactor activity by further proteolysis of the molecule.[147] High M_r kininogen has a high affinity for plasma prekallikrein[29,30,46,62,66,124] and Factor XI,[31,63,125] which explains why these zymogens circulate in plasma complexed with the cofactor.[62,63] Since in contrast to prekallikrein and Factor XI high M_r kininogen also has a high affinity for the surface,[124] it is thought that one of the main functions of the cofactor is to bring these zymogens to the negatively charged surface, thus making them available for proteolytic cleavage by surface-bound Factor XII_a.[123] This view is supported by the observations that prekallikrein and Factor XI bind with higher affinity to negatively charged surfaces in the presence of high M_r kininogen.[84,123] When the concentration of high M_r kininogen becomes too high, it will, however, inhibit contact activation, presumably by competition with Factor XII (α-Factor XII_a) for binding sites at the procoagulant surface.[39,97,98,140,145,148] Detailed kinetic studies concerning the effect of high M_r kininogen on the contact activation reactions are only scarcely available, and as a consequence the molecular mechanism via which this cofactor stimulates contact activation is still not fully understood.

Using bovine proteins, Sugo et al.[140] reported that high M_r kininogen causes a considerable increase of the rate of kallikrein-dependent Factor XII activation and of the activation of prekallikrein by α-Factor XII_a in the presence of kaolin. In the case of prekallikrein activation, this stimulation was mainly due to a decrease in the K_m for prekallikrein (see also Table 5). This can be regarded to support the earlier hypothesis of Wiggins et al.[123] that high M_r kininogen promotes the binding of prekallikrein to the surface, where it is subsequently activated by surface-bound Factor XII_a. In the case of human Factor XII activation at procoagulant surfaces such as sulfatides or dextran sulfate, others have failed to find a substantial stimulation of the rate of the reaction by high M_r kininogen, and at higher concentrations marked inhibition was observed.[97,98]

No detailed kinetic data are available concerning the effect of high M_r kininogen on the activation of Factor XI. Since the activation of Factor XI in plasma shows an absolute requirement for the presence of the cofactor, there is, in this case, little doubt that high M_r kininogen will have a tremendous effect on the rate of Factor XI_a formation by α-Factor XII_a in the presence of a negatively charged surface.

An interesting alternative function for high M_r kininogen was put forward by Schapira et al.,[149,150] who reported that this protein cofactor protects kallikrein from inhibition by Cl inhibitor and α_2-macroglobulin. Such a mechanism will increase the amount of kallikrein available for Factor XII activation in plasma. In the case of inhibition of kallikrein by α_2-macroglobulin, this finding was confirmed,[143] but for kallikrein inhibition by Cl inhibitor (the major inhibitor of kallikrein in plasma), others have failed to find a protecting effect of high M_r kininogen.[142,151]

VI. PLATELET INVOLVEMENT IN CONTACT ACTIVATION

Although in vitro contact activation can initiate major pathways (intrinsic blood coagulation and fibrinolysis, complement and the kinin-forming pathways) that aid in the defense of the human body against injury (see References 1 to 3), the in vivo function of contact activation remains as yet to be elucidated. Individuals deficient in Factor XII (Hageman trait), prekallikrein (Fletcher trait), or high M_r kininogen (Flaujeac, Fitzgerald, or Williams trait) appear clinically asymptomatic. Factor XI deficiency is, however, frequently associated with mild bleeding problems. One of the reasons why individuals lacking a single contact factor are asymptomatic may be that there are a number of bypass reactions available for the activation of contact factors. This will result in contact activation to occur when necessary, albeit slower than normal. An example of retarded contact activation in the apparent absence of a coagulation factor is the slow generation of clot-promoting activity in prekallikrein-deficient plasma. Furthermore, it is not known whether individuals who lack a certain contact factor in plasma will be completely deficient in this protein or whether the deficiency is only apparent in plasma. Finally, another reason why the function of contact activation is as yet not understood is the lack of a well-defined physiological surface for contact activation in vivo. Sulfatides, for example, may have potential physiological significance, but it is as yet not clearly shown that this lipid actually participates in in vivo contact activation.

Another surface with potential physiological significance for contact activation is the platelet membrane. In 1972, Walsh[81] reported that ADP-stimulated platelets could promote contact activation. Although this observation was challenged by others[152,153] Walsh and Griffin[90] showed in later studies, with purified proteins and isolated platelets, that platelets can promote Factors XII and XI cleavage. Whether the platelets functioned in these experiments as a contact-promoting surface or whether they provided proteins (proteases) that enhanced the contact activation reactions is as yet unclear. Platelets appear to contain high M_r kininogen[154-156] and a protein with a M_r of approximately 200,000 daltons, which is immunologically related to Factor XI.[157] Binding studies have shown that Factors XI, XI_a, and high M_r kininogen can bind specifically and with high affinity to stimulated platelets. [158-160] Factor XI binding requires the presence of high M_r kininogen, as well as zinc and calcium ions at concentrations normally present in plasma.[158] Factor XI_a, on the other hand, appears to bind to different sites on activated platelets, since in this case no calcium or zinc ions are needed. The presence of high M_r kininogen is, however, also required.[160] Thus, it seems plausible that Factors XI and XI_a bind to platelets complexed with high M_r kininogen. The dissociation constants for the platelet-Factor XI-high M_r kininogen complex (1 to 10 n*M*) are well below the plasma concentrations of Factor XI (25 n*M*) and high M_r kininogen (80 n*M*), indicating that the platelet binding sites can be easily saturated. The number of binding sites is, however, rather limited. About 1500 sites per platelet were reported for Factor XI[158] and 150 to 550 for Factor XI_a.[160]

Platelets also appear to contain a number of highly positively charged polypeptides (e.g., platelet Factor 4) which are released during platelet activation and efficiently inhibit surface-dependent contact activation.[161-163] Moreover, platelets will release inhibitors of activated contact factors, such as α_1-antitrypsin,[164,165] Cl inhibitor,[166] α_2-macroglobulin,[165] and an as yet unidentified inhibitor of Factor XI_a, which effectively inhibits the activation of Factor IX.[167]

It will be clear that all these experimental data produce a rather incomplete picture for the possible involvement of platelets in contact activation. The data, however, seem to suggest that if platelets play a role in contact activation it appears to be a specific one with specific binding sites for high M_r kininogen and Factor XI/XI_a complexes, instead of providing a negatively charged surface at which the contact activation proteins bind and interact and react. The thought that platelets can function in contact activation remains an attractive hypothesis though, since it will strictly limit the process of contact activation and coagulation to the site of injury where the platelets are stimulated and aggregate.

REFERENCES

1. **Cochrane, C. G. and Griffin, J. H.,** The biochemistry and pathophysiology of the contact system of plasma, *Adv. Immunol.*, 33, 241, 1982.
2. **Bouma, B. N. and Griffin, J. H.,** Initiation mechanisms: the contact activation system in plasma, in *Blood Coagulation*, Zwaal, R. F. A. and Hemker, H. C., Eds., Elsevier, Amsterdam, 1986, 103.
3. **Colman, R. W.,** Surface mediated defense reactions. The plasma contact activation system, *J. Clin. Invest.*, 73, 1249, 1984.
4. **Fujikawa, K. and Davie, E. W.,** Human factor XII (Hageman factor), *Methods Enzymol.*, 80, 198, 1981.
5. **Revak, S. D., Cochrane, C. G., Johnston, A. R., and Hugli, T. E.,** Structural changes accompanying enzymatic activation of human Hageman factor, *J. Clin. Invest.*, 54, 619, 1974.
6. **Saito, H., Ratnoff, O. D., and Pensky, J.,** Radioimmunoassay of human Hageman factor (Factor XII), *J. Lab. Clin. Med.*, 88, 506, 1976.
7. **Fujikawa, K. and McMullen, B. A.,** Amino acid sequence of human β-Factor XII_a, *J. Biol. Chem.*, 258, 10924, 1983.
8. **McMullen, B. A. and Fujikawa, K.,** Amino acid sequence of the heavy chain of human α-Factor XII_a (activated Hageman factor), *J. Biol. Chem.*, 260, 5328, 1985.
9. **Cool, D. E., Edgell, C. S., Louie, G. V., Zoller, M. J., Brayer, G. D., and MacGillivray, R. T. A.,** Characterization of human blood coagulation Factor XII cDNA. Prediction of the primary structure of Factor XII and the tertiary structure of β-Factor XII_a, *J. Biol. Chem.*, 260, 13666, 1985.
10. **Petersen, T. E., Thogersen, H. C., Skorstengaard, K., Vibe-Petersen, K., Sahl, P., Sottrup-Jenssen, L., and Magnusson, S.,** Partial primary structure of bovine plasma fibronectin. Three types of internal homology, *Proc. Natl. Acad. Sci. U.S.A.*, 80, 137, 1983.
11. **Savage, C. R., Inagami, T., and Cohen, S.,** The primary structure of epidermal growth factor, *J. Biol. Chem.*, 247, 7612, 1972.
12. **Savage, C. R., Hash, J. H., and Cohen, S.,** Epidermal growth factor. Location of disulfide bonds, *J. Biol. Chem.*, 248, 7669, 1973.

13. **Magnusson, S., Petersen, T. E., Sottrup-Jensen, L., and Claeys, H.,** Complete primary structure of prothrombin, in *Proteases and Biological Control,* Reich, E., Rifkin, D. B., and Shaw, W., Eds., Cold Spring Harbor Laboratory, Cold Spring Harbor, N.Y., 1975, 123.
14. **Magnusson, S., Sottrup-Jensen, L., Petersen, T. E., Dudek-Wojciechowska, G., and Claeys, H.,** *Proteolysis and Physiological Regulation,* Robbins, D. W. and Brew, K., Eds., Academic Press, New York, 1976, 202.
15. **Pennica, D., Holmes, W. E., Kohr, W. J., Harkins, R. N., Vehar, G. A., Ward, C. A., Bennet, W. F., Yelverton, E., Seeburg, P. H., Heyneker, H. L., Goeddell, D. V., and Collen, D.,** Cloning and expression of human tissue-type plasminogen activator cDNA in E. coli, *Nature (London),* 301, 214, 1983.
16. **Pohl, G., Källström, M., Bergsdorf, N., Wallén, P., and Jörnvall, H.,** Tissue plasminogen activator: peptide analyses confirm an indirectly derived amino acid sequence, identify the active site serine residue, establish glycosylation sites and localize variant differences, *Biochemistry,* 23, 3701, 1983.
17. **Günzler, W. A., Steffens, G. J., Otting, F., Kim, S.-M. A., Frankus, E., and Flohé, L.,** The primary structure of high molecular mass urokinase from human urine. The complete amino acid sequence of the A chain, *Hoppe Seyler's Z. Physiol. Chem.,* 363, 1155, 1982.
18. **Steffens, G. J., Günzler, W. A., Otting, F., Frankus, E., and Flohé, L.,** The complete amino acid sequence of low molecular mass urokinase from human urine, *Hoppe Seyler's Z. Physiol. Chem.,* 363, 1043, 1982.
19. **Verde, P., Stoppelli, M. P., Galeffi, P., DiNocera, P., and Blasi, F.,** Identification and primary sequence of an unspliced human urokinase poly(A^+)RNA, *Proc. Natl. Acad. Sci. U.S.A.,* 81, 4727, 1984.
20. **Revak, S. D. and Cochrane, C. G.,** The relationship of structure and function in human Hageman factor. The association of enzymatic and binding activities with separate regions of the molecule, *J. Clin. Invest.,* 57, 852, 1976.
21. **Revak, S. D., Cochrane, C. G., and Griffin, J. H.,** The binding and cleavage characteristics of human Hageman factor during contact activation. A comparison of normal plasma with plasmas deficient in Factor XI, prekallikrein, or high molecular weight kininogen, *J. Clin. Invest.,* 59, 1167, 1977.
22. **Dunn, J. T., Silverberg, M., and Kaplan, A. P.,** The cleavage and formation of activated human Hageman factor by autodigestion and by kallikrein, *J. Biol. Chem.,* 257, 1779, 1982.
23. **Dunn, J. T. and Kaplan, A. P.,** Formation and structure of human Hageman factor fragments, *J. Clin. Invest.,* 70, 627, 1982.
24. **Bouma, B. N., Miles, L. A., Beretta, G., and Griffin, J. H.,** Human plasma prekallikrein. Studies of its activation by activated Factor XII and its inactivation by diisopropyl phosphofluoridate, *Biochemistry,* 19, 1151, 1980.
25. **Mandle, R. and Kaplan, A. P.,** Hageman factor substrates. Human plasma prekallikrein: mechanism of activation by Hageman factor and participation in Hageman factor-dependent fibrinolysis, *J. Biol. Chem.,* 252, 6097, 1977.
26. **Saito, H., Poon, M. C., Vicic, W., Goldsmith, G. H., and Menitove, J. E.,** Human plasma prekallikrein (Fletcher factor) clotting activity and antigen in health and disease, *J. Lab. Clin. Med.,* 92, 84, 1978.
27. **Bouma, B. N., Kerbiriou, D. M., Vlooswijk, R. A. A., and Griffin, J. H.,** Immunological studies of prekallikrein, kallikrein, and high molecular-weight kininogen in normal and deficient plasmas and in normal plasma after cold-dependent activation, *J. Lab. Clin. Med.,* 96, 693, 1980.
28. **Chung, D. W., Fujikawa, K., McMullen, B. A., and Davie, E. W.,** Human plasma prekallikrein, a zymogen to a serine protease that contains four tandem repeats, *Biochemistry,* 25, 2410, 1986.
29. **van der Graaf, F., Tans, G., Bouma, B. N., and Griffin, J. H.,** Isolation and functional properties of the heavy and light chains of human plasma kallikrein, *J. Biol. Chem.,* 257, 14300, 1982.
30. **Bock, P. E., Shore, J. D., Tans, G., and Griffin, J. H.,** Protein-protein interactions in contact activation of blood coagulation. Binding of high molecular weight kininogen and the 5-(iodoacetamide)fluorescein-labeled kininogen light chain to prekallikrein, kallikrein and the separated kallikrein heavy and light chains, *J. Biol. Chem.,* 260, 12434, 1985.
31. **van der Graaf, F., Greengard, J. S., Bouma, B. N., Kerbiriou, D. M., and Griffin, J. H.,** Isolation and functional characterization of the active light chain of activated human blood coagulation Factor XI, *J. Biol. Chem.,* 258, 9669, 1983.
32. **Bouma, B. N. and Griffin, J. H.,** Human blood coagulation Factor XI. Purification, properties and mechanism of activation by activated Factor XII, *J. Biol. Chem.,* 252, 6432, 1977.
33. **Kurachi, K. and Davie, E. W.,** Activation of human factor XI (plasma thromboplastin antecedent) by Factor XII_a (activated Hageman factor), *Biochemistry,* 16, 5831, 1977.
34. **Saito, H. and Goldsmith, G. H.,** Plasma thromboplastin antecedent (PTA, Factor XI): a specific and sensitive radioimmunoassay, *Blood,* 50, 377, 1977.
35. **Fujikawa, K., Chung, D. W., Hendrickson, L. E., and Davie, E. W.,** Amino acid sequence of human Factor XI, a blood coagulation factor with four tandem repeats that are highly homologous with plasma prekallikrein, *Biochemistry,* 25, 2417, 1986.

36. **Colman, R. W., Bagdasarian, A., Talamo, R. C., Scott, C. F., Seavey, M., Guimaraes, J. A., Pierce, J. V., and Kaplan, A. P.**, Williams trait. Human kininogen defiency with diminished levels of plasminogen proactivator and prekallikrein associated with abnormalities of the Hageman factor-dependent pathways, *J. Clin. Invest.*, 56, 1650, 1975.
37. **Wuepper, K. D., Miller, D. R., and Lacombe, M. J.**, Flaujeac trait: deficiency of human plasma kininogen, *J. Clin. Invest.*, 56, 1663, 1975.
38. **Griffin, J. H. and Cochrane, C. G.**, Mechanisms for the involvement of high molecular weight kininogen in surface-dependent reactions of Hageman factor, *Proc. Natl. Acad. Sci. U.S.A.*, 73, 2554, 1976.
39. **Meier, H. L., Pierce, J. V., Colman, R. W., and Kaplan, A. P.**, Activation and function of human Hageman factor. The role of high molecular weight kininogen and prekallikrein, *J. Clin. Invest.*, 60, 18, 1977.
40. **Schiffman, S., Lee, P., and Waldmann, R.**, Identity of contact activation cofactor and Fitzgerald factor, *Thromb. Res.*, 6, 451, 1976.
41. **Kerbiriou, D. M. and Griffin, J. H.**, Human high molecular weight kininogen. Studies of structure-function relationships and of proteolysis of the molecule occuring during contact activation of plasma, *J. Biol. Chem.*, 254, 12020, 1979.
42. **Kleniewski, J. and Donaldson, V. H.**, Quantification of human high molecular weight kininogen (HMW-KGN) by specific hemagglutination inhibition reaction, *Proc. Soc. Exp. Biol. Med.*, 156, 113, 1977.
43. **Proud, D., Pierce, J. V., and Pisano, J. J.**, Radioimmunoassay of human high molecular weight kininogen in normal and deficient plasmas, *J. Lab. Clin. Med.*, 95, 563, 1980.
44. **Schiffman, S., Mannhalter, C., and Tyner, K. D.**, Human high molecular weight kininogen. Effects of cleavage by kallikrein on protein structure and procoagulant activity, *J. Biol. Chem.*, 255, 6433, 1980.
45. **Mori, K. and Nagasawa, S.**, Studies on human high molecular weight (HMW) kininogen. II. Structural changes of HMW kininogen by the action of human plasma kallikrein, *J. Biochem.*, 89, 1465, 1981.
46. **Bock, P. E. and Shore, J. D.**, Protein-protein interactions in contact activation of blood coagulation. Characterization of fluorescein-labeled human high molecular weight kininogen-light chain as a probe, *J. Biol. Chem.*, 258, 15079, 1983.
47. **Sugo, T., Kato, H., Iwanaga, S., and Fujii, S.**, The accelerating effect of bovine plasma HMW Kininogen on the surface-mediated activation of Factor XII: generation of a derivative form (active kininogen) with maximal cofactor activity by limited proteolysis, *Thromb. Res.*, 24, 329, 1981.
48. **Scott, C. F., Silver, L. D., Schapira, M., and Colman, R. W.**, Cleavage of human high molecular weight kininogen markedly enhances its coagulant activity. Evidence that this molecule exists as a pro-cofactor, *J. Clin. Invest.*, 73, 954, 1984.
49. **Takagaki, Y., Kitamura, N., and Nakanishi, S.**, Cloning and sequence analysis of cDNA's for human high molecular weight and low molecular weight prekininogens. Primary structures of two human prekininogens, *J. Biol. Chem.*, 260, 8601, 1985.
50. **Lottspeich, F., Kellerman, J., Henschen, A., Foertsch, B., and Müller-Esterl, W.**, The amino acid sequence of the light chain of human high-molecular-mass kininogen, *Eur. J. Biochem.*, 152, 307, 1985.
51. **Kellerman, J., Lottspeich, F., Henschen, A., and Müller-Esterl, W.**, Completion of the primary structure of human high-molecular-mass kininogen. The amino acid sequence of the entire heavy chain and evidence for its evolution by gene triplication, *Eur. J. Biochem.*, 154, 471, 1986.
52. **Sueyoshi, T., Enjyoji, K.-I., Shimada, T., Kato, H., Iwanaga, S., Bando, Y., Kominami, E., and Katunuma, N.**, A new function of kininogens as thiol proteinase inhibitors: inhibition of papain and cathepsins B, H, and L by bovine, rat and human plasma kininogens, *FEBS Lett.*, 182, 193, 1985.
53. **Müller-Esterl, W., Fritz, H., Machleidt, W., Ritonja, A., Brzin, J., Kotnik, M., Turk, V., Kellerman, J., and Lottspeich, F.**, Human plasma kininogens are identical with α-cysteine proteinase inhibitors. Evidence from immunological, enzymological and sequence data, *FEBS Lett.*, 182, 310, 1985.
54. **Higashiyama, S., Ohkubo, I., Ishiguro, H., Kunimatsu, M., Sawaki, K., and Sasaki, M.**, Human high molecular weight kininogen as a thiol proteinase inhibitor: presence of the entire inhibition capacity in the native form of heavy chain, *Biochemistry*, 25, 1669, 1986.
55. **Thompson, R. E., Mandle, R., Jr., and Kaplan, A. P.**, Characterization of human high molecular weight kininogen. Procoagulant activity associated with the light chain of kinin-free high molecular weight kininogen, *J. Exp. Med.*, 147, 488, 1978.
56. **Sugo, T., Ikari, N., Kato, H., Iwanaga, S., and Fujii, S.**, Functional sites of bovine high molecular weight kininogen as a cofactor in kaolin-mediated activation of Factor XII (Hageman factor), *Biochemistry*, 19, 3215, 1980.
57. **Han, Y. N., Komiya, M., Iwanaga, S., and Suzuki, T.**, Studies on the primary structure of bovine high-molecular-weight kininogen. Amino acid sequence of a fragment ("histidine-rich peptide") released by plasma kallikrein, *J. Biochem.*, 77, 55, 1975.
58. **Han, Y. N., Kato, H., Iwanaga, S., and Suzuki, T.**, Primary structure of bovine plasma high-molecular-weight kininogen. The amino acid sequence of a glycopeptide portion (fragment 1) following the C-terminus of the bradykinin moiety, *J. Biochem.*, 79, 1201, 1976.

59. **Waldmann, R., Scicli, A. G., McGregor, R. K., Carretero, O. A., Abraham, J. P., Kato, H., Han, Y. N., and Iwanaga, S.,** Effect of bovine high molecular weight kininogen and its fragments on Fitzgerald trait plasma, *Thromb. Res.*, 8, 785, 1976.
60. **Matheson, R. T., Miller, D. R., Lacombe, M., Han, Y. N., Iwanaga, S., Kato, H., and Wuepper, K. D.,** Flaujeac factor deficiency. Reconstitution with highly purified bovine high molecular weight kininogen and delineation of a new permeability peptide released by plasma kallikrein from bovine high molecular weight kininogen, *J. Clin. Invest.*, 58, 1395, 1976.
61. **Scicli, A. G., Waldmann, R., Guimaraes, J. A., Scicli, G., Carretero, O. A., Kato, H., Han, Y. N., and Iwanaga, S.,** Relationship between structure and correcting activity of bovine high molecular weight kininogen upon the clotting time of Fitzgerald trait plasma, *J. Exp. Med.*, 149, 847, 1979.
62. **Mandle, R. J., Colman, R. W., and Kaplan, A. P.,** Identification of prekallikrein and high-molecular-weight kininogen as a complex in human plasma, *Proc. Natl. Acad. Sci. U.S.A.*, 73, 4179, 1976.
63. **Thompson, R. E., Mandle, R., Jr., and Kaplan, A. P.,** Association of Factor XI and high molecular weight kininogen in human plasma, *J. Clin. Invest.*, 60, 1376, 1977.
64. **Bouma, B. N., Vlooswijk, R. A. A., and Griffin, J. H.,** Immunologic studies of human coagulation Factor XI and its complex with high molecular weight kininogen, *Blood,* 62, 1123, 1983.
65. **Kerbiriou, D. M., Bouma, B. N., and Griffin, J. H.,** Immunochemical studies of human high molecular weight kininogen and of its complexes with plasma prekallikrein or kallikrein, *J. Biol. Chem.*, 255, 3952, 1980.
66. **Tait, J. F. and Fujikawa, K.,** Identification of the binding site for plasma prekallikrein in human high molecular weight kininogen. A region from residues 185 to 224 of the kininogen light chain retains full binding activity, *J. Biol. Chem.*, 261, 15396, 1986.
67. **Margolis, J.,** The interrelationship of coagulation of plasma and release of peptides, *Ann. N.Y. Acad. Sci.*, 104, 133, 1963.
68. **Ratnoff, O. D.,** The biology and pathology of the initial stages of blood coagulation, *Prog. Hematol.*, 5, 204, 1966.
69. **Ratnoff, O. D. and Crum, J. D.,** Activation of Hageman factor by solutions of ellagic acid, *J. Lab. Clin. Med.*, 63, 359, 1964.
70. **Kluft, C.,** Determination of prekallikrein in human plasma: optimal conditions for activating prekallikrein, *J. Lab. Clin. Med.*, 91, 83, 1978.
71. **Shimada, T., Sugo, T., Kato, H., Yoshido, K., and Iwanaga, S.,** Activation of Factor XII and prekallikrein with polysaccharide sulfates and sulfatides: comparison with kaolin-mediated activation, *J. Biochem.*, 97, 429, 1985.
72. **Moskowitz, R. W., Schwartz, H. J., Michel, B., Ratnoff, O. D., and Astrup, T.,** Generation of kinin-like agents by chondroitin sulfate, heparin, chitin sulfate and human articular cartilage: possible pathophysiologic implications, *J. Lab. Clin. Med.*, 76, 790, 1970.
73. **Ratnoff, O. D.,** Activation of Hageman factor by L-homocystine, *Science,* 162, 1007, 1968.
74. **Kellermeyer, R. W. and Breckenridge, R. T.,** The inflammatory process in acute gouty arthritis. I. Activation of Hageman factor by sodium urate crystals, *J. Lab. Clin. Med.*, 65, 307, 1965.
75. **Morrisson, D. C. and Cochrane, C. G.,** Direct evidence for Hageman factor (Factor XII) activation by bacterial lipopolysaccharides (endotoxins), *J. Exp. Med.*, 140, 797, 1974.
76. **Fujikawa, K., Heimark, R. L., Kurachi, K., and Davie, E. W.,** Activation of bovine Factor XII (Hageman factor) by plasma kallikrein, *Biochemistry,* 19, 1322, 1980.
77. **Shimada, T., Kato, H., Iwanaga, S., Iwamori, M., and Nagai, Y.,** Activation of Factor XII and prekallikrein with cholesterol sulfate, *Thromb. Res.*, 38, 21, 1985.
78. **Didisheim, P. and Mibashan, R. S.,** Activation of Hageman factor (Factor XII) by long-chain saturated fatty acids, *Thromb. Diathes. Haemorrh.*, 9, 346, 1963.
79. **Margolis, J.,** Activation of Hageman factor by saturated fatty acids, *Aust. J. Exp. Biol. Med. Sci.*, 40, 505, 1962.
80. **Connor, W. E.,** The acceleration of thrombus formation by certain fatty acids, *J. Clin. Invest.*, 41, 1199, 1962.
81. **Walsh, P. N.,** The role of platelets in the contact phase of blood coagulation, *Br. J. Haematol.*, 22, 237, 1972.
82. **Wiggins, R. C., Loskutoff, D. J., Cochrane, C. G., Griffin, J. H., and Edgington, T. S.,** Activation of rabbit Hageman factor by homogenates of cultured rabbit endothelial cells, *J. Clin. Invest.*, 65, 197, 1980.
83. **Griep, M. A., Fujikawa, K., and Nelsestuen, G. L.,** Possible basis for the apparent surface selectivity of the contact activation of human blood coagulation Factor XII, *Biochemistry,* 25, 6688, 1986.
84. **Silverberg, M., Nicoll, J. E., and Kaplan, A. P.,** The mechanism by which the light chain of cleaved HMW-kininogen augments the activation of prekallikrein, Factor XI and Hageman factor, *Thromb. Res.*, 20, 173, 1980.

85. **Bock, P. E., Srinivasan, K. R., and Shore, J. D.,** Activation of intrinsic blood coagulation by ellagic acid: insoluble ellagic acid-metal ion complexes are the activating species, *Biochemistry,* 20, 7258, 1981.
86. **Hojima, Y., Cochrane, C. G., Wiggins, R. C., Austen, K. F., and Stevens, R. L.,** In vitro activation of the contact (Hageman factor) system of plasma by heparin and chondroitin sulfate E, *Blood,* 63, 1453, 1984.
87. **Soulier, J. P. and Gozin, D.,** Contact activation of prekallikrein and of fibrinolysis by heparinoids and heparin, *Haematologia,* 13, 117, 1980.
88. **Kellermeijer, R. W. and Breckenridege, R. T.,** The inflammatory process in acute gouty arthritis. II. The presence of Hageman factor and plasma thromboplastin antecedent in synovial fluid, *J. Lab. Clin. Med.,* 67, 455, 1966.
89. **Ginsberg, M. H., Jacques, B., Cochrane, C. G., and Griffin, J. H.,** Urate crystal-dependent cleavage of Hageman factor in human plasma and synovial fluid, *J. Lab. Clin. Med.,* 95, 497, 1980.
90. **Walsh, P. N. and Griffin, J. H.,** Contributions of human platelets to the proteolytic activation of blood coagulation Factors XII and XI, *Blood,* 57, 106, 1981.
91. **Mason, J. W., Kleeberg, U., Dolan, P., and Colman, R. W.,** Plasma kallikrein and Hageman factor in gram-negative bacteremia, *Ann. Intern. Med.,* 73, 545, 1970.
92. **Kimball, H. R., Melmon, K. L., and Wolff, S. M.,** Endotoxin-induced kinin production in man, *Proc. Soc. Exp. Biol. Med.,* 139, 1078, 1972.
93. **Hase, S. and Rietschell, E. Th.,** Isolation and analysis of the lipid A backbone. Lipid A structure of lipopolysaccharides from various bacterial groups, *Eur. J. Biochem.,* 63, 101, 1976.
94. **Tans, G. and Griffin, J. H.,** Properties of sulfatides in Factor XII-dependent contact activation, *Blood,* 59, 69, 1982.
95. **Espana, F. and Ratnoff, O. D.,** Activation of Hageman factor (factor XII) by sulfatides and other agents in the absence of plasma proteases, *J. Lab. Clin. Med.,* 102, 31, 1983.
96. **Tans, G., Rosing, J., and Griffin, J. H.,** Sulfatide-dependent autoactivation of human blood coagulation Factor XII (Hageman factor), *J. Biol. Chem.,* 258, 8215, 1983.
97. **Espana, F. and Ratnoff, O. D.,** The role of prekallikrein and high molecular weight kininogen in the contact activation of Hageman factor (Factor XII) by sulfatides and other agents, *J. Lab. Clin. Med.,* 102, 487, 1983.
98. **Rosing, J., Tans, G., and Griffin, J. H.,** Surface-dependent activation of human Factor XII (Hageman factor) by kallikrein and its light chain, *Eur. J. Biochem.,* 151, 531, 1985.
99. **Tans, G., Rosing, J., Berrettini, M., Lämmle, B., and Griffin, J. H.,** Autoactivation of human plasma prekallikrein, *J. Biol. Chem.,* 262, 11308, 1987.
100. **Karlsson, K.-A.,** Glycosphingolipids and surface membranes, in *Biological Membranes,* Vol. 4, Chapman, D., Ed., Academic Press, New York, 1982, 1.
101. **Svennerholm, L. and Ställberg-Stenhagen, S.,** Changes in the fatty acid composition of cerebrosides and sulfatides of human nervous tissue with age, *J. Lipid Res.,* 9, 215, 1968.
102. **Dopouey, P., Zalc, B., Lefroit-Joly, M., and Gomes, D.,** Localization of galactosylceramide and sulfatide at the surface of the myelin sheath: an immunofluorescence study in liquid medium, *Cell. Mol. Biol.,* 25, 269, 1979.
103. **Karlsson, K.-A., Samuelsson, B. E., and Steen, G. O.,** The lipid composition and Na^+-K^+-dependent adenosine-triphosphatase activity of the salt(nasal) gland of eider duck and herring gull, *Eur. J. Biochem.,* 46, 243, 1974.
104. **Hansson, C. G., Karlsson, K.-A., and Samuelsson, B. E.,** The identification of sulphatides in human erythrocyte membrane and their relation to sodium-potassium dependent adenosine triphosphatase, *J. Biochem.,* 83, 813, 1978.
105. **Simon, J. and Hiller, J. M.,** The opiate receptors, *Ann. Rev. Pharmacol. Toxicol.,* 18, 371, 1978.
106. **Loh, H. H. and Law, P. Y.,** The role of membrane lipids in receptor mechanisms, *Ann. Rev. Pharmacol. Toxicol.,* 20, 201, 1980.
107. **Karlsson, K.-A.,** On the chemistry and occurrence of sphingolipid long-chain bases, *Chem. Phys. Lipids,* 5, 6, 1970.
108. **Abrahamsson, S., Pascher, I., Larsson, K., and Karlsson, K.-A.,** Molecular arrangements in glycosphingolipids, *Chem. Phys. Lipids,* 8, 152, 1972.
109. **Cestaro, B., Pistolesi, E., Hershkowitz, N., and Gatt, S.,** Preparation of asymetric, cerebroside sulfate containing phospholipid vesicles, *Biochim. Biophys. Acta,* 685, 13, 1982.
110. **Viani, P., Cervato, G., Marchesini, S., and Cestaro, B.,** Fluorospectroscopic studies of mixtures of distearoylphosphatidylcholine and sulfatides with defined fatty acid compositions, *Chem. Phys. Lipids,* 39, 41, 1986.
111. **Gammack, B. D., Perrin, J. H., and Saunders, L.,** The dispersion of cerebral lipids in aqueous media by ultrasonic irradiation, *Biochim. Biophys. Acta,* 84, 576, 1964.
112. **Jeffrey, H. J. and Roy, A. B.,** Micelles of cerebroside sulfate, *AJEBAK,* 55, 339, 1977.

113. **Verkleij, A. J. and Ververgaart, P. H. J. Th.,** Architecture of biological and artificial membranes as visualized by freeze etching, *Ann. Rev. Phys. Chem.,* 26, 101, 1975.
114. **Costello, M. J. and Gulik-Krzywicki, T.,** Correlated X-ray diffraction and freeze-fracture studies on membrane model systems. Perturbations induced by freeze-fracture preparative procedures, *Biochim. Biophys. Acta,* 455, 412, 1976.
115. **Ranck, J. L., Mateu, L., Sadler, D. M., Tardieu, A., Gulick-Krzywicki, T., and Luzatti, V.,** Order-disorder conformational transitions of the hydrocarbon chains of lipids, *J. Mol. Biol.,* 85, 249, 1974.
116. **Koshy, K. M. and Boggs, J. M.,** Partial synthesis and physical properties of cerebroside sulfate containing palmitic acid or α-hydroxy palmitic acid, *Chem. Phys. Lipids,* 34, 41, 1983.
117. **McMillin, C. R., Saito, H., Ratnoff, O. D., and Walton, A. G.,** The secondary structure of human Hageman factor (Factor XII) and its alteration by activating agents, *J. Clin. Invest.,* 54, 1312, 1974.
118. **Fair, B. D., Saito, H., Ratnoff, O. D., and Rippon, W. B.,** Detection by fluorescence of structural changes accompanying the activation of Hageman factor (Factor XII), *Proc. Soc. Exp. Biol. Med.,* 155, 199, 1977.
119. **Kirby, E. P. and Devitt, P. J.,** The binding of bovine Factor XII to kaolin, *Blood,* 61, 652, 1983.
120. **Griffin, J. H.,** Role of surface in surface-dependent activation of Hageman factor (blood coagulation Factor XII), *Proc. Natl. Acad. Sci. U.S.A.,* 75, 1998, 1978.
121. **Mannhalter, C. and Schiffman, S.,** Surface adsorption of Factor XI. Association of adsorption sites with the heavy chain of activated Factor XI, *Thromb. Haemostas.,* 43, 124, 1980.
122. **Mannhalter, C. and Schiffman, S.,** Surface adsorption of Factor XI. II. Evidence that different mechanisms are involved in binding to glass and plastic materials, *Thromb. Haemostas.,* 47, 214, 1982.
123. **Wiggins, R. C., Bouma, B. N., Cochrane, C. G., and Griffin, J. H.,** Role of high-molecular-weight kininogen in surface-binding and activation of coagulation Factor XI and prekallikrein, *Proc. Natl. Acad. Sci. U.S.A.,* 74, 4636, 1977.
124. **Shimada, T., Kato, H., Maeda, H., and Iwanaga, S.,** Interaction of Factor XII, high-molecular-weight (HWM) kininogen and prekallikrein with sulfatide: analysis by fluorescence polarization, *J. Biochem.,* 97, 1637, 1985.
125. **Warn-Cramer, B. J. and Bajaj, S. P.,** Stoichiometry of binding of high molecular weight kininogen to Factor XI/XIa, *Biochem. Biophys. Res. Commun.,* 133, 417, 1985.
126. **Griep, M. A., Fujikawa, K., and Nelsestuen, G. L.,** Binding and activation properties of human Factor XII, prekallikrein and derived peptides with acidic lipid vesicles, *Biochemistry,* 24, 4124, 1985.
127. **Schiffman, S., Rosenfeld, R., and Retzios, A. D.,** Interaction of Factor XI and sulfatide, *Thromb. Res.,* 41, 575, 1986.
128. **Scott, C. F., Kirby, E. P., Schick, P. K., and Colman, R. W.,** Effect of surfaces on fluid-phase prekallikrein activation, *Blood,* 57, 553, 1981.
129. **Fujikawa, K., Kurachi, K., and Davie, E. W.,** Characterization of bovine Factor XII_a (activated Hageman factor), *Biochemistry,* 16, 4182, 1977.
130. **Bagdasarian, A., Lahiri, B., Talamo, R. C., Wong, P., and Colman, R. W.,** Immunochemical studies of plasma kallikrein, *J. Clin. Invest.,* 54, 1444, 1973.
131. **Cochrane, C. G., Revak, S. D., and Wuepper, K. D.,** Activation of Hageman factor in solid and fluid phases. A critical role of kallikrein, *J. Exp. Med.,* 138, 1564, 1973.
132. **Saito, H., Ratnoff, O. D., and Donaldson, V. H.,** Defective activation of clotting, fibrinolytic, and permeability enhancing systems in human Fletcher trait plasma, *Circ. Res.,* 34, 641, 1974.
133. **Weiss, A. S., Gallin, J. I., and Kaplan, A. P.,** Fletcher factor deficiency. A diminished rate of Hageman factor activation caused by absence of prekallikrein with abnormalities of coagulation, fibrinolysis, chemotactic activity, and kinin generation, *J. Clin. Invest.,* 53, 622, 1974.
134. **Wuepper, K. D.,** Prekallikrein deficiency in man, *J. Exp. Med.,* 138, 1345, 1973.
135. **Wiggins, R. C. and Cochrane, C. G.,** The autoactivation of rabbit Hageman factor, *J. Exp. Med.,* 150, 1122, 1979.
136. **Silverberg, M., Dunn, J. T., Garen, L., and Kaplan, A. P.,** Autoactivation of human Hageman factor. Demonstration utilizing a synthetic substrate, *J. Biol. Chem.,* 255, 7281, 1980.
137. **Tankersley, D. L. and Finlayson, J. S.,** Kinetics of activation and autoactivation of human Factor XII, *Biochemistry,* 23, 273, 1984.
138. **Ratnoff, O. D. and Saito, H.,** The evolution of clot-promoting and amidolytic activities in mixtures of Hageman factor (Factor XII) and ellagic acid. The enhancing effect of other proteins, *J. Lab. Clin. Med.,* 100, 248, 1982.
139. **Sugo, T., Hamaguchi, A., Shimada, T., Kato, H., and Iwanaga, S.,** Mechanism of surface-mediated activation of bovine Factor XII and plasma prekallikrein, *J. Biochem.,* 92, 689, 1982.
140. **Sugo, T., Kato, H., Iwanaga, S., Takada, K., and Sakakibara, S.,** Kinetic studies on surface mediated activation of bovine Factor XII and prekallikrein. Effects of kaolin and high-M_r kininogen on the activation reactions, *Eur. J. Biochem.,* 146, 43, 1985.

141. **Chan, J. Y. C., Habal, F. M., Burrowes, C. E., and Movat, H. Z.,** Interaction between Factor XII (Hageman factor), high molecular weight kininogen and prekallikrein, *Thromb. Res.*, 9, 432, 1976.
142. **van der Graaf, F., Koedam, J. A., Griffin, J. H., and Bouma, B. N.,** Interaction of human plasma kallikrein and its light chain with Cl-inhibitor, *Biochemistry*, 22, 4860, 1983.
143. **van der Graaf, F., Rietveld, A., Keus, F. J. A., and Bouma, B. N.,** Interaction of human plasma kallikrein and its light chain with α_2-macroglobulin, *Biochemistry*, 23, 1760, 1984.
144. **Tankersley, D. L., Fournel, M. A., and Schroeder, D. D.,** Kinetics of activation of prekallikrein by prekallikrein activator, *Biochemistry*, 19, 3121, 1980.
145. **Kurachi, K., Fujikawa, K., and Davie, E. W.,** Mechanism of activation of bovine Factor XI by Factor XII and Factor XII_a, *Biochemistry*, 19, 1330, 1980.
146. **Wiggins, R. C.,** Kinin release from high molecular weight kininogen by the action of Hageman factor in the absence of kallikrein, *J. Biol. Chem.*, 258, 8963, 1983.
147. **Scott, C. F., Silver, L. D., Purdon, D. A., and Colman, R. W.,** Cleavage of human high molecular weight kininogen by Factor XI_a in vitro. Effect on structure and function, *J. Biol. Chem.*, 260, 10856, 1985.
148. **Goldsmith, G. H.,** Contact-activated fibrinolysis: role of surface concentration and high molecular weight kininogen, *J. Lab. Clin. Med.*, 96, 222, 1980.
149. **Schapira, M., Scott, C. F., and Colman, R. W.,** Protection of human plasma kallikrein from inactivation by Cl inhibitor and other protease inhibitors. The role of high molecular weight kininogen, *Biochemistry*, 20, 2738, 1981.
150. **Schapira, M., Scott, C. F., James, A., Silver, L. D., Kueppers, F., James, H. L., and Colman, R. W.,** High molecular weight kininogen or its light chain protects human plasma kallikrein from inactivation by plasma protease inhibitors, *Biochemistry*, 21, 567, 1982.
151. **Silverberg, M., Longo, J., and Kaplan, A. P.,** Study of the effect of high molecular weight kininogen upon the fluid-phase inactivation of kallikrein by Cl-inhibitor, *J. Biol. Chem.*, 261, 14965, 1986.
152. **Vecchione, J. and Zucker, M. B.,** Procoagulant activity of platelets in recalcified plasma, *Br. J. Haematol.*, 31, 423, 1975.
153. **Vicic, W. J., Ratnoff, O. D., Saito, H., and Goldsmith, G. H.,** Platelets and surface-mediated clotting activity, *Br. J. Haematol.*, 43, 91, 1979.
154. **Kerbiriou-Nabias, D. M., Garcia, F. O., and Larrieu, M.-J.,** Radioimmunoassays of human high and low molecular weight kininogen in plasmas and platelets, *Br. J. Haematol.*, 56, 273, 1984.
155. **Schmaier, A. H., Zuckerberg, A., Silverman, C., Kuchibhotla, J., Tuszynski, G. P., and Colman, R. W.,** High molecular weight kininogen. A secreted platelet protein, *J. Clin. Invest.*, 71, 1477, 1983.
156. **Schmaier, A. H., Smith, P. M., Purdon, A. D., White, J. G., and Colman, R. W.,** High molecular weight kininogen: localization in the unstimulated and activated platelet, and activation by platelet calpain(s), *Blood*, 67, 119, 1986.
157. **Tuszynski, G. P., Bevacqua, S. J., Schmaier, A. H., Colman, R. W., and Walsh, P. N.,** Factor XI antigen and activity in human platelets, *Blood*, 59, 1148, 1982.
158. **Greengard, J. S., Heeb, M. J., Ersdal, E., Walsh, P. N., and Griffin, J. H.,** Binding of coagulation Factor XI to washed human platelets, *Biochemistry*, 25, 3884, 1986.
159. **Greengard, J. S. and Griffin, J. H.,** Receptors for high molecular weight kininogen on stimulated washed human platelets, *Biochemistry*, 23, 6863, 1984.
160. **Sinha, D., Seaman, F. S., Koshy, A., Knight, L. C., and Walsh, P. N.,** Blood coagulation Factor XIa binds specifically to a site on activated human platelets distinct from that for Factor XI, *J. Clin. Invest.*, 73, 1550, 1984.
161. **Kodama, K., Kato, H., and Iwanaga, S.,** Isolation of bovine platelet cationic proteins which inhibit the surface-mediated activation of factor XII and prekallikrein, *J. Biochem.*, 97, 139, 1985.
162. **Weerasinghe, K. M., Scully, M. F., and Kakkar, V. V.,** A platelet derived inhibitor of plasma prekallikrein activation, *Thromb. Res.*, 32, 519, 1983.
163. **Weerasinghe, K. M., Scully, M. F., and Kakkar, V. V.,** Inhibition of cerebroside sulfate (sulfatide)-induced contact activation reactions by platelet factor four, *Thromb. Res.*, 33, 625, 1984.
164. **Bagdasarian, A. and Colman, R. W.,** Subcellular localization and purification of platelet α_1-antitrypsin, *Blood*, 51, 139, 1978.
165. **Nachman, R. L. and Harpel, P. C.,** Platelet α_2-macroglobulin and α_1-antitrypsin, *J. Biol. Chem.*, 251, 4514, 1976.
166. **Schmaier, A. H., Smith, P. M., and Colman, R. W.,** Platelet Cl inhibitor: a secreted alpha-granule protein, *J. Clin. Invest.*, 75, 242, 1985.
167. **Soons, H., Janssen-Claessen, T., Hemker, H. C., and Tans, G.,** The effect of platelets in the activation of human blood coagulation Factor IX by Factor XIa, *Blood*, 68, 140, 1986.

168. **Tans, G. and Rosing, J.,** unpublished data.
169. **Tans, G., Verkleij, A. J., Yu, J., and Griffin, J. H.,** Sulfatides as a model surface for contact activation of human plasma, *Biochem. Biophys. Res. Commun.*, 149, 1002, 1987.
170. **Tans, G., Rosing, J., and Griffin, J. H.,** unpublished observations.

Chapter 6

TISSUE THROMBOPLASTIN AND THE INITIATION OF COAGULATION

Rogier M. Bertina, Anton M. H. P. van den Besselaar, and Victor J. J. Bom

TABLE OF CONTENTS

I. INTRODUCTION

It has been known for more than a century that the in vitro coagulation time of blood can be shortened by adding a sufficient amount of tissue extract. According to the classical theory of Morawitz,[1] a tissue factor called thrombokinase reacts with prothrombin and calcium to form thrombin, which converts fibrinogen to fibrin. Howell[2] introduced the term "thromboplastin" for the tissue factor, and the International Committee for the Nomenclature of Blood Coagulation Factors assigned the Roman numeral III to the tissue factor.[3] Factor III should not be confused with platelet factor 3.[4] In this chapter we will use both the term "tissue factor" and the term "tissue thromboplastin".

Further investigations revealed other plasma factors which are involved in thromboplastin action, namely, factor V,[5] factor VII,[6-8] and factor X.[9,10] The thromboplastin system for prothrombin conversion was called the extrinsic system, which had to be distinguished from the intrinsic system involving surface contact factors, factors V, VIII, IX, and X, phospholipids, and calcium.[11]

The extrinsic and intrinsic systems were thought to represent two independent pathways for the conversion of factor X into factor Xa. The first indication for a closer relationship between both systems was obtained by Biggs and Nossel[12] in experiments where they used very diluted tissue extracts. Their findings were substantiated biochemically by Østerud and Rapaport,[13] who demonstrated that the reaction product of tissue factor and factor VII functioned as a potent activator of factor IX.

After the development of new assays with which the activation of factor X and factor IX could be followed by measuring the release of radiolabeled activation peptides, it was possible to study the kinetics of the initial reactions of the extrinsic pathway in greater detail.[14-16]

Physicochemical characterization of the tissue factor as a lipoprotein was started by Chargaff and co-workers[17] and continued by research groups at Yale University[18] and the University of Oslo.[19,20] The specificity of tissue factor is localized in the apoprotein moiety, but its procoagulant activity is expressed only if the apoprotein is associated with phospholipids. Purification of tissue factor apoprotein (TFAP, apoprotein III) has been a laborious task because of a hydrophobic nature.[21]

Tissue factor is of widespread occurrence in the mammalian organism. In vitro, certain cells synthesize apoprotein III constitutively (fibroblasts, smooth muscle cells, glioma cells, and placental cells). Other cells which normally do not synthesize apoprotein III can be induced to do so by a number of pathophysiological agents such as immune complexes, endotoxins, and lymphokines. Such cells are monocytes, macrophages, and endothelial cells. Finally, there are cells (lymphocytes, granulocytes, erythrocytes, and platelets) in which so far no thromboplastin synthesis has been demonstrated, in spite of the use of several inducers.[22]

The monocyte tissue factor response has been shown to be an important effector response in the immunopathogenesis of delayed-type hypersensitivity, viral infections, disseminated intravascular coagulation, and allogeneic organ graft rejection.[23] Induction of tissue factor activity in monocytes and endothelial cells also has been frequently associated with the occurrence of thrombosis in the microcirculation.[24,25]

In this chapter we will review our present knowledge of the biochemistry and cell biology of tissue factor and discuss in more detail the initial reactions of extrinsic fibrin formation.

II. PURIFICATION OF TISSUE FACTOR APOPROTEIN

The history of tissue thromboplastin purification is closely related to that of its physicochemical characterization. In 1912, Howell[26] inferred from tissue extraction experiments with ether that the thromboplastic activity is dependent on the presence of both lipid and protein. The lipoprotein nature of tissue thromboplastin was confirmed by Mills,[27] who fractionated the procoagulant activity from beef lung tissue. Recombination of the less active lipid fraction with the inactive protein fraction restored most of the original activity.

Ultracentrifugation experiments by Chargaff et al.[17] showed that the sedimentation constant of beef lung thromboplastin corresponded to a particle weight of 167,000,000 daltons. Chargaff was the first to demonstrate the solubilization of tissue thromboplastin by the detergent sodiumdeoxycholate.[28] Human brain thromboplastin solubilized by deoxycholate (DOC) was separated into a protein component and a phospholipid moiety by gel filtration.[19,20] By this procedure a 20-fold purification was obtained.

Nemerson and Pitlick[29] achieved an 800- to 1500-fold purification of bovine lung thromboplastin by a procedure involving delipidation with heptane-butanol, solubilization with DOC, ammonium sulfate precipitation, ion exchange chromatography with DEAE-Sephadex®, and finally agarose chromatography. Pitlick showed in 1975 that bovine tissue factor activity can be inhibited completely by concanavalin A.[30] Subsequently, the purification steps after solubilization with DOC were replaced by one-step affinity chromatography on concanavalin A-Sepharose® yielding the same specific activity as earlier preparations.[31] Norwegian investigators introduced preparative electrophoresis in the presence of sodium dodecyl sulfate (SDS).[32,33] They achieved a 1000- to 2000-fold purification of human brain apoprotein III. SDS has a strong inhibitory effect on thromboplastin activity,[31,34] and renaturation of active tissue thromboplastin is not easily achieved, although Bjørklid et al.[32] claimed that SDS could be removed by dialysis. Bach et al.[21] developed a new procedure for recovery of TFAP activity after exposure to SDS. Furthermore, these investigators introduced Triton® X-100 as a nonionic detergent for thromboplastin solubilization. The apoprotein was purified by a combination of concanavalin-A Sepharose® chromatography and preparative SDS polyacrylamide-gel electrophoresis. Rabbit antibodies raised against the purified apoprotein were then used to construct an immunoadsorbent column by which the purification procedure could be simplified and scaled up. The apoprotein (M_r 43,000) was purified 142,000-fold, and homogeneity could be demonstrated by limited digestion with trypsin.[21]

In contrast to bovine tissue factor, only about half of human TFAP binds to concanavalin A because of heterogeneous glycosylation.[35] Purification of human thromboplastin by concanavalin A-Sepharose® chromatography will, therefore, yield only a selected population of molecules.[36]

Since tissue factor interacts specifically with factors VII and VIIa, purification by affinity chromatography should be possible. Recently, Broze et al.[37] reported a 53000-fold purification of human brain TFAP using affinity chromatography on factor VII-agarose. Binding of tissue factor solubilized with Triton® X-100 occurred in the presence of $CaCl_2$, and bound tissue factor was eluted with EDTA. The yield of the procedure was 41%. The homogeneity of the preparation was assessed by SDS-polyacrylamide gel electrophoresis and determination of the NH_2-terminal amino acid sequence. The apparent M_r was 44,000, and the NH_2-terminal sequence was Ser-X-Asn-Thr-Val-Ala-Val-Tyr-X-Tyr-X-Leu-Lys-(Ser)-Lys-Asn-Phe. The success of affinity chromatography for human tissue factor purification was confirmed by Bom et al.[38] and by Guha et al.,[39] who obtained 40,000- and 50,000-fold purification, respectively. Binding of tissue factor to factor VII appeared to be calcium-specific, and phospholipids seemed not to be required.[38]

In contrast to the findings of Broze et al.,[37] Guha et al.[39] reported that human brain apoprotein had a blocked amino terminus. Human placenta apoprotein purified by Guha et al.[39] yielded a unique sequence: X-Glu-X-Tyr-Asn-X-Pro-Asn-Pro-Thr-Ala-Asp-X-Lys-Thr-Ala-Val-X-X-Ser-Ser-Asp-Phe-X-Ala-X-Leu-Ile.

The recovery of TFAP from immunoaffinity columns has been increased by the application of monoclonal antibodies against bovine tissue factor.[40] These antibodies inhibit reconstituted bovine tissue factor activity and bind to the same region of the tissue factor molecule as factor VIIa. In contrast, another monoclonal antibody which inhibits the procoagulant activity of activated human monocytes does not block the activity of reconstituted tissue factor apoprotein,[41] and the specificity of this antibody for human tissue factor apoprotein has not been demonstrated to date.

III. RECONSTITUTION OF TISSUE FACTOR AND PHOSPHOLIPID REQUIREMENTS

Nemerson[18] demonstrated that phospholipids were required to restore the activity of delipidated tissue factor. In this work bovine brain particles were delipidated by butanol extraction. Relipidation with purified phospholipids was performed in butanol and by subsequent removal of butanol under reduced pressure. Phosphatidylethanolamine (PE) could restore the activity of the brain particles about twice as much as phosphatidylcholine (PC), while pure phosphatidylserine (PS) and lysophosphatidylcholine were inactive.

In a later study, Nemerson[42] relipidated purified apoprotein with phospholipids in the presence of 0.25% sodium deoxycholate. The excess of DOC was removed by dialysis.

Recombination of active tissue factor could also be effected by mixing the protein and phospholipids in the presence of Triton® X-100 and subsequent removal of Triton® X-100 by binding of the detergent to a styrene-divinylbenzene copolymer.[43]

In a recent study[44] it was deduced that TFAP reconstituted into phospholipid vesicles using octylglucoside as detergent is randomly orientated in the bilayer. Thus, the effective concentration in these vesicles was half the total concentration.[44]

Pitlick and Nemerson[45] investigated the recombination process by sucrose density gradient centrifugation. Complexes between phospholipid and purified protein were obtained in the presence of DOC. If DOC is omitted during the recombination, lipid does not bind to TFAP, nor is activity restored. Binding of TFAP to phospholipid is required for activity.[45] Inclusion of cadmium chloride in the relipidation mixture greatly increases the recovered activity of highly purified tissue factor from human placenta by promoting incorporation of tissue factor into phospholipid vesicles.[46,47] Calcium chloride and magnesium chloride do not enhance the reconstitution of tissue factor vesicle complexes nearly as efficiently as does cadmium chloride. Cadmium causes vesicle leakage under conditions which favor reconstitution of tissue factor-vesicle complexes.[48]

Purified phospholipids were not as effective as mixed brain lipids in restoring activity.[42] Other authors confirmed that optimal activity could be obtained by relipidation of the protein moiety with binary[49] or ternary phospholipid mixtures.[33] Although pure PS is inactive in restoring activity, this lipid appears to play a special role, since a limited amount of PS introduced into a PC + PE mixture increases the activity 100-fold.[33] These findings led the authors to believe that a particular electrostatic charge of the lipid moiety is a requirement for optimum exhibition of the activity of the tissue factor apoprotein.[33,49] It was recently suggested that acidic phospholipids accelerate the tissue factor pathway by enhancing the direct interaction of the catalytic complex (factor VII-tissue factor) with free factor X, rather than by concentrating substrate at the lipid surface.[44] Furthermore, factor VII binding to tissue factor is more effective by the introduction of PS in the phospholipid mixture.

The optimum pH for recombination is 4.0, as shown by Wijngaards et al.,[49] using sodium taurocholate for the solubilization-dialysis procedure. According to these authors, electrostatic repulsion between negatively charged groups of lipid and protein interferes with the reconstitution. Elimination of the electrostatic repulsion could be achieved by lowering the pH or by adding salt.[49]

The fatty acid moiety of phospholipid is critical in the restoration of the procoagulant activity of the reconstituted tissue factor. Increased unsaturation in the fatty acids correlated with an increase in the thromboplastin activity of the recombinant.[49] Complete saturation resulted in inactive preparations.[18] Another factor determining the activity of reconstituted tissue factor is the ratio of phospholipid to apoprotein. Optimal ratios of 1.1 (w/w),[33] 1.5,[42] 12,[51] 450,[21] 500,[36] and 600[37] have been reported. These wide variations probably reflect the purity of the protein, although differences between human and bovine apoprotein and the quality of the phospholipids also may account for the wide range. In some reports, an activity plateau was reached in the thromboplastin activity by increasing the phospholipid-to-protein ratio.[21,37,51] Other investigators observed a decrease of activity by further increasing the ratio.[33,36,42] The inhibitory effect of phospholipid was attributed to competition with factor VII for complexing the substrate (factor X) in a form that limits accessibility to the enzyme.[16]

IV. FACTOR VII

Factor VII (proconvertin, serum prothrombin conversion accelerator, SPCA, stable factor, or autoprothrombin I) is a trace protein in plasma which is synthesized by the liver.[52] The existence was first proposed by Alexander et al.[8] in 1951, after the identification of a patient who was deficient in this previously unknown coagulation protein. A hereditary deficiency of factor VII is associated with a severe to a very mild bleeding tendency in affected homozygotes or double heterozygotes,[53,54] thus establishing the importance of this protein for in vivo thrombin generation.

Factor VII is a vitamin K-dependent glycoprotein with a molecular weight of about 50,000. During the treatment of patients with oral anticoagulants, plasma factor VII activity decreases, while concomitantly partially and noncarboxylated forms of factor VII appear in the circulation.[55-58] It has been purified from both bovine[59-61] and human plasma.[69,70] Recently, the complete amino acid sequence of the human factor VII has been derived from the nucleotide sequence of the human factor VII cDNA.[62] The protein is secreted in the blood as a single chain protein of 406 amino acids. The amino-terminal sequence (Gla-domain) is highly homologous with those of prothrombin, factor IX, protein S, and with the amino-terminal sequences of the light chains of factor X and protein C.[62] It contains ten γ-carboxyglutamic acid residues (positions 6, 7, 14, 16, 19, 20, 25, 26, 29, and 35) and one β-hydroxy aspartic acid residue (position 63).[62-64] The γ-carboxyglutamic acid residues probably are involved in the binding of Ca^{2+} (Reference 65) and in the formation of Ca^{2+}-dependent conformational changes.[56,58] Apart from the Gla-domain we can identify two epidermal growth factor domains and one catalytic domain containing the three principal residues involved in the catalytic activity of this serine protease (His 193, Asp 242, and Ser 344). Residues 145 and 322 have been identified as potential attachment sites for carbohydrate side chains. Recently, Broze et al.[56] reported that 5 to 8% of plasma factor VII is of lower molecular weight (about 4500 less). They provided evidence that this FVII* lacks the Gla domain. FVII* is also produced by cultured Hep G-2 cells. Of interest is the observation that both in vivo and in vitro the production of FVII* is much less sensitive to warfarin than that of the intact factor VII.[56] The physiological significance of this constitutively produced FVII* is not known.

Factor VII is unique among the coagulation proteins in the sense that the zymogen has some esterase and protease activity.[66,67] After proteolytic cleavage at the Arg^{152}-Ile^{153} bond, two-chain factor VII or αFVIIa is formed.[62,68] The two chains which migrate on reduced gels as proteins of 29,500 daltons (heavy chain) and 23,500 daltons (light chain) are linked by one disulfide bond probably involving cysteine residues in position 135 and 262.[61,62] The proteolytic activation of factor VII can be catalyzed by several proteases. The most potent activator in vitro seems to be factor Xa.[60,69,70-72] For factor VII activation, factor Xa requires the presence of Ca^{2+} and phospholipids, while according to Nemerson and Repke,[73] the activation reaction is markedly accelerated by tissue factor. Less potent activators are factor IXa in the presence of Ca^{2+} and phospholipids,[72,74,75] factor XIIa,[69,74,76,77] thrombin,[60] and plasmin.[75] The specific coagulant activity of the FVIIa has been reported to be 25- to 120-fold higher than that of native factor VII.[61,69,70] Zur et al.[67] reported that in the bovine system the factor VII zymogen probably has 0.8% of the coagulant activity of the VIIa form.

Both native factors VII and VIIa can be inactivated by diisopropylfluorophosphate (DFP).[59,69,78,80,81] The rate of inactivation of FVIIa by DFP is 2.7 to 4.1 times higher than that of inactivation of factor VII.[67,69] The question of the existence of physiologic inhibitors of FVIIa has not yet been answered satisfactorily. Broze et al.[69] reported that under appropriate conditions both factors VII and VIIa can be neutralized by antithrombin III (only in the presence of heparin), and that factor VIIa is inhibited 25 times faster than the factor VII zymogen. Other authors, however, claim that factor VIIa is insensitive to antithrombin III-heparin.[82,83] Dahl et al.[84] claim that there is FVIIa-neutralizing activity in human plasma, and that antithrombin III accounts for about 30% of the inhibitory potential. Our own experience is that human factor VIIa, when added to plasma, is extremely stable even at prolonged incubation times (4 hr at 37°C). Many investigators have observed inactivation of FVIIa after prolonged incubation with the activator.[60,61,71] One possible explanation is that factor VIIa can be degraded by proteolytic removal of a carboxy-terminal fragment containing the active-site serine. Such a cleavage has been demonstrated to occur in bovine factor VIIa in the presence of factor Xa.[71] Factor Xa then cleaves an Arg-Gly bond in the heavy chain of factor VIIa, thus removing a 12,500-dalton fragment which contains the active site. However, Bajaj et al.[70] report that inactivation of human factor VIIa by prolonged incubation with factor Xa never gave rise to the appearance of a three-chain molecule after analysis by SDS-polyacrylamide gel electrophoresis. They suggest that the loss in factor VII activity is due to instability of the isolated factor VIIa.

Although the liver seems to be the main source of factor VII, recent reports suggest that factor VII also might be produced by other cells.[85-87] Chapman et al.[86] provided especially convincing data that human alveolar macrophages can produce factor VII, and that the synthesis of factor VII by those cells is sensitive to warfarin. Because these cells also produce tissue factor, these findings may provide us with new insights in the in vivo mechanisms for the initiation of blood coagulation.

V. FACTOR X

Factor X (Stuart factor) is a vitamin K-dependent plasma protein with a molecular weight of approximately 59,000,[63] which is involved in both the extrinsic and intrinsic pathway of coagulation.[88] It has been isolated both from bovine[89-91] and human plasma,[63,92,93] and the complete amino acid sequence is known.[94-97] In plasma factor X circulates as a two-chain molecule linked by a disulfide bridge. The amino-terminal part of the light chain (M_r 16,500) contains the γ-carboxyglutamic acid residues (Gla-domain), which are involved in the Ca^{2+}-dependent interaction of the molecule with phospholipid membranes.[98-100] The heavy chain (M_r 39,300) contains the serine protease part of the molecule. Upon activation by either factor VIIa-tissue factor or factor IXa-factor VIII, a peptide bond is cleaved in the amino-terminal region of the heavy chain: Arg^{51}-Ile^{52} in bovine factor X[79,101-103] and the Arg^{52}-Ile^{53} bond in human factor X.[97,104]

The product (αXa) is rapidly converted into βXa by the autocatalytic removal of a 4500-M_r peptide from the carboxy-terminal part of the heavy chain.[102,105] This reaction is dependent on the presence of both negatively charged phospholipids and Ca^{2+}. So far, no significant differences have been reported for the activities of these two forms of factor Xa.[79,102]

Product factor Xa can also hydrolyze other peptide bonds in the factor X zymogen (see Figure 1). In bovine factor X, factor Xa can cleave the same Arg-Ile bond as cleaved by the physiological activators, thus giving rise to additional factor Xa formation.[79,103] This reaction is not observed in human factor X.[105,106] However, in human factor X, factor Xa

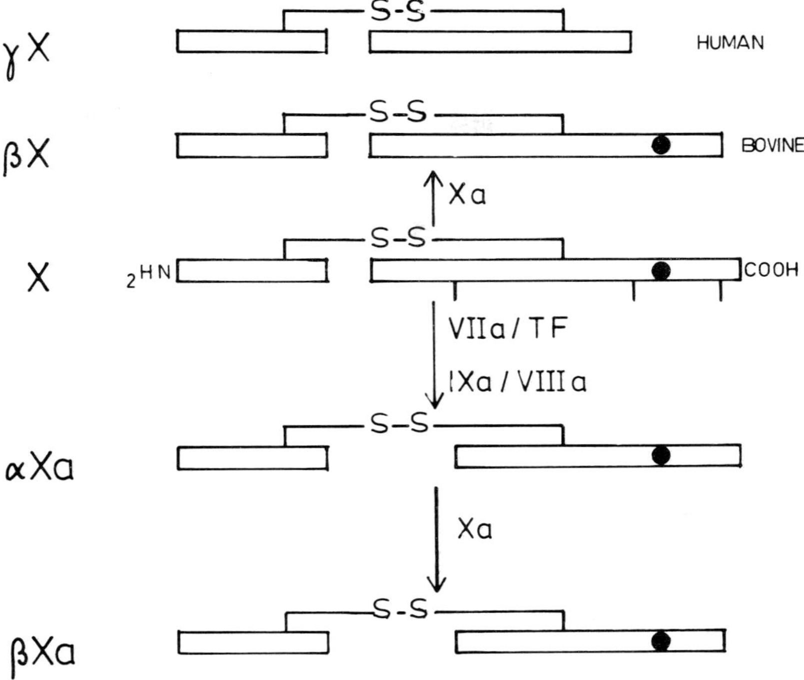

FIGURE 1. Activation of factor X.

can remove a carboxy-terminal fragment (M_r 13,000) from the heavy chain which contains the active site serine residue.[105,106] Both reactions require rather high concentrations of factor Xa, and it seems doubtful whether they have any physiological significance. On the other hand, they might influence kinetic studies with isolated coagulation factors. The occurrence of feedback activation of factor X in the bovine system has been one of the reasons that some of those studies have been performed in the presence of factor Xa-inhibitors.[14,107]

VI. FACTOR IX

Factor IX is a single-chain vitamin K-dependent glycoprotein with a molecular weight of 57,100 (for a recent review see Reference 108). It has been purified both from bovine and human plasma.[63,109-111] The complete amino acid sequence is known.[112,113,115] In factor IX we can recognize four functional domains: the Gla domain (residues 1 to 45), which contains 12 γ-carboxyglutaminc acid residues, the connecting peptide region (residues 46 to 145), the activation peptide region (residues 146 to 180), and the catalytic region (181 to 415). A hereditary defect in factor IX, which inherits as an X-linked recessive disorder (Hemophilia B), is associated with a severe to mild bleeding tendency.[108,116,117]

Upon activation by either factor XIa or factor VIIa-tissue factor, two peptide bonds are cleaved in the factor IX molecule (see Figure 2): Arg^{145}-Ala^{146} and Arg^{180}-Val^{181}. Cleavage of the first bond results in the formation of factor IXα, which still has no detectable enzymatic activity.[118] The subsequent cleavage of the Arg-Val bond will result in the release of an activation peptide and the formation of factor IXaβ, which is the catalytically active form of factor IX.[118] Factor IXaβ, in turn, can activate factor X, and the rate of this reaction is greatly enhanced by the presence of Ca^{2+} ions, phospholipids, and activated factor VIII.[119,120] Much attention has been paid to the problem of which of the two cleavages is the rate-limiting reaction. Bajaj et al.[121] reported that in the activation of human factor IX by either

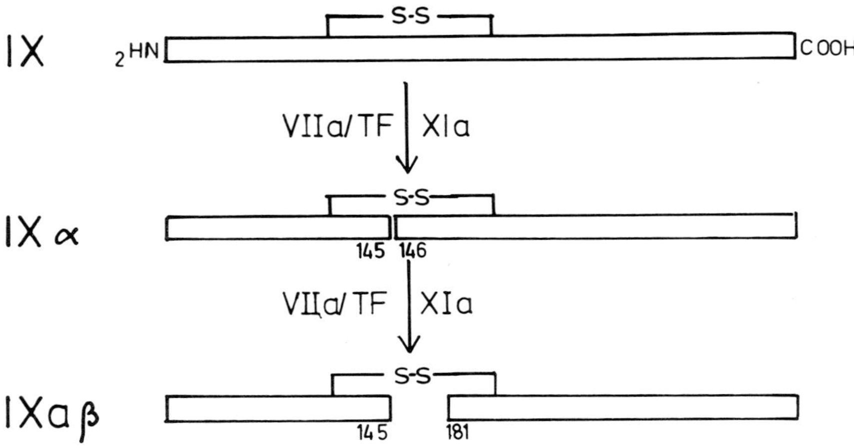

FIGURE 2. Activation of factor IX.

factor XIa or VIIa, the cleavage of the Arg-Val bond is the rate-limiting reaction. This conclusion confirmed earlier results of DiScipio et al.[118] and Østerud and Rapaport,[122] but was in disagreement with the findings of Zur and Nemerson[16] in the bovine system. Bajaj et al.[121] concluded that there was no concerted effect of factor VIIa-tissue factor and factor XIa in factor IX activation.

VII. INTERACTION BETWEEN FACTOR VII AND TISSUE FACTOR

The interaction between factor VII and tissue factor has been studied in two different ways: first, by assessment of the binding of factor VII to to tissue factor, and second, by analysis of the kinetics of the catalytic proteolysis of factor X or IX.

The reaction between tissue factor and factor VII is extremely rapid and requires the presence of calcium ions.[123] The coagulant activity generated by bovine tissue factor and bovine factor VII was tightly bound to the tissue particles and was not eluted from them by detergents or organic solvents.[123] Other investigators using human tissue factor and human factor VII originally claimed that binding of factor VII to tissue factor is not necessary for the activation of factor X by factor VII, provided that factor VII previously had been exposed to tissue factor.[124]

Factor VII coupled to Sepharose® proved to be an effective binding ligand for human TFAP.[37-39] This interaction is completely calcium dependent, and the calcium ions cannot be replaced by magnesium or barium ions.[38] One might expect that phospholipids play a role in the Ca^{2+}-dependent complex formation between TFAP and factor VII. However, binding of the apoprotein to the factor VII-Sepharose® was phospholipase C-insensitive, suggesting that a phospholipid surface was not involved in this interaction.[38] Monoclonal antibodies against bovine tissue factor have been prepared which inhibit tissue factor procoagulant activity and also inhibit factor VIIa binding to the tissue factor.[40] This strengthens the hypothesis that a factor VII-tissue factor complex is the enzymatically active species responsible for tissue factor-initiated coagulation.

The affinity constant for the binding of factor VII to tissue factor has been determined in equilibrium binding assays.[50] In 100% PC vesicles, one-chain factor VII binds to tissue factor with only slightly less affinity (K_H = 15 n*M*) than the more active two-chain enzyme (K_H = 5.5 n*M*).[50] Active site modification of factors VII and VIIa with DFP resulted in tighter binding of the derived molecules. In all binding experiments, 1 mol of factor VII was bound per mole of available tissue factor at saturation. This stoichiometry was not influenced by the form of the enzyme employed (FVII, FVIIa, DIP-FVII, DIP-FVIIa) or the phospholipid composition of the vesicles.

Inclusion of PS in the vesicles altered the binding both quantitatively and qualitatively.[50] With increasing acidic phospholipid, the concentration of enzyme required to occupy half the tissue factor sites was decreased. In addition, positive cooperativity was observed, the degree of which depended on the vesicle charge and the form of factor VII. An explicit two-site cooperative binding model was proposed in which tissue factor is at least a dimer with two interacting factor VII binding sites.[50]

Careful analysis of the catalytic properties of the factor VIIa-tissue factor complex resulted in the proposal of a model where factor VII undergoes two conformational transformations; one as a consequence of binding to tissue factor, resulting in a species which binds to and hydrolyzes its natural substrates,[125] and the other conformational change in factor VII is induced by substrate, resulting in a species which binds much more tightly to the tissue factor apoprotein. Thus, a "conformational cage" is hypothesized which precludes the dissociation of factor VII from tissue factor under conditions that significant concentrations of substrate are present.[125]

Human coagulation factors VII and VIIa have been reported to bind with equal affinity to monocytes stimulated with endotoxin.[126] The monocyte binding sites appear to represent tissue factor, and the rate of conversion of factor X to Xa in mixtures containing factor VIIa and monocytes was directly related to the quantity of factor VIIa bound to the monocyte surface.

VIII. EXTRINSIC ACTIVATION OF FACTOR X

In 1957 Hjort postulated the existence of a reaction product between factor VII, tissue factor, and calcium, which was responsible for extrinsic prothrombinase activity. Later, Hougie[127] attributed enzymatic properties to factor VII. He proposed that factor X was the natural substrate of factor VII. Many studies have since been devoted to the resolution of the kinetic principles involved in the interactions between tissue factor, factor VII, factor X, and Ca^{2+} ions.[14,29,79,123,124,128,129]

Straub and Duckert[128] were the first to report that the presence of all components in a ternary complex was required to form a product (presently known as factor Xa) with prothrombinase activity. In subsequent studies a concept has been developed in which factor VII is the zymogen of an enzyme that can hydrolyze a peptide bond in the protein substrate factor X, while tissue factor and Ca^{2+} are obligatory cofactors for this reaction.[80] For the study of the kinetics of the activation of factor X by the factor VII-tissue factor complex, it is necessary to follow the time course of the reaction. Basically, two methods have been used. Most authors use factor X in which the carbohydrate has been labeled with tritium.[14,15,130] In factor X most of the carbohydrate is covalently linked to the activation peptide. Therefore, activation of ^{3}H-factor X will be accompanied by the release of ^{3}H-activation peptide, which can be readily quantitated by the assessment of the amount of radioactivity in a 5% trichloroacetic acid supernatant.[14] One of the advantages of this method is that rates of factor X activation can be measured in the presence of factor Xa-inhibitors (suppression of feedback interactions).

In the other method factor X activation is followed by assessing the amount of factor Xa produced with a chromogenic assay specific for factor Xa.[131-133] The advantage of this method is extreme sensitivity, which allows the measurement of activation of factor X by factors VIIa or IXa in the absence of cofactors.[132,133]

The presently available information clearly indicates that tissue factor is an essential cofactor for the activation of factor X by factor VIIa. In the past many authors even concluded that there is an absolute requirement for this cofactor.[60,123,134] Only after the successful

Table 1
CONTRIBUTIONS OF COFACTORS TO THE INITIAL RATE OF ACTIVATION OF FACTOR X BY FACTOR VIIa

	V_i(mol $X_a$mol VIIa/min)	Relative rate
VIIa	4.2×10^{-7}	1
VIIa + Ca^{2+}	3.2×10^{-6}	8
VIIa + Ca^{2+} + PS/PC	9.2×10^{-4}	2.10^3
VIIa + Ca^{2+} + PS/PC + TFAP	18.6	4.10^7

Note: Factor X = 50 n*M*, $CaCl_2$ = 10 m*M*, PS/PC(50/50) = 100 μ*M*, tissue factor apoprotein = 0.4 n*M*.

Table 2
EFFECTS OF Ca^{2+}, PHOSPHOLIPID (PL), AND TISSUE FACTOR APOPROTEIN (TFAP) ON THE KINETIC CONSTANTS FOR THE ACTIVATION OF FACTOR X BY FACTOR VIIa

	Km (n*M*)	kcat (min^{-1})
$+Ca^{2+}$	11.4×10^3	1.1×10^{-3}
$+Ca^{2+}$ + 10 μ*M* PL	59	1.0×10^{-3}
+ 25 μ*M* PL	77	2.04×10^{-3}
+ 100 μ*M* PL	290	7.12×10^{-3}
$+Ca^{2+}$ + TFAP	180	3.4
$+Ca^{2+}$ + PL[a] + TFAP	55	81

[a] 25 μ*M* PS/PC (50/50).

purification of TFAP[21,37-39] could one answer this question successfully. In our laboratory we were able to demonstrate that factor VIIa in the absence of any cofactors can activate factor X, and that the rate of factor Xa formation was linear in time, proportional with the factor VIIa concentration, and sensitive to antibodies specific for human factor VII.[133] By the subsequent addition of Ca^{2+} ions, phospholipid membranes and highly purified TFAP, we were able to assess the contributions of each of the cofactors to the activation of factor X by factor VIIa (Tables 1 and 2). Addition of Ca^{2+} ions alone results in an eight-fold stimulation of the reaction rate, which is mainly caused by a decrease in the Km of factor X. In the presence of 6 m*M* $CaCl_2$, factor X activation follows Michaelis-Menten kinetics: Km factor X, 11.4 μ*M* and kcat, 1.1×10^{-3} min^{-1}. The addition of phospholipids (PS/PC 50/50) results in a further 250-fold stimulation of the initial reaction rate. This stimulation is caused by a decrease in the apparent Km of factor X and an increase in the V_{max} and might be explained from the accumulation of enzyme and substrate in the perivesicular shell surrounding the phospholipid membrane (see Reference 114). In agreement with such a hypothesis is the finding that the apparent Km of factor X increases with increasing phospholipid concentrations (see Table 2). So far there is only one other kinetic study reporting on the activation of factor X by factor VIIa in the absence of tissue factor. Using bovine coagulation factors, Silverberg et al.[14] reported that in the presence of 0.75 mg/mℓ cephalin and 5 m*M* Ca^{2+}, the apparent Km of factor X is 4.8 μ*M* and the kcat = 3.95×10^{-4} sec^{-1}. The value for kcat is of the same order of magnitude as found in our studies using the human proteins (see Table 2). The relatively high Km of factor X can be explained by the high concentration of phospholipid used by Silverberg et al.[14]

The addition of TFAP to a system containing factor VIIa, phospholipid, and Ca^{2+} results in a further 20,000-fold stimulation of the rate of factor X activation (see Table 1), which clearly establishes the importance of this protein in the extrinsic factor X activation.

Taken together, the results of Table 1 show that the addition of tissue factor, i.e., phospholipid plus TFAP will result in a six million-fold stimulation of the rate of activation of factor X by factor VIIa in the presence of $CaCl_2$. Although it is difficult to analyze the separate contributions of the phospholipids and the TFAP, we will discuss a number of important observations that might help us to understand this complex reaction.

First, it has been clearly demonstrated that in the absence of phospholipids, TFAP can bind to factor VIIa.[37-39] Ca^{2+} ions are required for this interaction. Guha et al[39] reported that in the presence of the nonionic detergent Triton® X-100, TFAP can stimulate the activation of factor X by factor VIIa. They report that the kcat of this reaction is 0.6% of that in the presence of PC. These data strongly suggest that a ternary complex consisting of factor VIIa, factor X, and TFAP can be formed even in the absence of phospholipids. Preliminary data from our own laboratory indicate that the catalytic capacity of TFAP-factor VIIa is about 3000-fold higher than that of factor VIIa alone (see Table 2).

On the other hand, it has been demonstrated that TFAP can be incorporated in phospholipid vesicles (see paragraph on reconstitution of TFAP in phospholipid vesicles). Bach et al.[50] showed that varying the PC content of PS/PC vesciles from 100 to 40% has no major effect on the amount of TFAP incorporated into the membranes, but had a clear effect on the binding affinity of the factor VIIa to the membrane-bound TFAP. The binding of factor VIIa to membrane-bound TFAP is completely dependent on the presence of Ca^{2+} ions.[50,126] The introduction of negatively charged phospholipids (PS) decreased the apparent affinity of factor VIIa for binding to tissue factor about twofold and introduced positive cooperativity in the binding isotherms (the Hill coefficient changed from 1.1 to 1.6). From these data we must conclude that TFAP can be incorporated in phospholipid membranes independent of the actual composition, and that the apoprotein exposed on the outside of the vesicle can be saturated with factor VIIa, while the binding constant is only slightly dependent on the phospholipid composition.[50]

The situation becomes more complicated when we consider the effects of substrate addition. It is well known that acidic phospholipids such as PS are essential for the binding of factor X to phospholipid membranes.[98-100] This means that depending on the actual composition of the phospholipid vesicles, a variable fraction of the total factor X added will be bound to the surface. In the absence of TFAP we had to conclude that factor X activation occurs predominantly at the phospholipid surface, i.e., phospholipid-bound factor X will be the major substrate (see Table 2). In the presence of TFAP, however, the situation is completely different. Forman and Nemerson[44] showed very elegantly that under such conditions free factor X is the substrate of choice. When using 100% PC vesicles, they calculated a Km for FX of 791 n*M* and a kcat of 6.2 sec^{-1}. Under these conditions the reaction rates were not influenced by the presence of prothrombin fragment 1 (F_1), which is known to bind to negatively charged phospholipids. Using, however, vesicles containing 30% PS, they found that F1 stimulates the rate of factor X activation, suggesting that free factor X is the substrate for the reaction. Indeed, they found identical Kms for factor X of about 50 n*M* both in the absence and in the presence of F_1 when they used the calculated free factor X concentrations for their analysis. The kcat (6.5 sec^{-1}) was in both cases identical to that found in the 100% PC system.[44]

In summary, we may conclude that in the presence of Ca^{2+} ions factor VIIa can catalyze the activation of factor X. However, this reaction is very slow and probably will not occur under physiological conditions. Binding of factor VIIa to TFAP is accompanied by an increase in the kcat of the reaction — about 3000-fold in the presence of Triton® micelles and about 75,000-fold in the presence of phospholipids. At the same time, there is a decrease in the

Km of factor X, which is more pronounced when the molar fraction of negatively charged phospholipid increases. Finally, negatively charged phospholipids will allow binding of factor X to the membranes and thus will lower the concentration of substrate (free factor X) in the solution. This will result in an increase in the apparent Km of factor X for the reaction, as has been reported by several authors. In the presence of a molar excess of factor VIIa (when compared to the apoprotein), phospholipid-bound factor X might be cleaved by factor VIIa via the tissue factor independent pathway. However, the kcat of this reaction is so low (see Table 2) that it is doubtful whether this reaction will contribute significantly to the overall factor Xa formation.

IX. INITIATION AND CONTROL OF EXTRINSIC FACTOR X ACTIVATION

When factor VII zymogen is incubated with tissue factor, factor X, and Ca^{2+} ions, the rate of factor Xa formation rapidly increases after a short lag period.[83] This has been explained by the rapid activation of factor VII by product factor Xa.[67] Preincubation of the factor VII-tissue factor complex with low concentrations of factor Xa shortens the lag phase.[83] From binding studies we know that there is only a slight difference in the affinities of tissue factor for binding to factor VII or VIIa.[50,67,126] The important question is whether the initial rate of factor X activation reflects the activity of the factor VII zymogen or is due to the presence of low concentrations of factor VIIa in the factor VII preparations used. In 1978 it was reported that bovine factor VII zymogen has significant esterase activity, and that this activity is only doubled after complete activation of factor VII.[66] This finding suggests that factor VII zymogen itself is an active enzyme. A similar conclusion was reached after careful analysis of the inactivation of factors VII and VIIa by DFP.[67] The pseudo-first-order rate constant for the inactivation of factor VIIa (0.130 min^{-1}) was four times higher than that for the inactivation of factor VII (0.032 min^{-1}). Using this type of analysis, Zur et al.[67] could estimate the factor VIIa content of the factor VII preparation, and from these data they could calculate that zymogen factor VII has about 0.8% of the activity of two-chain factor VIIa. Independent evidence for the enzymatic activity of factor VII was obtained from data reported by Jesty and Morrison.[107] They found that in bovine plasma the factor VII-tissue factor complex has a 3-fold lower Km for factor IX (17.3 n*M*) than the factor VIIa-tissue factor complex (53.3 n*M*), while the V_{max} for the second reaction is about 40-fold higher.

In the extrinsic factor X activation, the initial event then probably is the formation of a tissue factor-factor VII complex, which catalyzes the proteolytic activation of factor X. Product factor Xa then cleaves factor VII into its two-chain form (factor VIIa). Recently, Nemerson and Gentry[125] proposed an ordered addition model for the assembly of the catalytic complex in which factor VIIa undergoes two different conformational changes. A first one was due to the binding of tissue factor (see also Reference 67) and a second one was due to the binding of factor X to the factor VIIa-tissue factor complex. The second conformational change will induce a 100-fold increase in the affinity of factor VIIa for tissue factor and prevents the rapid dissociation of factor VIIa from the catalytic complex.

Interestingly, the activity of the factor VIIa-tissue factor complex can decrease during the course of the reaction (either factor X or IX activation). This self-dampening of the reaction is especially notable in a plasma system.[83,135,223] Morrison and Jesty[135] provided evidence that in the bovine plasma system the inhibition was caused by the inactivation of factor VIIa (presumably by factor Xa). However, in the human system Rao et al.[136] could not demonstrate appreciable degradation of the factor VIIa-heavy chain during thromboplastin-induced coagulation of whole plasma. In systems using purified coagulation factors, inhibition of factor VIIa by factor Xa is either completely absent or much less pronounced.[69,70,72] Recent studies suggest that for the inactivation of the factor VIIa-tissue factor complex both factor X (Xa) and the lipoprotein fraction of barium-absorbed plasma are required.[137,223] Indeed, purified lipoprotein fractions have been found to inhibit the activation of factor X by the factor VIIa-tissue factor complex.[138,139] and to bind factor Xa.[140] However, no definite mechanism has been proposed for the rapid inactivation of the factor VIIa-tissue factor complex. Sanders et al.[223] argue that the tissue factor moiety of the complex may be affected, but it still cannot be excluded that a plasma inhibitor of factor VIIa[84] is involved.

X. EXTRINSIC ACTIVATION OF FACTOR IX

In 1977 Østerud and Rapaport[13] reported the first evidence that the factor VIIa-tissue factor complex also can activate factor IX. Until then it was believed that factor IX could be activated only via factor XIa, which is generated via the intrinsic pathway.[141] Although there had been reports on the possible involvement of factor IX in the extrinsically triggered factor X activation,[12,142,143] the existence of an additional activation pathway raised a number of questions with respect to the physiological significance of both pathways.

In most studies the activation of factor IX is followed by measuring the release of activation peptide from ^{3}H-factor IX.[16,67,83,107,121,135] Recently, we introduced a very sensitive immunoradiometric assay specific for factor IXa[144] that has been used succesfully for the study of factor IX activation in a system of purified proteins.

So far, most kinetic studies have been aimed at the determination of the kinetic constants for the activation of factor IX by the factor VIIa-tissue factor complex (Km factor IX, kcat) in order to compare them with the kinetic constants obtained for the extrinsic factor X activation.[16,83,135] Such studies have been performed both in a system of purified coagulation factors and in plasma systems (see Tables 3 and 4). In general, the results indicate that the Km of factor IX is rather similar to that of factor X and that, as has been found for factor X, the Km of factor IX will increase with increasing phospholipid concentration.[16,121] Most studies report that the kcat for factor IX activation is slightly lower than that for factor X activation.

As in the case of factor X activation, a lag is observed in the activation of factor IX by factor VII-tissue factor, which confirms that factor IXa is also an activator of the factor VII zymogen.[107,223] This lag, which is appreciably longer than that for factor X activation, can be shortened by preincubation of the factor VII-tissue factor complex with low concentrations of factor Xa.[67] Factor IXa seems to be a much less potent activator of factor VII than factor Xa.[72,107,135] So far, no evidence has been obtained that, in plasma, factor IXa also can inactivate factor VIIa.[135,136]

XI. RELATIVE CONTRIBUTIONS OF EXTRINSIC ACTIVATION OF FACTOR X AND FACTOR IX TO FIBRIN FORMATION

In 1977 Østerud et al.[13] clearly demonstrated that the tissue factor-factor VII complex can activate factor IX. This finding has been confirmed now in other laboratories, as has been previously discussed.[16,43,83,107,121,135] The tissue factor-factor VII complex then will contribute to the activation of factor X via two different pathways (see Figure 3). First, it can activate factor X directly, and second, it can activate factor IX, after which factor IXa will activate factor X. The latter reaction is controlled by the availability of activated factor VIII (factor VIIIa).[119,120] The intriguing question is what the relative contribution of these two pathways is to extrinsically triggered factor X activation.

From in vitro observations we know that the prothrombin time of citrated plasma is hardly affected by the plasma factors IX and VIII concentration.[146] Even when high dilutions of a partially purified tissue factor preparation were used, clotting times were found to be independent of the presence or absence of factors IX and VIII.[43] Therefore, it is not surprising

Table 3
REPORTED VALUES FOR THE KINETIC CONSTANTS FOR THE ACTIVATION OF FACTOR X AND FACTOR IX BY FACTOR VII-TISSUE FACTOR IN SYSTEMS OF PURIFIED COAGULATION FACTORS

	FX		FIX		
B/H[a]	Km (n*M*)	kcat (sec^{-1})	Km (n*M*)	kcat (sec^{-1})	Ref.
B	—	—	49	0.036[b]	67
H			254	0.23[c]	121
			352	0.25[d]	
			540	0.55[e]	
B	88	2.2	87	0.15[f]	16
	230	5.2	177	0.40[g]	
	300	3.8	191	0.42[h]	
	433	2.6	243	0.26[i]	
	450	1.15	—	—	14
	791	6.2[j]	—	—	44
	16	1.5[k]	—	—	125
H	55	1.4	15	0.44	145[l]

[a] B: bovine system, H: human system.
[b] Excess FVIIa over tissue factor.
[c] 0.17 vol tissue factor, 1.24 m*M* phospholipid.
[d] 0.17 vol tissue factor, 2.18 m*M* phospholipid.
[e] 0.51 vol tissue factor, 3.72 m*M* phospholipid.
[f] 2.5% tissue factor.
[g] 10% tissue factor.
[h] 20% tissue factor.
[i] 50% tissue factor.
[j] PC as phospholipid source.
[k] PS/PC (10/90).
[l] 25 μ*M* PS/PC (50/50), excess tissue factor over FVIIa.

Table 4
REPORTED VALUES FOR THE KINETIC CONSTANTS FOR THE ACTIVATION OF FACTOR X AND FACTOR IX BY FACTOR VIIa IN PLASMA SYSTEMS

	FX		FIX		
B/H[a]	Km (n*M*)	V_{max} (n*M* Xa/min/U tpl)	Km (n*M*)	V_{max} (n*M* Xa/min/U tpl)	Ref.
H	380	903	410	680	135
B	430	815	73	115	83
	—	—	53	25[b]	107

[a] B: bovine system, H: human system.
[b] In the presence of protease inhibitor.

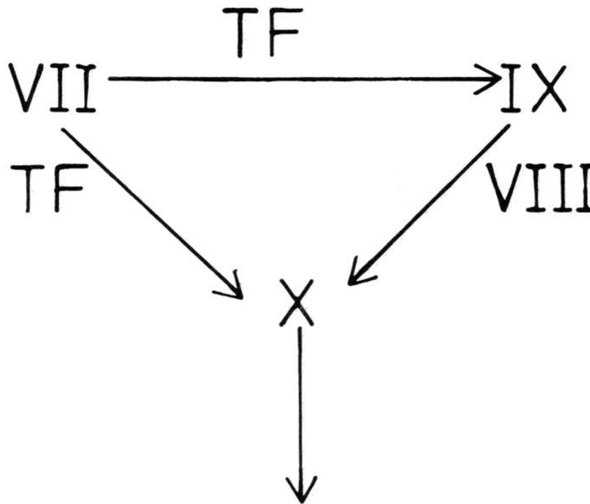

FIGURE 3. Extrinsic activation of factor X.

that most of the patients with severe hemophilia A or B have a completely normal prothrombin time. Only in patients with hemophilia B_m is the ox brain prothrombin time severely prolonged,[147] which is probably due to the increased affinity of an abnormal factor IX molecule for the factor VII/tissue factor complex.[148] These in vitro observations are consistent with the results of detailed kinetic studies, which show that the kinetic constants (Km, V_{max}) for the activation of factors X and IX are rather similar (see Tables 3 and 4). At present it is not known whether the microenvironment of the tissue factor in the biological membrane will have much influence on these parameters. Theoretically, it is possible that they create a preference of the factor VII-tissue factor for either factor IX or X activation.[149]

On the other hand, there have been several reports which indicate that at low tissue factor concentrations the rate of factor X or II activation becomes dependent on the presence of factors VIII and IX.[12,142,143,150] The important difference between these studies and the forementioned prothrombin time studies is the time scale of the experiment. For instance, Marlar et al.[150] followed the activation of factor X over a period of time much longer than necessary for clot formation, the end point of the prothrombin time determination. Therefore, it might be that factors IX and VIII are not involved in the formation of the first traces of thrombin (necessary for fibrin formation), but do contribute to the subsequent steady-state rate of factor X activation (at least at low tissue factor concentrations). In this respect, it is of interest that Mertens and Bertina[150a] reported that trace amounts of factor Xa, formed by extrinsic activation of factor X, can stimulate the factor IXa-dependent factor Xa formation by the efficient activation of factor VIII. In their experiments factor Xa formation at prolonged time intervals is almost completely sensitive to both antifactor VII serum and antifactor VIII serum.

Apart from the results of these in vitro experiments, we should also consider the available information on the behavior of the coagulation system in vivo. For instance, the classical coagulation pathways (see Figure 4) provide no satisfactory explanation for the observation that patients with severe factors XI or XII deficiency have only a very mild bleeding tendency when compared to patients with severe deficiencies of factors VIII or IX. Those observations can only be explained by assuming that during in vivo coagulation the factor VII-IX-X pathway is the predominant pathway leading to the hemostatic response. Such a hypothesis would mean that the factor XI-IX-X pathway and the factor VII-X pathway are only of minor importance. Indeed, there is some evidence that during in vivo coagulation, the factor VII-X pathway is relatively unimportant. Bertina et al.[150b] have described a patient with an abnormal factor X molecule (Factor X Utrecht), which can be normally activated by the factor IXa-VIII complex, but cannot be activated by the factor VII-tissue complex. In agreement with these findings is that the patient has a strongly prolonged prothrombin time

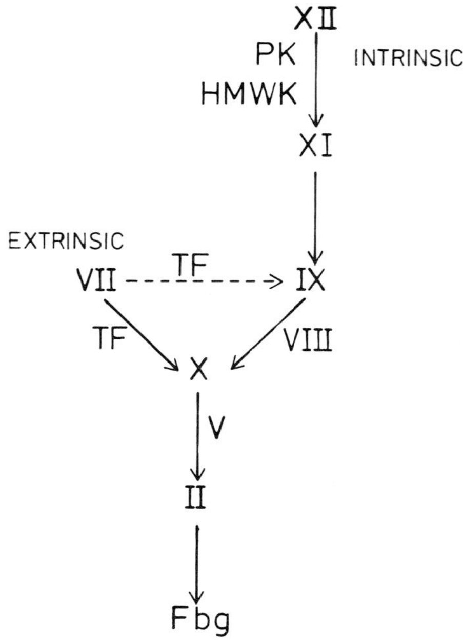

FIGURE 4. Classical coagulation scheme. HMWK: high molecular weight kininogen, PK: prekallikrein, TF: tissue factor, Fbg: fibrinogen.

and a normal activated partial thromboplastin time. Interestingly, this patient (presently 56 years old) never experienced clinically significant bleeding. More recently, Girolami et al.[151] described a patient with a similar abnormality, and this patient also showed no bleeding symptoms.

A completely different line of evidence for the relative importance of the factor VII-IX-X pathway comes from transfusion experiments in normal and hemophilic dogs.[152] Mertens et al.[152] found that the infusion of purified human factor VIIa in dogs with hemophilia A (with or without an inhibitor against factor VIII) did not result in an increase in plasma fibrinopeptide A levels, while similar infusions in nonhemophilic dogs resulted in a more than 100-fold increase in plasma fibrinopeptide A. Together, such observations strongly suggest that in vivo the direct activation of factor X by the factor VII-tissue factor complex is only of minor importance.

Recently, it has become increasingly clear that endothelial cells play an important role in the maintenance of the hemostatic balance in vivo.[149,153,154] Perturbation of the endothelial membrane induces a transition of the membrane from an anticoagulant into a procoagulant state. This transition is marked by a reduction in anticoagulant membrane proteins (thrombomodulin and protein S receptor) and an increase in procoagulant membrane proteins (tissue factor and factor IX receptor).[149] The discovery of the presence of a specific factor IX receptor on the endothelial cell membrane[161,166] has especially revived the discussions on the role of factor IX in tissue factor-dependent coagulation. Under equilibrium conditions factors IX and IXa bind with equal affinity to the membrane receptor (K_D = 2 n*M*).[166] However, under turnover conditions, when the catalytic IXa-VIII-X complex is assembled on the receptor, the affinity of the receptor for factor IXa is tenfold higher than that for factor IX.[155] Nawroth and co-workers[149] speculate that in the perturbed membrane, the effective assembly of the factor IXa-VIII-X complex (on the factor IX-receptor) close to the tissue factor (site of factors IX and X activation) might contribute to the relative importance of the factor VII-IX-X pathway.

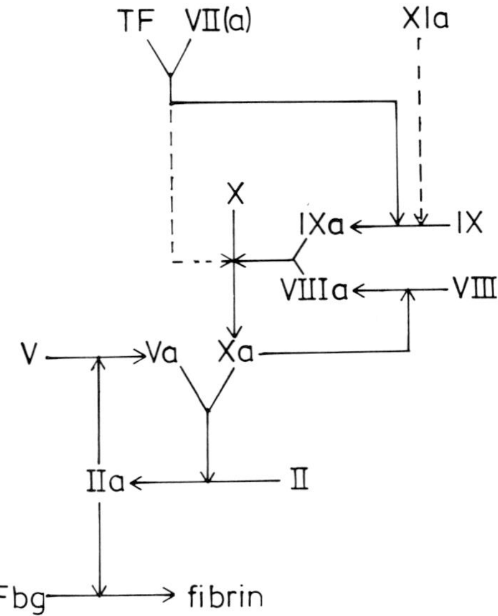

FIGURE 5. Extrinsic pathway of coagulation. TF: tissue factor, Fbg: fibrinogen.

Based on the aforementioned considerations, we would propose the following model for tissue factor-induced coagulation. When tissue factor is exposed to the blood, it will bind factor VII and subsequently activate trace amounts of factors X and IX at about similar rates. Formed factor Xa will rapidly activate factors VII, VIII, and II, causing clot formation in vitro and the deposition of fibrin in vivo. Factor X activation then will continue by the catalytic action of both the factor VIIa/tissue factor complex and the factor IXa-VIIIa complex. The rate of the first reaction will be efficiently suppressed by the inhibition of the factor VIIa-tissue factor by factor Xa, while the rate of the second reaction is controlled by the availability of factor VIIIa and will continue to go on until the factor VIIIa has been inactivated, for instance, by the proteolytic action of the activated protein C-protein S complex.[156] In this model the direct activation of factor X by the factor VII-tissue factor complex functions as an amplification loop for the factor IXa-dependent reaction by the efficient activation of factor VIII (see Figure 5). However, when the activity of this amplification loop is strongly reduced, as, for instance, in the patient with factor X Utrecht, this will not lead to impaired fibrin formation, because activation of factor VIII still can be catalyzed by the Xa generated by factor IXa or by thrombin.

So far we have only discussed tissue factor-initiated coagulation and contribution to *intravascular* fibrin formation, reactions that play a pivotal role in haemostasis and wound repair, but also in the pathogenesis of hypercoagulable states[23,157-160] and diffuse intravascular coagulation.[23,162] However, extrinsic factor X activation may have a completely different role in extravascular fibrin formation. Evidence is accumulating that, for instance, macrophages can be induced to synthesize not only tissue factor, but also factors VII, II, X, and V.[85-87,163,164] Under suitable conditions macrophages may, therefore, produce all the necessary components to initiate local fibrin formation, a process which seems to be intimately involved in inflammatory immune disorders[23,165] and in the growth and metastasis of malignant tumors.[24,167] However, we will need much more information before we can fully appreciate the role of extrinsic factor X activation in these processes.

XII. CELL BIOLOGY OF TISSUE FACTOR

Tissue factor is present in most mammalian tissues. High tissue factor contents have been

Table 5
STIMULATION OF PRODUCTION OF TISSUE FACTOR IN VITRO IN MONOCYTES, MACROPHAGES, OR ENDOTHELIAL CELLS

Stimulus	Ref.
Antigen	184—186
Immune complexes	187—190
Complement products	191—195
Allogeneic cells	196, 197
Lymphokines	197—201
Phagocytosis	202—204
Lipoproteins	205
Serum component	206
Phorbol esters	181, 207—209
Endotoxin	175, 178, 179, 208—218
Amines	214
Ionophore A23187	219
Lectins/mitogens	174, 177, 179, 181, 187
Thrombin	208, 221
Interleukin-1	222

reported for lung, placenta, brain (both in the white and gray matter), thyroid gland, arterial intima, and intraperitoneal and bone marrow fat.[22,168,169] Very low tissue factor activity was found in synovial membrane and fibrous capsular tissue.[170] It is not known whether tissue factors from different organs have identical structures,[37,39] but they do cross-react with heterologous antibodies against tissue factor[169] and show the same degree of heterogeneous glycosylation.[35] On the other hand, it has been reported that tissue factors from different species differ largely in their clot-promoting activity in heterologous plasma systems.[171]

In vitro we can distinguish three types of cells with respect to tissue factor production: (1) cells that produce tissue factor constitutively, such as placental throphoblasts[172] and glioma cells,[22] (2) cells that do not produce tissue factor, such as lymphocytes, granulocytes, and platelets,[173-175] and (3) cells that show an inducible tissue factor synthesis such as monocytes,[173,175-177] macrophages,[165,178,179] and certain kinds of endothelial cells.[180-182] Most of the information on the cell biology of tissue factor has been derived from experiments where cellular tissue factor production could be induced in vitro. Because mononuclear cells have been reported to produce a variety of procoagulant factors,[165,183] it is important to use assay systems that are specific for tissue factor (see discussion in Reference 22). In general, investigators use one- or two-stage coagulation or spectrophotometric assays in which the accelerating effect of tissue factor on the factor VII-catalyzed factor X activation is evaluated. The procoagulant activity needs to be dependent on the presence of both factors VII and X. Additional criteria that have been used for identifying tissue factor are insensitivity to DFP, sensitivity to antibodies against purified bovine or human tissue factor, sensitivity to treatment with phospholipase C, and binding of the procoagulant concanavalin A.

In vitro induction of tissue factor activity can be affected by a variety of stimuli (see Table 5). Most of these stimuli can also trigger other immune responses. Some of them are products of activation of the immune system. Table 5 presents a list of those stimuli most frequently discussed in the literature. Most of these stimuli are effective both on monocytes/macrophages and on endothelial cells. It should be remembered, however, that major differences may be found with cells from different species or different anatomical sites.[216,217]

In general, two major pathways for the induction of tissue factor activity can be recognized: (1) the T-cell-independent pathway, activated by direct perturbation of monocytes or endothelial cells and (2) the T-cell-dependent pathway, activated by immune recognition and mediated at least in part by lymphokines. Many studies have been devoted to elucidate the role of lymphocyte cooperation in the induction of tissue factor activity.[165,178,189,200,212,224-228] Specific questions that have been addressed are whether there is an absolute requirement for lymphocytes,[178,212,224-226] whether special subpopulations of T lymphocytes are required,[196,225,229] whether immunogenetic restrictions for lymphocyte cooperation occur,[165,199,226] whether lymphocyte cooperation is dependent on cell-cell interactions,[227,229,230] or whether products of activated lymphocytes (lymphokines) are the obligatory mediators.[200,201] Apart from lymphocytes, other cells (especially thrombocytes) have been found to play an important regulatory role in tissue factor induction.[231-233]

Most stimuli used for the induction of tissue factor activity are supposed to induce perturbation of the plasma membrane. In general, tissue factor production can be demonstrated within 2 hr after stimulation and reaches a maximum after 2 to 4 hr (endotoxin) or 16 to 20 hr (immune complexes, phorbolesters), depending on the inducer.[22] The induction of tissue factor activity requires m-RNA and protein synthesis[181,187,207,234] and probably involves direct transport of vesicular TFAP from the cytosol to the plasma membrane,[235] although it cannot be excluded that intracellular pools of TFAP may exist.[203,236,237] At prolonged incubation times, tissue factor activity may be found in the cell-conditioned medium, probably by shedding of membrane vesicles.[238,239] At present no information is available on the cellular mechanism that triggers the expression of the tissue factor gene.[22,235,240] There is, however, strong evidence that high intracellular c-AMP levels may suppress tissue factor expression. For instance, dibutyryl c-AMP, PGE, and phosphodiesterase inhibitors inhibit tissue factor production in cells stimulated by immune complexes.[219,241] However, not all stimuli that induce tissue factor activity do affect the intracellular c-AMP level.[219,241] Initial transient changes in c-AMP, however, may contribute to the lag in the induction time.[207] Another intracellular process that might be involved in the modulation of tissue factor synthesis is phospholipid transmethylation.[240] Most stimuli will induce an increase in the PC content of the plasma membrane,[237] but the precise role of these changes is not well understood. Also, arachidonic acid metabolites have been implicated to play an important role. Inhibition of lipoxygenase and phospholipase A2 have especially been found to inhibit tissue factor synthesis.[242] Inhibitors of cyclooxygenase had no effect on tissue factor synthesis.[242] The observation that the Ca^{2+} ionophore A23187 is a potent stimulus of tissue factor induction suggests that intracellular Ca^{2+} may also play an important role.[219] Such a hypothesis could explain the modulating influence of intracellular c-AMP and is supported by our understanding of the effects of amines and phorbolesters on intracellular Ca^{2+} concentrations. It also would explain the inhibitory effects of Ca^{2+} antagonists on tissue factor induction.[240]

Although we presently have no detailed knowledge of the intracellular mechanisms secondary to membrane perturbation that are involved in the expression of TFAP, it is clear that many physiological stimuli can induce tissue factor synthesis and thus may provide plasma membranes with a receptor for coagulation factor VII. Under the appropriate conditions, the tissue factor-factor VII complex may initiate the activation of the coagulation process, thus giving rise to fibrin formation — either intravascular (endothelial cells, monocytes) or extravascular (macrophages at sites of inflammatory lesions).

REFERENCES

1. **Morawitz, P.,** Die Chemie der Blutgerinnung, *Ergeb. Physiol.*, 4, 307, 1905.
2. **Howell, W. H.,** The role of antithrombin and thromboplastin (thromboplastic substance) in the coagulation of blood, *Am. J. Physiol.*, 29, 187, 1911.
3. **Wright, I. S.,** The nomenclature of blood clotting factors, *Thromb. Diath. Haemorrh.*, 7, 381, 1962.

4. **Weiss, H. J.,** Platelet physiology and abnormalities of platelet function, *N. Engl. J. Med.*, 293, 531, 1975.
5. **Owren, P. A.,** The coagulation of blood. Investigation on a new clotting factor, *Acta Med. Scand.*, 194 (Suppl.), 1947.
6. **de Vries, A., Alexander, B., and Goldstein, R.,** A factor in serum which accelerates the conversion of prothrombin to thrombin. I. Its determination and some physiologic and biochemical properties, *Blood,* 4, 247, 1949.
7. **Koller, F., Loeliger, A., and Duckert, F.,** Experiments on a new clotting factor (Factor VII), *Acta Haematol.*, 6, 1, 1951.
8. **Alexander, B., Goldstein, R., Landwehr, G., and Cook, C. D.,** Congenital SPCA deficiency: a hitherto unrecognized coagulation defect with hemorrhage rectified by serum and serum fractions, *J. Clin. Invest.*, 30, 596, 1951.
9. **Telfer, T. P., Denson, K. W., and Wright, D. R.,** A "new" coagulation defect, *Br. J. Haematol.*, 2, 308, 1956.
10. **Hougie, C., Barrow, E. M., and Graham, J. B.,** Stuart clotting defect. Segregation of an hereditary hemorrhagic state from the heterogeneous group heretofore called "stable factor" (SPCA, proconvertin, Factor VII) deficiency, *J. Clin. Invest.*, 36, 485, 1957.
11. **Davie, E. W. and Ratnoff, O. D.,** Waterfall sequence for intrinsic blood clotting, *Science,* 145, 1310, 1964.
12. **Biggs, R. and Nossel, H. L.,** Tissue extract and the contact reaction in blood coagulation, *Thromb. Diath. Haemorrh.*, 6, 1, 1961.
13. **Østerud, B. and Rapaport, S. I.,** Activation of factor IX by the reaction product of tissue factor and factor VII: additional pathway for initiating blood coagulation, *Proc. Natl. Acad. Sci. U.S.A.*, 74, 5260, 1977.
14. **Silverberg, S. A., Nemerson, Y., and Zur, M.,** Kinetics of the activation of bovine coagulation factor X by components of the extrinsic pathway. Kinetic behaviour of two chain factor VII in the presence and absence of tissue, *J. Biol. Chem.*, 252, 8481, 1977.
15. **Zur, M. and Nemerson, Y.,** Radiometric assays for blood coagulation factors, *Methods Enzymol.*, 80, 237, 1982.
16. **Zur, M. and Nemerson, Y.,** Kinetics of factor IX activation via the extrinsic pathway. Dependence of Km on tissue factor, *J. Biol. Chem.*, 255, 5703, 1980.
17. **Chargaff, E., Moore, D. H., and Bendich, A.,** Ultracentrifugal isolation from lung tissue of a macromolecular protein component with thromboplastic properties, *J. Biol. Chem.*, 145, 593, 1942.
18. **Nemerson, Y.,** The phospholipid requirement of tissue factor in blood coagulation, *J. Clin. Invest.*, 47, 72, 1968.
19. **Hvatum, M. and Prydz, H.,** Studies on tissue thromboplastin. Solubilization with sodium deoxycholate, *Biochim. Biophys. Acta,* 130, 92, 1966.
20. **Hvatum, M. and Prydz, H.,** Studies on tissue thromboplastin. Its splitting into two separable parts, *Thromb. Diath. Haemorrh.*, 21, 217, 1969.
21. **Bach, R., Nemerson, Y., and Konigsberg, W.,** Purification and characterization of bovine tissue factor, *J. Biol. Chem.*, 256, 8324, 1981.
22. **Prydz, H.,** Triggering of the extrinsic blood coagulation system, in *Blood Coagulation and Haemostasis. A Practical Guide,* Thomson, J. M., Ed., Churchill Livingstone, Edinburgh, 1985, 1.
23. **Lyberg, T.,** Clinical significance of increased thromboplastin activity on the monocyte surface. A brief review, *Haemostasis,* 14, 430, 1984.
24. **Rickles, F. R. and Edwards, R. L.,** Activation of blood coagulation in cancer: Trousseau's syndrome revisited, *Blood,* 62, 14, 1983.
25. **Miller, C. L., Graziano, C., Lim, R. C., and Chin, M.,** Generation of tissue factor by patient monocytes: correlation to thromboembolic complications, *Thromb. Haemostasis,* 46, 489, 1981.
26. **Howell, W. H.,** The nature and action of the thromboplastic (zymoplastic) substance of the tissues, *Am. J. Physiol.*, 31, 1, 1912.
27. **Mills, C. A.,** Chemical nature of tissue coagulins, *J. Biol. Chem.*, 46, 135, 1921.
28. **Chargaff, E.,** Studies on the mechanism of the thromboplastic effect, *J. Biol. Chem.*, 173, 253, 1948.
29. **Nemerson, Y. and Pitlick, F. A.,** Purification and characterization of the protein component of tissue factor, *Biochemistry,* 9, 5100, 1970.
30. **Pitlick, F. A.,** Concanavalin A inhibits tissue factor coagulant activity, *J. Clin. Invest.*, 55, 175, 1975.
31. **Pitlick, F. A. and Nemerson, Y.,** Purification and characterization of tissue factor apoprotein, *Methods Enzymol.*, 45, 37, 1976.
32. **Bjørklid, E., Storm, E., and Prydz, H.,** The protein component of human brain thromboplastin, *Biochem. Biophys. Res. Commun.*, 55, 969, 1973.
33. **Bjørklid, E. and Storm, E.,** Purification and some properties of the protein component of tissue thromboplastin from human brain, *Biochem. J.*, 165, 89, 1977.

34. **Wijngaards, G., Hemker, H. C., and van Deenen, L. L. M.,** Partial purification of the protein moiety of porcine tissue thromboplastin, *Haemostasis,* 6, 269, 1977.
35. **van den Besselaar, A. M. H. P. and Bertina, R. M.,** Interaction of thromboplastin apoprotein of different tissues with concanavalin A. Evidence for heterogeneous glycosylation of the human apoprotein, *Thromb. Haemostasis,* 52, 192, 1984.
36. **Tanaka, H., Janssen, B., Preissner, K. T., and Müller-Berghaus, G.,** Purification of glycosylated apoprotein of tissue factor from human brain and inhibition of its procoagulant activity by a specific antibody, *Thromb. Res.,* 40, 745, 1985.
37. **Broze, G. J., Leykam, J. E., Schwartz, B. D., and Miletich, J. P.,** Purification of human brain tissue factor, *J. Biol. Chem.,* 260, 10917, 1985.
38. **Bom, V. J. J., Ram, I. E., Alderkamp, G. H. J., Reinalda-Poot, H. H., and Bertina, R. M.,** Application of factor VII-Sepharose affinity chromatography in the purification of human tissue factor apoprotein, *Thromb. Res.,* 42, 635, 1986.
39. **Guha, A., Bach, R., Konigsberg, W., and Nemerson, Y.,** Affinity purification of human tissue factor: interaction of factor VII and tissue factor in detergent micelles, *Proc. Natl. Acad. Sci. U.S.A.,* 83, 299, 1986.
40. **Carson, S. D., Bach, R., and Carson, S. M.,** Monoclonal antibodies against bovine tissue factor, which block interaction with factor VIIa, *Blood,* 66, 152, 1985.
41. **Ewan, V. A., Cieplinski, W., Hancock, W. W., Goldschneider, I., Boyd, A. W., and Rickles, F. R.,** Production and characterization of a monoclonal antibody (A1-3) that binds selectively to activated monocytes and inhibits monocyte procoagulant activity, *J. Immunol.,* 136, 2408, 1986.
42. **Nemerson, Y.,** Characteristics and lipid requirements of coagulant proteins extracted from lung and brain: the specificity of the protein component of tissue factor, *J. Clin. Invest.,* 48, 322, 1969.
43. **van den Besselaar, A. M. H. P., Ram, I. E., Alderkamp, G. H. J., and Bertina, R. M.,** The role of factor IX in tissue thromboplastin induced coagulation, *Thromb. Haemostasis,* 48, 54, 1982.
44. **Forman, S. D. and Nemerson, Y.,** Membrane-dependent coagulation reaction is independent of the concentration of phospholipid-bound substrate: fluid phase factor X regulates the extrinsic system, *Proc. Natl. Acad. Sci. U.S.A.,* 83, 4675, 1986.
45. **Pitlick, F. A. and Nemerson, Y.,** Binding of the protein component of tissue factor to phospholipids, *Biochemistry,* 9, 5105, 1970.
46. **Carson, S. D. and Konigsberg, W. H.,** Lipid activation of coagulation factor III apoprotein (tissue factor). Reconstitution of the protein-membrane complex, *Thromb. Haemostasis,* 44, 12, 1980.
47. **Carson, S. D. and Konigsberg, W. H.,** Cadmium increases tissue factor (coagulation factor III) activity by facilitating its reassociation with lipids, *Science,* 208, 307, 1980.
48. **Carson, S. D.,** Cadmium causes vesicle leakage under conditions which favor reconstitution of tissue factor-vesicle complexes, *J. Membr. Biol.,* 75, 123, 1983.
49. **Wijngaards, G., van Deenen, L. L. M., and Hemker, H. C.,** Reconstitution and lipid requirements of porcine tissue thromboplastin, *Biochim. Biophys. Acta,* 488, 161, 1977.
50. **Bach, R., Gentry, R., and Nemerson, Y.,** Factor VII binding to tissue factor in reconstituted phospholipid vesicles: induction of cooperativity by phosphatidylserine, *Biochemistry,* 25, 4007, 1986.
51. **Liu, D. I. H. and McCoy, L. E.,** Tissue extract thromboplastin: quantitation, fractionation and characterization of protein components, *Thromb. Res.,* 7, 199, 1975.
52. **Fair, D. S. and Marlar, R. A.,** Biosynthesis and secretion of factor VII, protein C, protein S, and the protein C inhibitor from a human hepatoma cell line, *Blood,* 67, 64, 1986.
53. **Mariani, G. and Mazzucconi, M. G.,** Factor VII congenital deficiency, *Haemostasis,* 13, 169, 1983.
54. **Triplett, D. A., Brandt, J. T., McGann Batard, M. A., Schaeffer Dixon, J. L., and Fair, D. S.,** Hereditary factor VII deficiency: heterogeneity defined by combined functional and immunochemical analysis, *Blood,* 66, 1284, 1985.
55. **Fair, D. S.,** Quantitation of factor VII in the plasma of normal and warfarin-treated individuals by radioimmunoassay, *Blood,* 62, 784, 1983.
56. **Broze, G. J., Hickman, S., and Miletich, J. P.,** Monoclonal anti-human factor VII antibodies. Detection in plasma of a second protein antigenically and genetically related to factor VII, *J. Clin. Invest.,* 76, 937, 1985.
57. **Mariani, G., Mazzucconi, M. G., Solinas, S., Avvisati, G., Chistolini, A., and Moretti, T.,** Studies on PIVKA VII, *Haemostasis,* 14, 238, 1984.
58. **Bom, V. J. J., van Tilburg, N. H., Krommenhoek-van Es, C., and Bertina, R. M.,** Immunoradiometric assays for human coagulation factor VII using polyclonal antibodies against the Ca(II)-dependent and Ca(II)-independent conformation, *Thromb. Haemostasis,* 56, 343, 1986.
59. **Kisiel, W. and McMullen, B. A.,** Isolation and characterization of human factor VIIa, *Thromb. Res.,* 22, 375, 1981.
60. **Radcliffe, R. and Nemerson, Y.,** Activation and control of factor VII by activated factor X and thrombin. Isolation and characterization of a single chain form of factor VII, *J. Biol. Chem.,* 250, 388, 1975.

61. **Bach, R., Oberdick, J., and Nemerson, Y.,** Immunoaffinity purification of bovine factor VII, *Blood,* 63, 393, 1984.
62. **Hagen, F. S., Gray, C. L., O'Hara, P., Grant, F. J., Saari, G. C., Woodbury, R. G., Hart, C. E., Insley, M., Kisiel, W., Kurachi, K., and Davie, E. W.,** Characterization of a cDNA coding for human factor VII, *Proc. Natl. Acad. Sci. U.S.A.,* 83, 2412, 1986.
63. **DiScipio, R. G., Hermodson, M. A., Yates, S. G., and Davie, E. W.,** A comparison of human prothrombin, factor IX (Christmas factor), factor X (Stuart factor) and protein S, *Biochemistry,* 16, 698, 1977.
64. **McMullen, B. A., Fujikawa, K., and Kisiel, W.,** The occurrence of beta-hydroxyaspartic acid in the vitamin K-dependent blood coagulation zymogens, *Biochem. Biophys. Res. Commun.,* 115, 8, 1983.
65. **Strickland, D. K. and Castellino, F. J.,** The binding of calcium to bovine factor VII, *Arch. Biochem.,* 199, 61, 1980.
66. **Zur, M. and Nemerson, Y.,** The esterase activity of coagulation factor VII. Evidence for intrinsic activity of the zymogen, *J. Biol. Chem.,* 253, 2203, 1978.
67. **Zur, M., Radcliffe, R. D., Oberdick, J., and Nemerson, Y.,** The dual role of factor VII in blood coagulation. Initiation and inhibition of a proteolytic system by a zymogen, *J. Biol. Chem.,* 257, 5623, 1982.
68. **Nemerson, Y., Jackson, C. M., and Aronson, D. L.,** Nomenclature recommendations for factor VII, *Thromb. Haemostasis,* 44, 175, 1980.
69. **Broze, G. J. and Majerus, P. W.,** Purification and properties of human coagulation factor VII, *J. Biol. Chem.,* 255, 1242, 1980.
70. **Bajaj, S. P., Rapaport, S. I., and Brown, S. F.,** Isolation and characterization of human factor VII. Activation of factor VII by factor Xa, *J. Biol. Chem.,* 256, 253, 1981.
71. **Radcliffe, R. and Nemerson, Y.,** Mechanism of activation of bovine factor VII. Products of cleavage by factor Xa, *J. Biol. Chem.,* 251, 4797, 1976.
72. **Masys, D. R., Bajaj, S. P., and Rapaport, S. I.,** Activation of human factor VII by activated factors IX and X, *Blood,* 60, 1143, 1982.
73. **Nemerson, Y. and Repke, D.,** Tissue factor accelerates the activation of coagulation factor VII: the role of a bifunctional coagulation cofactor, *Thromb. Res.,* 40, 351, 1985.
74. **Seligsohn, U., Østerud, B., Brown, S. F., Griffin, J. H., and Rapaport, S. I.,** Activation of human factor VII in plasma and in purified systems. Roles of activated factor IX, kallikrein and activated factor XII, *J. Clin. Invest.,* 64, 1056, 1979.
75. **Laake, K. and Østerud, B.,** Activation of purified plasma factor VII by human plasmin, plasma kallikrein and activated components of the human intrinsic blood coagulation system, *Thromb. Res.,* 5, 759, 1974.
76. **Kisiel, W., Fujikawa, K., and Davie, E. W.,** Activation of bovine factor VII (Proconvertin) by factor XIIa (activated Hageman factor), *Biochemistry,* 16, 4189, 1977.
77. **Radcliffe, R., Bagdasarian, A., Colman, R., and Nemerson, Y.,** Activation of bovine factor VII by Hageman factor fragments, *Blood,* 50, 611, 1977.
78. **Jesty, J. and Nemerson, Y.,** Purification of factor VII from bovine plasma. Reaction with tissue factor and activation of factor X, *J. Biol. Chem.,* 249, 509, 1974.
79. **Jesty, J., Spencer, A. K., and Nemerson, Y.,** The mechanism of activation of factor X. Kinetic control of alternative pathways leading to the formation of activated factor X, *J. Biol. Chem.,* 249, 5614, 1974.
80. **Østerud, B., Bjørklid, E., and Brown, S. F.,** The interaction of human blood coagulation factor VII and tissue factor: the effect of anti-factor VII, anti-tissue factor and diisopropylfluorophosphate, *Biochem. Biophys. Res. Commun.,* 88, 59, 1979.
81. **Wijngaards, G. and Immerzeel, J.,** Divalent cations and complex formation between tissue thromboplastin and factor VII, *Biochem. Biophys. Res. Commun.,* 77, 658, 1977.
82. **Jesty, J.,** The inhibition of activated bovine coagulation factors X and VII by antithrombin III, *Arch. Biochem. Biophys.,* 185, 165, 1978.
83. **Jesty, J. and Silverberg, S. A.,** Kinetics of the tissue factor-dependent activation of coagulation factors IX and X in a bovine plasma system, *J. Biol. Chem.,* 254, 12337, 1979.
84. **Dahl, P. E., Abildgaard, U., Larsen, M. L., and Tjensvoll, L.,** Inhibition of activated coagulation factor VII by normal human plasma, *Thromb. Haemostasis,* 48, 253, 1982.
85. **Godfrey, H. P., Angadi, C. V., Haak-Frendscho, M., and Kaplan, A. P.,** Concurrent production of macrophage agglutination factor and factor VII by antigen-stimulated human peripheral blood mononuclear cells, *Immunology,* 57, 77, 1986.
86. **Chapman, H. A., Allen, C. L., and Stone, O. L.,** Human alveolar macrophages synthesize factor VII in vitro. Possible role in interstitial lung disease, *J. Clin. Invest.,* 75, 2030, 1985.
87. **Tsao, B. P., Fair, D. S., Curtiss, L. K., and Edgington, T. S.,** Monocytes can be induced by lipopolysaccharide-triggered T lymphocytes to express functional factor VII/VIIa protease activity, *J. Exp. Med.,* 159, 1042, 1984.
88. **Jackson, C. M.,** Factor X, *Prog. Haemostasis Thromb.,* 7, 55, 1984.

89. **Esnouf, M. P., Lloyd, P. H., and Jesty, J.,** A method for the simultaneous isolation of factor X and prothrombin from bovine plasma, *Biochem. J.,* 131, 781, 1973.
90. **Fujikawa, K., Coan, M. H., Legaz, M. E., and Davie, E. W.,** The mechanism of activation of bovine factor X (Stuart factor) by intrinsic and extrinsic pathways, *Biochemistry,* 13, 5290, 1974.
91. **Jackson, C. M. and Hanahan, D.,** Studies on bovine factor X. I. Large scale purification of the bovine plasma protein possessing factor X activity, *Biochemistry,* 7, 4492, 1968.
92. **Rosenberg, J. S., Beeler, D. L., and Rosenberg, R. D.,** Activation of human prothrombin by highly purified human factors V and Xa in the presence of human antithrombin, *J. Biol. Chem.,* 250, 1607, 1975.
93. **Kosow, D. P.,** Purification and activation of human factor X: cooperative effect of Ca^{2+} on the activation reaction, *Thromb. Res.,* 9, 565, 1976.
94. **Enfield, D. L., Ericsson, L. H., Walsh, K. A., Neurath, H., and Titani, K.,** Bovine factor X_1 (Stuart factor). Primary structure of the light chain, *Proc. Natl. Acad. Sci. U.S.A.,* 72, 16, 1975.
95. **Titani, K., Fujikawa, K., Enfield, D. L., Ericsson, L. H., Walsh, K. A., and Neurath, H.,** Bovine factor X_1 (Stuart factor): amino acid sequence of heavy chain, *Proc. Natl. Acad. Sci. U.S.A.,* 72, 3082, 1975.
96. **Fung, M. R., Hay, C. W., and MacGillivray, R. T.,** Characterization of an almost full-length cDNA coding for human blood coagulation factor X, *Proc. Natl. Acad. Sci. U.S.A.,* 82, 3591, 1985.
97. **Leytus, S. P., Chung, D. W., Kisiel, W., Kurachi, K., and Davie, E. W.,** Characterization of a cDNA coding for human factor X, *Proc. Natl. Acad. Sci. U.S.A.,* 81, 3699, 1984.
98. **Nelsestuen, G. L. and Lim, T. K.,** Equilibria involved in prothrombin- and blood clotting factor X-membrane binding, *Biochemistry,* 16, 4164, 1977.
99. **Nelsestuen, G. L., Kisiel, W., and DiScipio, R. G.,** Interaction of vitamin K-dependent proteins with membranes, *Biochemistry,* 17, 2134, 1978.
100. **Zwaal, R. F. A.,** Membrane and lipid involvement in blood coagulation, *Biochim. Biophys. Acta,* 515, 163, 1978.
101. **Fujikawa, K., Legaz, M. E., and Davie, E. W.,** Bovine factors X_1 and X_2 (Stuart factor). Isolation and characterization, *Biochemistry,* 11, 4882, 1972.
102. **Fujikawa, K., Titani, K., and Davie, E. W.,** Activation of bovine factor X (Stuart factor): conversion of factor Xa-alpha to factor Xa-beta, *Proc. Natl. Acad. Sci. U.S.A.,* 72, 3359, 1975.
103. **Jesty, J., Spencer, A. K., Nakashima, Y., Nemerson, Y., and Konigsberg, W.,** The activation of coagulation factor X. Identity of cleavage sites in the alternative activation pathways and characterization of the COOH-terminal peptide, *J. Biol. Chem.,* 250, 4497, 1975.
104. **DiScipio, R. G., Hermodson, M. A., and Davie, E. W.,** Activation of human factor X (Stuart factor) by a protease from Russell's viper venom, *Biochemistry,* 16, 5253, 1977.
105. **Mertens, K. and Bertina, R. M.,** Pathways in the activation of human coagulation factor X, *Biochem. J.,* 185, 647, 1980.
106. **Mertens, K., Wortelboer, M., van Dieijen, G., and Bertina, R. M.,** Proteolysis of blood coagulation factor X by activated factor X. Difference between the bovine and human proteins, *FEBS Lett.,* 139, 174, 1982.
107. **Jesty, J. and Morrison, S. A.,** The activation of factor IX by tissue factor-factor VII in a bovine plasma system lacking factor X, *Thromb. Res.,* 32, 171, 1983.
108. **Thompson, A. R.,** Structure, function and molecular defects of factor IX, *Blood,* 67, 565, 1986.
109. **Andersson, L. O., Borg, H., and Miller-Andersson, M.,** Purification and characterization of human factor IX, *Thromb. Res.,* 7, 451, 1975.
110. **Bajaj, S. P., Rapaport, S. I., and Prodanos, C.,** A simplified procedure for purification of human prothrombin, factor IX and factor X, *Prep. Biochem.,* 11, 397, 1981.
111. **Fujikawa, K., Thompson, A. R., Legaz, M. E., Meyer, R. G., and Davie, E. W.,** Isolation and characterization of bovine factor IX (Christmas factor), *Biochemistry,* 12, 4938, 1973.
112. **Kurachi, K. and Davie, E. W.,** Isolation and characterization of a cDNA coding for human factor IX, *Proc. Natl. Acad. Sci. U.S.A.,* 79, 6461, 1982.
113. **Jaye, M., de la Salle, H., Schamber, F., Balland, A., Kohli, V., Findeli, A., Tolstoshev, P., and Lecocq, J. P.,** Isolation of a human anti-haemophilic factor IX cDNA clone using a unique 52-base synthetic oligonucleotide probe deduced from the amino acid sequence of bovine factor IX, *Nucl. Acids Res.,* 11, 2325, 1983.
114. **Nesheim, M. E., Tracy, R. P., and Mann, K. G.,** "Clotspeed", a mathematical simulation of the functional properties of prothrombinase, *J. Biol. Chem.,* 259, 1447, 1984.
115. **Anson, D. S., Choo, K. H., Rees, D. J. G., Giannelli, F., Gould, K., Huddleston, J. A., and Brownlee, G. G.,** The gene structure of human anti-hemophilic factor IX, *EMBO J.,* 3, 1053, 1984.
116. **Aggeler, P. M., White, S. G., Glendenning, M. B., Page, E. W., Leake, T. B., and Bates, G.,** Plasma thromboplastin component (PTC) deficiency: a new disease resembling haemophilia, *Proc. Soc. Exp. Biol. Med.,* 79, 692, 1952.

117. **Biggs, R., Douglas, A. S., MacFarlane, R. G., Dacie, J. V., Pitney, W. R., Merskey, C., and O'Brien, J. R.,** Christmas disease: a condition previously mistaken for haemophilia, *Br. Med. J.*, 2, 1378, 1952.
118. **DiScipio, R. G., Kurachi, K., and Davie, E. W.,** Activation of human factor IX (Christmas Factor), *J. Clin. Invest.*, 61, 1528, 1978.
119. **van Dieijen, G., Tans, G., Rosing, J., and Hemker, H. C.,** The role of phospholipid and factor VIIIa in the activation of bovine factor X, *J. Biol. Chem.*, 256, 3433, 1981.
120. **Mertens, K., van Wijngaarden, A., and Bertina, R. M.,** The role of factor VIII in the activation of human blood coagulation factor X by activated factor IX, *Thromb. Haemostasis*, 54, 654, 1985.
121. **Bajaj, S. P., Rapaport, S. I., and Russell, W. A.,** Redetermination of the rate-limiting step in the activation of factor IX by factor XIa and by factor VIIa/tissue factor. Explanation for different electrophoretic radioactivity profiles obtained on activation ^{3}H- and ^{125}I-labeled factor IX, *Biochemistry*, 22, 4047, 1983.
122. **Østerud, B. and Rapaport, S. I.,** Activation of ^{125}I- factor IX and ^{125}I-factor X: effect of tissue factor and factor VII, factor Xa and thrombin, *Scand. J. Haematol.*, 24, 213, 1980.
123. **Nemerson, Y.,** The reaction between bovine brain tissue factor and factors VII and X, *Biochemistry*, 5, 601, 1966.
124. **Østerud, B., Berre, A., Otnaess, A. B., Bjørklid, E., and Prydz, H.,** Activation of the coagulation factor VII by tissue thromboplastin and calcium, *Biochemistry*, 11, 2853, 1972.
125. **Nemerson, Y. and Gentry, R.,** An ordered addition, essential activation model of the tissue factor pathway of coagulation: evidence for a conformational cage, *Biochemistry*, 25, 4020, 1986.
126. **Broze, G. J.,** Binding of human factor VII and VIIa to monocytes, *J. Clin. Invest.*, 70, 526, 1982.
127. **Hougie, C.,** Reactions of Stuart factor and factor VII with brain and factor V, *Proc. Soc. Exp. Biol. (N.Y.)*, 101, 132, 1959.
128. **Straub, W. and Duckert, F.,** The formation of the extrinsic prothrombin activator, *Thromb. Diath. Haemorrh.*, 5, 402, 1961.
129. **Williams, W. J. and Norris, D. G.,** Purification of a bovine plasma protein (factor VII) which is required for the activity of lung microsomes in blood coagulation, *J. Biol. Chem.*, 241, 1847, 1966.
130. **van Lenten, L. and Ashwell, G.,** Studies on the chemical and enzymatic modification of glycoproteins, *J. Biol. Chem.*, 246, 1889, 1971.
131. **Aurell, L., Friberger, P., Karlsson, G., and Claeson, G.,** A new sensitive and highly specific chromogenic peptide substrate for factor Xa, *Thromb. Res.*, 11, 595, 1977.
132. **Mertens, K. and Bertina, R. M.,** The contribution of Ca^{2+} and phospholipids to the activation of human blood coagulation factor X by activated factor IX, *Biochem. J.*, 223, 607, 1984.
133. **Bom, V. J. J. and Bertina, R. M.,** The contributions of Ca^{2+}, phospholipid (PL) and tissue factor apoprotein (TFAP) to the activation of factor X (FX) by activated factor VII (FVIIa), *Thromb. Haemostasis*, 54, 215, 1985.
134. **Kisiel, W. and Davie, E. W.,** Isolation and characterization of bovine factor VII, *Biochemistry*, 14, 4928, 1975.
135. **Morrison, S. A. and Jesty, J.,** Tissue factor-dependent activation of tritium-labeled factor IX and factor X in human plasma, *Blood*, 63, 1338, 1984.
136. **Rao, I. V. M., Bajaj, S. P., and Rapaport, S. I.,** Activation of human factor VII during clotting in vitro, *Blood*, 65, 218, 1985.
137. **Hubbard, A. R. and Jennings, C. A.,** Inhibition of tissue thromboplastin-mediated blood coagulation, *Thromb. Res.*, 42, 489, 1986.
138. **Kondo, S. and Kisiel, W.,** Isolation of an inhibitor of the factor VIIa-tissue factor mediated activation of factor X, *Fed. Proc.*, 45, 1073, 1986.
139. **Carson, S. D.,** Plasma high density lipoproteins inhibit the activation of coagulation factor X by factor VIIa and tissue factor, *FEBS Lett.*, 132, 37, 1981.
140. **Duthille, P. and Comijn, J.,** Apoprotein B from low-density lipoproteins and factor X. Approaches to their interaction, *Ann. Pharmacol.*, F 41, 31, 1983.
141. **Østerud, B., Laake, K., and Prydz, H.,** The activation of human factor IX, *Thromb. Diath. Haemorrh.*, 33, 553, 1975.
142. **Josso, F. and Prou-Wartelle, O.,** Interaction of tissue factor and factor VII at the earliest phase of coagulation, *Thromb. Diath. Haemorrh.*, 17 (Suppl.), 35, 1965.
143. **Rapaport, S. I., Hjort, P. F., Patch, M. J., and Jeremic, M.,** Consumption of serum factors and prothrombin during intravascular clotting in rabbits, *Scand. J. Haematol.*, 3, 59, 1966.
144. **Bom, V. J. J., Reinalda-Poot, H. H., Poort, S. R., Cupers, R., and Bertina, R. M.,** Solid phase immunoradiometric assay of activated human coagulation factor IX, *Thromb. Res.*, 45, 661, 1987.
145. **Bom, V. J. J. and Bertina, R. M.,** unpublished observations.
146. **Ørstavik, K. H. and Laake, K.,** Antiserum against factor IX shortens the bovine thromboplastin coagulation time of human plasma, *Thromb. Res.*, 12, 455, 1978.
147. **Hougie, C. and Twomey, J. J.,** Haemophilia B_m: a new type of factor IX deficiency, *Lancet*, 1, 698, 1967.

148. **Østerud, B., Kasper, C. K., Lavine, K. K., Prodanos, C., and Rapaport, S. I.,** Purification and properties of an abnormal blood coagulation factor IX (factor IX B_m)/kinetics of its inhibition of factor X activation by factor VII and bovine tissue factor, *Thromb. Haemostasis,* 45, 55, 1981.
149. **Nawroth, P. P., Handley, D., and Stern, D. M.,** The multiple levels of endothelial cell-coagulation factor interactions, *Clin. Haematol.,* 15, 293, 1986.
150. **Marlar, R. A., Kleiss, A. J., and Griffin, J. H.,** An alternative extrinsic pathway of human blood coagulation, *Blood,* 60, 1353, 1982.
150a. **Mertens, K. and Bertina, R. M.,** Activation of human coagulation factor VIII by activated factor X, the common product of the intrinsic and the extrinsic pathway of blood coagulation, *Thromb. Haemostasis,* 47, 96, 1982.
150b. **Bertina, R. M., Alderkamp, G. H. J., and de Nooy, E.,** A variant of factor X that is defective only in extrinsic coagulation, *Thromb. Haemostasis,* 46, 88, 1981.
151. **Girolami, A., Vicarioto, M., Ruzza, G., Cappellato, G., and Vergolani, A.,** Factor-X Padua — a new congential factor X abnormality with a defect only in the extrinsic system, *Acta Haematol.,* 73, 31, 1985.
152. **Mertens, K., Giles, A. R., and Briët, E.,** Assessment of factor VIII-bypassing activity of factor VIIa in a canine model of hemophilia, *Thromb. Haemostasis,* 54, 258, 1985.
153. **Stern, D. M., Bank, I., Nawroth, P. P., et al.,** Self-regulation of procoagulant events on the endothelial cell surface, *J. Exp. Med.,* 162, 1223, 1985.
154. **Nawroth, P., Kisiel, W., and Stern, D.,** The role of endothelium in the homeostatic balance of haemostasis, *Clin. Haematol.,* 14, 531, 1985.
155. **Stern, D. M., Nawroth, P. P., Kisiel, W., Vehar, G., and Esmon, C. T.,** The binding of factor IXa to cultured bovine aortic endothelial cells, *J. Biol. Chem.,* 260, 6717, 1985.
156. **Clouse, L. H. and Comp, P. C.,** The regulation of hemostasis: the protein C system, *N. Engl. J. Med.,* 314, 1298, 1986.
157. **Balleisen, L., Bailey, J., Epping, P. H., Schulte, H., and Van de Loo, J.,** Epidemiological study on factor VII, factor VIII and fibrinogen in an industrial population. I. Baseline data on the relation to age, gender, body-weight, smoking, alcohol, pill-using and menopause, *Thromb. Haemostasis,* 54, 475, 1985.
158. **Dalaker, K. and Prydz, H.,** The coagulation factor VII in pregnancy, *Br. J. Haematol.,* 56, 233, 1984.
159. **Meade, T. W.,** Factor VII and ischaemic heart disease: epidemiological evidence, *Haemostasis,* 13, 178, 1983.
160. **Meade, T. W., Chakrabarti, R., Haines, A. P., North, W. R. S., Stirling, Y., and Thompson, S. G.,** Haemostatic function and cardiovascular death: early results of a prospective study, *Lancet,* 1, 1050, 1980.
161. **Heimark, R. L. and Schwartz, S.,** Binding of coagulation factors IX and X to the endothelial cell surface, *Biochem. Biophys. Res. Commun.,* 111, 723, 1983.
162. **Østerud, B. and Flaegstad, T.,** Increased tissue thromboplastin activity in monocytes of patients with meningococcal infection: related to an unfavourable prognosis, *Thromb. Haemostasis,* 49, 5, 1983.
163. **Østerud, B., Lindahl, U., and Seljelid, R.,** Macrophages produce blood coagulation factors, *FEBS Lett.,* 120, 41, 1980.
164. **Østerud, B., Bogwald, J., Lindahl, U., and Seljelid, R.,** Production of blood coagulation factor V and tissue thromboplastin by macrophages in vitro, *FEBS Lett.,* 127, 154, 1981.
165. **Edwards, R. L. and Rickles, F. R.,** Macrophage procoagulants, *Prog. Haemostasis Thromb.,* 7, 183, 1984.
166. **Stern, D. M., Drillings, M., Nossel, H. L., Hurlet-Jensen, A., LaGamma, K. S., and Owen, J.,** Binding of factors IX and IXa to cultured vascular endothelial cells, *Proc. Natl. Acad. Sci. U.S.A.,* 80, 4119, 1983.
167. **Donati, M. B. and Semeraro, N.,** Cancer cell procoagulants and their pharmacological modulation, *Haemostasis,* 14, 422, 1984.
168. **Astrup, T.,** Assay and content of tissue thromboplastin in different organs, *Thromb. Diath. Haemorrh.,* 14, 401, 1965.
169. **Bjørklid, E., Storm-Mathisen, J., Storm, E., and Prydz, H.,** Localization of tissue thromboplastin in the human brain, *Thromb. Haemostasis,* 37, 91, 1977.
170. **Astrup, T. and Sjolin, K. E.,** Thromboplastic and fibrinolytic activity of human synovial membrane and fibrous capsular tissue, *Proc. Soc. Exp. Biol. (N.Y.),* 97, 852, 1958.
171. **Janson, T. L., Stormorken, H., and Prydz, H.,** Species specificity of tissue thromboplastin, *Haemostasis,* 14, 440, 1984.
172. **Dalaker, K., Kaplun, A., Lyberg, T., and Prydz, H.,** Synthesis of thromboplastin (factor III) in mouse placental cells in vitro, *Gynaecol. Obstet. Invest.,* 15, 351, 1983.
173. **Prydz, H. and Allison, A. C.,** Tissue thromboplastin activity of isolated human moncoytes, *Thromb. Haemostasis,* 39, 582, 1978.
174. **Johnsen, U. L. H., Lyberg, T., Galdal, K. S., and Prydz, H.,** Platelets stimulate thromboplastin synthesis in human endothelial cells, *Thromb. Haemostasis,* 49, 69, 1983.

175. **Rivers, R. P., Hathaway, W. E., and Weston, W. L.,** The endotoxin-induced coagulant activity of human monocytes, *Br. J. Haematol.*, 30, 311, 1975.
176. **Rickles, F. R., Rick, P. D., and van Why, M.,** Structural features of Salmonella typhimurium lipopolysaccharide required for activation of tissue factor in human mononuclear cells, *J. Clin. Invest.*, 59, 1188, 1957.
177. **Edwards, R. L., Rickles, F. R., and Bobrove, A. M.,** Mononuclear cell tissue factor: cell of origin and requirements for activation, *Blood,* 54, 359, 1979.
178. **Semeraro, N., Biondi, A., Lorenzet, R., Locati, D., Mantovani, A., and Donati, M. B.,** Direct induction of tissue factor synthesis by endotoxin in human macrophages from divers anatomical sites, *Immunology,* 50, 529, 1983.
179. **Amlie, E., Lyberg, T., Kaplun, A., Hetland, Ø., and Prydz, H.,** Thromboplastin activity of mouse peritoneal macrophages, *Thromb. Res.*, 24, 61, 1981.
180. **Maynard, J. R., Dreyer, B. E., Stemerman, M. B., and Pitlick, F. A.,** Tissue factor coagulant activity of cultured human endothelial and smooth muscle cells and fibroblasts, *Blood,* 50, 387, 1977.
181. **Lyberg, T., Galdal, K. S., Evensen, S. A., and Prydz, H.,** Cellular cooperation in endothelial cell thromboplastin synthesis, *Br. J. Haematol.*, 53, 85, 1983.
182. **Stern, D. M., Drillings, M., Kisiel, W., Nawroth, P., Nossel, H. L., and LaGamma, K. S.,** Activation of factor IX bound to cultured bovine aortic endothelial cells, *Proc. Natl. Acad. Sci. U.S.A.*, 81, 913, 1984.
183. **Shands, J. W., Jr.,** Macrophage procoagulants, *Haemostasis,* 14, 373, 1984.
184. **Geczy, C. L. and Meyer, P. A.,** Leukocyte procoagulant activity in man: an in vitro correlate of delayed-type hypersensitivity, *J. Immunol.*, 128, 331, 1982.
185. **Rickles, F. R. and Edwards, R. L.,** Activation of monocyte tissue factor (MTF) in response to antigen recognition, *Blood,* 58 (Suppl.), 225, 1981.
186. **van Ginkel, C. J. W., Zeijlemaker, W. P., Stricker, L. A. M., Oh, J. I., and van Aken, W. G.,** Enhancement of monocyte thromboplastin activity by antigenically stimulated lymphocytes: a link between immune reactivity and blood coagulation, *Eur. J. Immunol.*, 11, 579, 1981.
187. **Prydz, H., Lyberg, T., Deteix, P., and Allison, A. C.,** In vitro stimulation of tissue thromboplastin (factor III) activity in human monocytes by immune complexes and lectins, *Thromb. Res.*, 15, 465, 1979.
188. **Rothberger, H., Zimmerman, T. S., Spiegelberg, H. L., and Vaughan, J. H.,** Leukocyte procoagulant activity. Enhancement of production in vitro by IgG and antigen-antibody complexes, *J. Clin. Invest.*, 59, 549, 1977.
189. **Schwartz, B. S. and Edgington, T. S.,** Lymphocyte collaboration is required for induction of murine monocyte procoagulant activity by immune complexes, *J. Immunol.*, 127, 438, 1981.
190. **Lyberg, T. and Prydz, H.,** Thromboplastin (factor III) activity in human monocytes induced by immune complexes, *Eur. J. Clin. Invest.*, 12, 229, 1982.
191. **Muhlfelder, T. W., Niemetz, J., Kreutzer, D., Beebe, D., Ward, P. A., and Rosenfeld, S. I.,** C5 chemotactic fragment induces leukocyte production of tissue factor activity. A link between complement and coagulation, *J. Clin. Invest.*, 63, 147, 1979.
192. **Prydz, H., Allision, A. C., and Schorlemmer, H. U.,** Further link between complement activation and blood coagulation, *Nature,* 270, 173, 1977.
193. **Janco, R. L. and Morris, P.,** Serum augments the generation of monocyte procoagulant stimulated by bacterial lipopolysaccharide or chemotactic fragments of C5, *Thromb. Res.*, 32, 73, 1983.
194. **Østerud, B., Olsen, J. O., and Benjaminsen, A. W.,** The role of complement in the induction of thromboplastin synthesis, *Haemostasis,* 14, 386, 1984.
195. **Østerud, B. and Eskeland, T.,** The mandatory role of complement in the endotoxin-induced synthesis of tissue thromboplastin in blood monocytes, *FEBS Lett.*, 149(1), 75, 1982.
196. **Helin, H. J. and Edgington, T. S.,** Allogenic induction of the human T cell-instructed monocyte procoagulant response is rapid and is elicited by HLA-DR, *J. Exp. Med.*, 158, 962, 1983.
197. **Rothberger, H., Zimmerman, T. S., and Vaughan, J. H.,** Increased production and expression of tissue thromboplastin-like procoagulant activity in vitro by allogeneically stimulated human leukocytes, *J. Clin. Invest.*, 62, 649, 1978.
198. **Edwards, R. L. and Rickles, F. R.,** The role of monocyte tissue factor in immune response, *Lymphokine Rep.*, 1, 181, 1981.
199. **Helin, H. and Edgington, T. S.,** A distinct ''slow'' cellular pathway involving soluble mediators for the T-cell instructed induction of monocyte tissue factor activity in an allogeneic immune response, *J. Immunol.*, 132, 2457, 1984.
200. **Geczy, C. L. and Hopper, K. E.,** A mechanism of migration inhibition in delayed-type hypersensitivity reactions. II. Lymphokines promote procoagulant activity of macrophages in vitro, *J. Immunol.*, 126, 1059, 1981.
201. **Geczy, C. L.,** Induction of macrophage procoagulant by products of activated lymophocytes, *Haemostasis,* 14, 400, 1984.

202. **van Ginkel, C. J. W., Thörig, L., Thompson, J., Oh, J. I. H., and van Aken, W. G.,** Enhancement of generation of moncoyte tissue thromboplastin by bacterial phagocytosis: possible pathway for fibrin formation on infected vegetations in bacterial endocarditis, *Infect. Immun.*, 25, 388, 1979.
203. **Dean, R. T. and Prydz, H.,** Inflammatory particles stimulate thromboplastin production by human monocytes, *Thromb. Res.*, 30, 357, 1983.
204. **Levy, G. A., Leibowitz, J. L., and Edgington, T. S.,** Induction of monocyte procoagulant activity by murine hepatitis virus type 3 parallels disease susceptibility in mice, *J. Exp. Med.*, 154, 1150, 1981.
205. **Levy, G. A., Schwartz, B. S., Curtiss, L. K., and Edgington, T. S.,** Plasma lipoprotein induction and suppression of the generation of cellular procoagulant activity in vitro, *J. Clin. Invest.*, 67, 1614, 1981.
206. **Edwards, R. L. and Perla, D.,** The effect of serum on monocyte tissue factor generation, *Blood*, 64, 707, 1984.
207. **Lyberg, T. and Prydz, H.,** Phorbol esters induce synthesis of thromboplastin activity in human monocytes, *Biochem. J.*, 194, 699, 1981.
208. **Galdal, K. S.,** Thromboplastin synthesis in endothelial cells, *Haemostasis*, 14, 378, 1984.
209. **Nawroth, P. P., Stern, D. M., Kisiel, W., and Bach, R.,** Cellular requirements for tissue factor generation by bovine aortic endothelial cells in culture, *Thromb. Res.*, 40, 677, 1985.
210. **Rickles, F. R., Levin, J., and Hardin, J. A.,** Tissue factor generation by human mononuclear cells: effects of endotoxin and dissociation of tissue factor generation from the mitogenic response, *J. Lab. Clin. Med.*, 89, 792, 1977.
211. **Levy, G. A., Schwartz, B. S., and Edgington, T. S.,** The kinetics and metabolic requirements for direct lymphocyte induction of human procoagulant monokines by bacterial lipopolysaccharide, *J. Immunol.*, 127, 357, 1981.
212. **Lyberg, T. and Prydz, H.,** Is lymphocyte co-operation necessary for thromboplastin synthesis by human monocytes?, *Clin. Exp. Immunol.*, 53, 731, 1983.
213. **Rothberger, H., Dove, F. B., Lee, T. K., McGee, M. P., and Kardon, B.,** Procoagulant activity of lymphocyte-macrophage populations in rabbits: selective increases in marrow, blood, and spleen cells during Shwartzman reactions, *Blood*, 61, 712, 1983.
214. **Dean, R. I. and Prydz, H.,** Amines induce increased thromboplastin activity in human monocytes, *Eur. J. Biochem.*, 131, 655, 1983.
215. **Colucci, M., Balconi, G., Lorenzet, R., Pietra, A., Locati, D., Donati, M. B., and Semeraro, N.,** Cultured human endothelial cells generate tissue factor in response to endotoxin, *J. Clin. Invest.*, 71, 1893, 1983.
216. **Lyberg, T., Amlie, E., Kaplun, A., and Prydz, H.,** Macrophage heterogeniety in thromboplastin response, *Scand. J. Immunol.*, 18, 235, 1983.
217. **Semeraro, N., Colucci, M., Mussoni, L., and Donati, M. B.,** Rat blood leucocytes, unlike rabbit leucocytes, do not generate procoagulant activity on exposure to endotoxin, *Br. J. Exp. Pathol.*, 62, 638, 1981.
218. **Goodnough, L. T., Kleinhenz, M. E., Goldsmith, G. H., Ziats, N. P., and Robertson, A. L.,** Bovine aortic endothelial cells elaborate an inhibitor of the generation of lipopolysaccharide-stimulated human blood monocyte procoagulant activity, *J. Clin. Invest.*, 74, 75, 1984.
219. **Prydz, H. and Lyberg, T.,** Effect of some drugs on thromboplastin (factor III) activity of human monocytes in vitro, *Biochem. Pharmacol.*, 29, 9, 1980.
220. **Lyberg, T. and Prydz, H.,** Lectin stimulation of tissue thromboplastin activity in human monocytes in vitro, *Thromb. Haemostasis*, 42, 1574, 1979.
221. **Brox, J. H., Østerud, B., Bjørklid, E., and Fenton, J. W.,** Production and availability of thromboplastin in endothelial cells: the effects of thrombin, endotoxin and platelets, *Br. J. Haematol.*, 57, 239, 1984.
222. **Bevilacqua, M. P., Pober, J. S., Majeau, G. R., Cotran, R. S., and Gimbrone, M. A.,** Interleukin 1 (IL-1) induced biosynthesis and cell surface expression of procoagulant activity in human vascular endothelial cells, *J. Exp. Med.*, 160, 618, 1984.
223. **Sanders, N. L., Bajaj, S. P., Zivelin, A., and Rapaport, S. I.,** Inhibition of tissue factor/factor VIIa activity in plasma requires factor X and an additional plasma component, *Blood*, 66, 204, 1985.
224. **Edwards, R. L. and Rickles, F. R.,** The role of human T cells (and T cell products) for monocyte tissue factor generation, *J. Immunol.*, 125, 606, 1980.
225. **Helin, H. J., Fox, R. I., and Edgington, T. S.,** The instructor cell for the human procoagulant monocyte response to bacterial lipopolysaccharide is a Leu-3a$^+$ T cell by fluorescence-activated cell sorting, *J. Immunol.*, 131, 749, 1983.
226. **Levy, G. A. and Edgington, T. S.,** The major histocompatibility complex requirement for cellular collaboration in the murine lymphoid procoagulant response stimulated by bacterial lipopolysaccharide, *J. Immunol.*, 128, 1284, 1982.
227. **Farram, E., Geczy, C. L., Moon, D. K., and Hopper, K.,** The ability of lymphokine and lipopolysaccharide to induce procoagulant activity in mouse macrophage cell lines, *J. Immunol.*, 130, 2750, 1983.

228. **Nakamura, S., Gotoh, S., Takenaka, O., and Takahashi, K.,** Monocyte thromboplastin (tissue factor): complementary effect of lymphocytes upon its generation by endotoxin-stimulated monkey (Macaca fuscata) cells, *J. Biochem.,* 97, 1603, 1985.
229. **Edgington, T. S., Levy, G. A., Schwartz, B. S., and Fair, D. S.,** An unidirectional pathway of lymphocyte instructed macrophage and monocyte function characterized by the generation of procoagulant monokines, in *Advances in Immunopathology,* Weigle, Ed., Elsevier/North-Holland, New York, 1981, 173.
230. **Schwartz, B. S. and Edgington, T. S.,** Immune complex-induced human monocyte procoagulant activity. I. A rapid unidirectional lymphocyte-instructed pathway, *J. Exp. Med.,* 154, 892, 1981.
231. **Østerud, B. and Bjørklid, E.,** The production and availability of tissue thromboplastin in cellular populations of whole blood exposed to various concentrations of endotoxin. An assay for detection of endotoxin, *Scand. J. Haematol.,* 29, 175, 1982.
232. **Pinder, P. B., Hunt, J. A., and Zacharski, L. R.,** In vitro stimulation of monocyte tissue factor activity by autologous platelets, *Am. J. Hematol.,* 19, 317, 1985.
233. **Smariga, P. E. and Maynard, J. R.,** Platelet effects on tissue factor and fibrinolytic inhibition of cultured human fibroblasts and vascular cells, *Blood,* 60, 140, 1982.
234. **Niemetz, J. and Herbert, V.,** The role of protein synthesis on the generation of tissue factor activity by leukocytes, *Proc. Soc. Exp. Biol. Med.,* 139, 1276, 1972.
235. **Dean, R. T., Leoni, P., and Rossi, B. C.,** Regulation of procoagulant factors in mononuclear phagocytes, *Haemostasis,* 14, 412, 1984.
236. **Leoni, P. and Dean, R. T.,** An intracellular pool of the procoagulant thromboplastin in human monocytes, *Thromb. Res.,* 40, 199, 1985.
237. **Hetland, O., Brovold, A. B., Holme, R., Gaudernack, G., and Prydz, H.,** Thromboplastin (tissue factor) in plasma membranes of human monocytes, *Biochem. J.,* 228, 735, 1985.
238. **Dvorak, H. F., Van de Water, L., Dvorak, A. M., Harvey, V. S., Anderson, D., De Wolf, W., and Bach, R.,** Human tumor cells and guinea pig macrophages shed plasma membrane derived vesicles with procoagulant activity (PCA), *Fed. Proc.,* 41, 270, 1982.
239. **Bastida, E., Ordinas, A., Escolar, G., and Jamieson, G. A.,** Tissue factor in microvesicles shed from U87MG human glioblastoma cells induces coagulation, platelet aggregation, and thrombogenesis, *Blood,* 64, 177, 1984.
240. **Lyberg, T.,** Intracellular signal mechanisms in induction of thromboplastin synthesis, *Haemostasis,* 14, 393, 1984.
241. **Lyberg, T.,** Effect of cyclic AMP and cyclic GMP on thromboplastin (factor III) synthesis in human monocytes in vitro, *Thromb. Haemostasis,* 50, 804, 1983.
242. **Crutchley, D. J.,** Effects of inhibitors of arachidonic acid metabolism on thromboplastin activity in human monocytes, *Biochem. Biophys. Res. Commun.,* 119, 179, 1984.
243. **Morrissey, J. H., et al.,** *Cell,* 50, 129, 1987.
244. **Spicer, E. K., et al.,** *Proc. Natl. Acad. Sci. U.S.A.,* 84, 5148, 1987.
245. **Scarpati, et al.,** *Biochemistry,* 26, 5234, 1987.
246. **Fisher, K. L., et al.,** *Thromb. Res.,* 48, 89, 1987.

Chapter 7

THE ROLE OF PHOSPHOLIPIDS IN THE ACTIVATION OF FACTOR X AND PROTHROMBIN

Jan Rosing and Guido Tans

TABLE OF CONTENTS

I. INTRODUCTION

During blood coagulation a number of circulating plasma proteins are converted into active proteolytic enzymes, which subsequently participate in a complex reaction sequence finally resulting in the conversion of fibrinogen into fibrin and in clot formation. All enzymatically active coagulation factors are serine proteases which are formed by proteolysis of one or two specific peptide bonds in a precursor or zymogen molecule. In that respect, the activation process is similar to that of the zymogens chymotrypsinogen and trypsinogen of the GI proteinases chymotrypsin and trypsin. There is, however, one major difference between the activations of chymotrypsinogen and trypsinogen and the activation of blood coagulation factors. The activations of the GI zymogens are rather efficient reactions, while blood coagulation factor activation occurs at a very low rate. Therefore, additional components (protein cofactors, metal ions, and so-called procoagulant surfaces) are required to accelerate the activation of zymogens during in vivo blood coagulation. The activation of the so-called contact factors (Factor XII, prekallikrein, and Factor XI) is stimulated by negatively charged surfaces and by the protein cofactor high molecular weight kininogen, while in vivo activation of prothrombin and Factor X requires the presence of negatively charged phospholipids, calcium ions, and a protein cofactor (Factor Va in prothrombin activation, Factor VIIIa in intrinsic Factor X activation, and tissue factor apoprotein in extrinsic Factor X activation).

In this paper we will review the role of phospholipids in the activation of Factor X and prothrombin. For full appreciation of the mode of action of phospholipids in the activation of these coagulation factors, it is necessary to have some insight into the structural and functional properties of the proteins involved in these reactions and also some understanding of structural aspects of lipids and procoagulant membranes. These topics will, however, be only briefly reviewed, since they are subject of more detailed discussion in other review papers[1-6] and in other chapters of this book.

II. STRUCTURAL AND FUNCTIONAL PROPERTIES OF THE PROTEINS INVOLVED IN PROTHROMBIN AND FACTOR X ACTIVATION

In the last decade much information has been obtained regarding the proteins that are involved in the prothrombinase complex and in the extrinsic and intrinsic Factor X-activating complexes. All proteins that participate in these reactions have been purified to homogeneity, and for many of them information is available about the secondary and tertiary structures. A schematic representation of the proteins picturing the structural properties pertinent to the discussions in this paper is presented in Figure 1.

An essential feature of four of these proteins, the so-called vitamin K-dependent coagulation factors (prothrombin, Factor X, Factor IX, and Factor VII), is the presence of γ-carboxyglutamic acid in the polypeptide chain (Figure 2). The occurrence of this amino acid is the result of a postribosomal carboxylation of a number of specific glutamic acid residues present in these proteins.[1-3] It is thought that the γ-carboxyglutamic acid residues play an essential role in the calcium-dependent binding of vitamin K-dependent coagulation factors to negatively charged phospholipid surfaces. This phenomenon will be discussed in more detail in paragraph V of this chapter. In addition to γ-carboxyglutamic acid, the vitamin K-dependent coagulation factors contain one other modified amino acid, i.e., β-hydroxyaspartic acid[7,8] (Figure 2). The biological function of this amino acid is not yet known.

The carboxyterminal region of the vitamin K-dependent coagulation factors is highly homologous to trypsin,[1-3] and the amino-terminal region comprises domains that appear to contain the structural information for interaction with protein cofactors, metal ions, and phospholipid membranes.

The protein cofactors have no structural and functional relationship with the vitamin K-

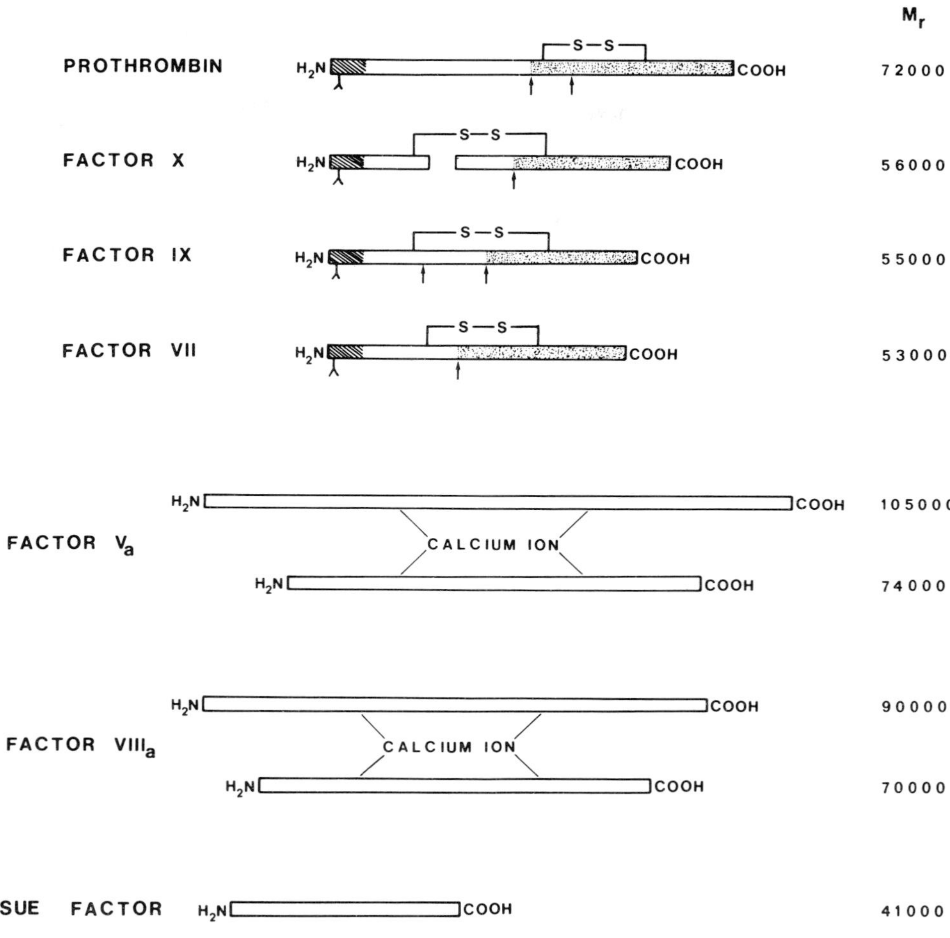

FIGURE 1. Proteins involved in prothrombin and Factor X activation. The amino-terminal (striped) region contains the γ-carboxyglutamic acid residues thought to be involved in the Ca^{2+}-dependent binding of the vitamin K-dependent proteins to phospholipids. The nonshaded areas of the vitamin K-dependent coagulation factors presumably contain the domains that interact with the protein cofactors. The gray-shaded carboxy-terminal part is highly homologous to trypsin and contains the active site region of the proteins.

dependent coagulation factors. Factors V and VIII are, however, functionally and structurally similar. Both proteins accelerate the activation of a coagulation factor, and recently it has been shown that there exists a high degree of amino acid sequence homology between Factors V and VIII.[9] There is, however, no structural relationship or known sequence homology of these protcins with tissue factor apoprotein.

A. Proteins Involved in Extrinsic Factor X Activation

In extrinsic Factor X activation the zymogen Factor X is converted into Factor Xa by the serine protease Factor VIIa in a reaction that is drastically stimulated by phospholipids plus calcium ions and by tissue factor apoprotein. Factor VIIa is a two-chain glycoprotein (M_r = 53,000) consisting of a light chain of 23,000 daltons that is linked via a disulfide bridge to a heavy chain of 30,000 daltons.[10] The light chain of Factor VIIa contains approximately

```
      H O                          H O
      | ||                         | ||
   H2N-C-C-OH                   H2N-C-C-OH
      |                            |
      CH2                        H-C-OH
      |                            |
      CH                           COOH
     /\
  HOOC COOH

γ-carboxyglutamic acid       β-hydroxyaspartic acid
```

FIGURE 2. Chemical structures of γ-carboxyglutamic acid and β-hydroxyaspartic acid.

ten γ-carboxyglutamic acid residues,[11] while the active site of this enzyme is located on the heavy chain.[12] Tissue factor apoprotein is a 41,000-dalton glycoprotein that has been purified to homogeneity from bovine[13] and human sources.[14,15] It requires lipidation to obtain functional activity in Factor X activation. The substrate Factor X is a glycoprotein that consists of two polypeptide chains. The bovine protein has a molecular weight of 56,000 daltons and is composed of a heavy chain of 38,000 daltons that is disulfide-linked to a light chain of 18,000 daltons.[16] The human protein has a molecular weight of 59,000 daltons and consists of a heavy chain of 42,000 daltons and a light chain of 17,000 daltons.[17,18] The amino acid sequence of both bovine[19,20] and human[21,22] Factor X is known, and it has further been established that the light chain of Factor X contains 12 to 14 γ-carboxyglutamic acid residues.[11,23,24] Activation of Factor X is the result of cleavage of a single peptide bond in the heavy chain, releasing an activation peptide of 11,000 daltons and producing Factor Xa (M_r = 45,000 daltons), which has an unaltered light chain that is linked via a disulfide bridge to a heavy chain of 27,000 daltons that contains the active site.[25,26]

B. Proteins Involved in Intrinsic Factor X Activation

Intrinsic Factor X activation is catalyzed by the serine protease Factor IXa and is stimulated by phospholipids plus calcium ions and by the protein cofactor VIIIa. Factors IXa and VIIa cleave the same peptide bond in Factor X, so the Factor Xa molecules produced by intrinsic and extrinsic Factor X activation have the same structural and functional properties. Factor IXa is a vitamin K-dependent protein (M_r = 44,000) consisting of a light chain of 17,000 daltons[27,28] that contains 12 γ-carboxyglutamic acid residues.[11,29] The light chain of Factor IXa is disulfide-linked to a heavy chain of 27,000 daltons,[27,28] which contains the active-site region of the molecule.[30] The entire amino acid sequences of both bovine[29] and human[30,31] Factor IXa have been established by conventional protein techniques[29] and by characterization of a cDNA coding for Factor IX.[30,31]

Efficient activation of Factor X via the intrinsic pathway requires the presence of the protein cofactor Factor VIII:C. Factor VIII:C is a glycoprotein[32] with a molecular weight of about 330,000 daltons.[33-35] The amino acid sequence of Factor VIII:C has been deduced from cDNA clones encoding the entire protein.[33-35] Limited proteolysis of Factor VIII:C by thrombin results in the disappearance of the high molecular weight forms[36-39] and the generation of 90,000- and 70,000-dalton polypeptides with concomitant increase of cofactor activity.[36,37] Prolonged incubation with thrombin gives rise to a further cleavage of the 90,000-dalton subunit yielding 55,000- and 40,000-dalton polypeptides. Fass et al.[39] have suggested that the polypeptide chains of activated Factor VIII:C are associated through interactions with calcium ion(s).

C. Proteins Involved in Prothrombin Activation

Prothrombin is a single-chain glycoprotein of 72,000 daltons.[1] It was the first coagulation zymogen for which the amino acid sequence was solved.[40] Three domains with different

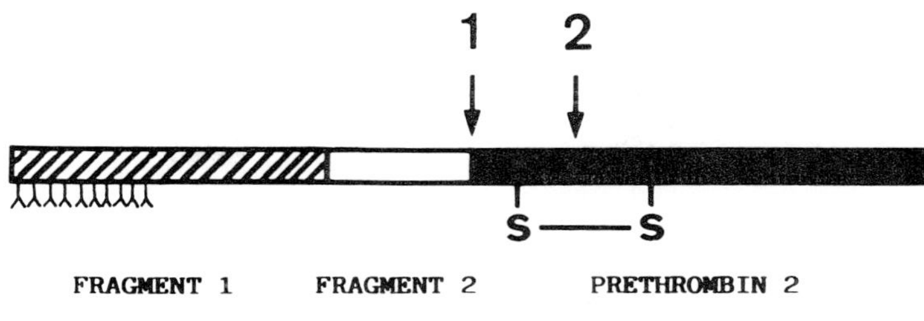

FIGURE 3. The prothrombin molecule. This figure depicts the three functional domains of prothrombin. The peptide bonds susceptible to cleavage by Factor Xa are indicated by arrows. λ is γ-carboxyglutamic acid.

functions can be distinguished in prothrombin (Figure 3). The fragment 1 region contains ten γ-carboxyglutamic acid residues[41,42] that presumably function in the calcium-dependent binding of prothrombin to negatively charged phospholipid surfaces. The fragment 2 region is thought to interact with the protein cofactor Factor V_a,[43] while the prethrombin 2 region contains the active site domain.[44] Conversion of prothrombin into thrombin is catalyzed by Factor Xa, a proteolytic enzyme that cleaves two peptide bonds in the prothrombin molecule (Figure 2). Depending upon the order of cleavage, prethrombin 2 (peptide bond 1 cleaved first) or so-called meizothrombin (peptide bond 2 cleaved first) can occur as intermediates. Since both prethrombin 2 [45,46] and meizothrombin[47,48] have been observed during prethrombin activation by Factor Xa, both pathways (cleavage order 1-2 or 2-1) are theoretically possible.

Factor Xa-catalyzed prothrombin activation is greatly stimulated by phospholipids plus calcium and by the protein cofactor Factor Va. Factor Va is a glycoprotein with a molecular weight of 180,000 daltons.[49-51] It is composed of a heavy chain of 105,000 daltons which is noncovalently associated through a calcium bridge[50,52] with a light chain of 74,000 daltons.

III. STRUCTURAL ASPECTS OF LIPIDS AND MEMBRANES

Phospholipids are amphipathic molecules, which means that they have a hydrophylic (or polar) and a hydrophobic (or nonpolar) end. The chemical structures of the major phospholipids that occur in biological membranes are presented in Figure 4. Phospholipids readily dissolve in organic solvents, but are insoluble in water. When phospholipids are suspended in an aqueous environment, they tend to form aggregates. Depending upon the type of lipid, the organization can either be in a micellar, bilayer, or hexagonal phase[4-6] (Figure 5). Micelles are spherical structures in which the phospholipids have the polar head groups exposed to water and the nonpolar hydrocarbon tails directed inward. The phospholipid molecules in bilayer structures are oriented such that the hydrocarbon chains are sandwiched between the molecules aggregate into cylindrical structures (Figure 5), with the polar head groups of the phospholipids directed inward, forming aqueous pores with a diameter of 2 nm or larger. From the physiologically occurring phospholipids (Figure 4), phosphatidylethanolamine preferentially adopts the hexagonal phase. Micelles are generally formed from phospholipid with hydrocarbon tails of short chain length or from lysophospholipids which are phospholipid molecules that lack the acyl chain esterified at the 2-position of glycerol. Phospholipids with long hydrocarbon chains (among which are most of the biologically occurring phospholipids) tend to form bilayers, which are generally organized in multilamellar structures called liposomes.

Upon sonication of liposomes, small unilamellar vesicles are obtained with diameters that are less than 50 nm.[53] Single bilayer vesicles are also obtained when solutions of phospho-

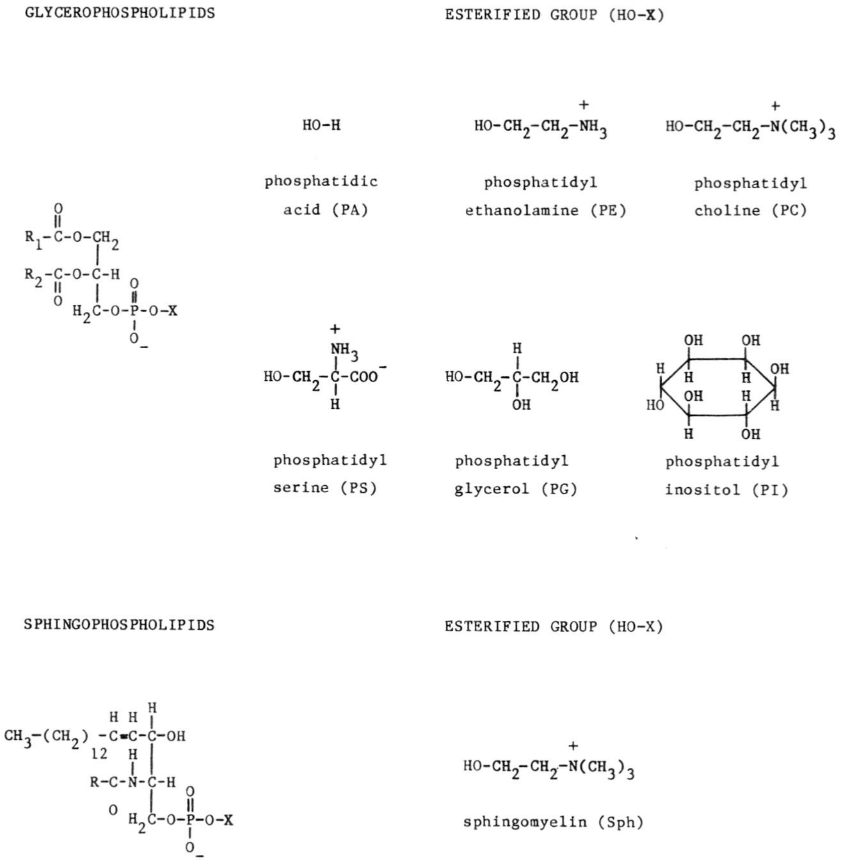

GLYCEROPHOSPHOLIPIDS

ESTERIFIED GROUP (HO-X)

HO-H — phosphatidic acid (PA)

$HO\text{-}CH_2\text{-}CH_2\text{-}\overset{+}{N}H_3$ — phosphatidyl ethanolamine (PE)

$HO\text{-}CH_2\text{-}CH_2\text{-}\overset{+}{N}(CH_3)_3$ — phosphatidyl choline (PC)

$R_1\text{-}C(=O)\text{-}O\text{-}CH_2$ / $R_2\text{-}C(=O)\text{-}O\text{-}C\text{-}H$ / $H_2C\text{-}O\text{-}P(=O)(O^-)\text{-}O\text{-}X$

$HO\text{-}CH_2\text{-}C(H)(\overset{+}{N}H_3)\text{-}COO^-$ — phosphatidyl serine (PS)

$HO\text{-}CH_2\text{-}C(H)(OH)\text{-}CH_2OH$ — phosphatidyl glycerol (PG)

inositol ring (OH, H substituents) — phosphatidyl inositol (PI)

SPHINGOPHOSPHOLIPIDS

ESTERIFIED GROUP (HO-X)

$CH_3\text{-}(CH_2)_{12}\text{-}C(H)=C(H)\text{-}C(H)\text{-}OH$ / $R\text{-}C(=O)\text{-}N(H)\text{-}C\text{-}H$ / $H_2C\text{-}O\text{-}P(=O)(O^-)\text{-}O\text{-}X$

$HO\text{-}CH_2\text{-}CH_2\text{-}\overset{+}{N}(CH_3)_3$ — sphingomyelin (Sph)

FIGURE 4. Chemical structures of biologically occurring phospholipids. Esterification of glycerophospholipid or sphingophospholipid with XOH yields the phospholipids: phosphatidic acid, phosphatidylethanolamine, phosphatidylcholine, phosphatidylserine, phosphatidylglycerol, phosphatidylinositol, and sphingomyeline.

lipids in ethanol[54] or ether[55] are injected into water, or when from a micellar phospholipid suspension in a water-detergent mixture the detergent is slowly removed.[56] Such unilamellar vesicles are commonly used as model membranes in studies of lipid-dependent activation of coagulation factors.

An artificial membrane that is composed of a single type of phospholipid will either be in the liquid crystalline (or fluid) state or in the gel (or solid) state. Such a membrane has a characteristic freezing point at which the phase transition from fluid into gel state occurs. The transition temperature is dependent on the kind of phospholipid (length and degree of saturation of the hydrocarbon tails and nature of the polar head group) that comprises the membrane bilayer. When a membrane contains a mixture of phospholipids with different transition temperatures, phase separations can occur. In that case, phospholipid molecules of the same type may cluster together and form areas with different freezing points. Such processes are, however, uncommon to biological membranes. Due to the fact that biologically occurring phospholipids contain a wide variety of fatty acids with different chain length and degree of saturation, most biological membranes are in the liquid crystalline (fluid) state, and phase separations do usually not occur in vivo. In membranes with homogeneous phospholipid distribution, the association with proteins,[57,58] or the addition of calcium ions[59,60] may, however, cause phase separation of phospholipid molecules. For instance, the addition

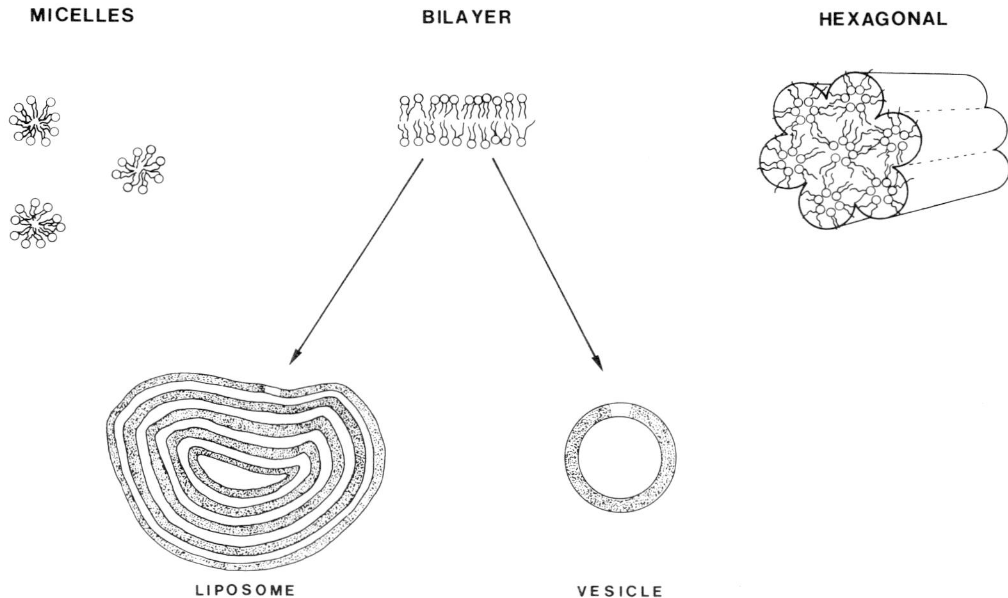

FIGURE 5. Polymorphic phases of phospholipids in aqueous environment.

of calcium ions to mixtures of phosphatidylcholine with phosphatidylserine or phosphatidic acid can induce phase separations between the two types of phospholipid molecules that form the membrane.[59,60] Such lateral phase separations may lead to fusion of vesicles and formation of large bilayer membranes.[61,62]

IV. PHOSPHOLIPID REQUIREMENTS OF COAGULATION FACTOR ACTIVATION

It has been recognized for many years that phospholipids play a crucial role in blood coagulation by accelerating the rate of Factor X and prothrombin activation. Early studies on phospholipid involvement dealt with questions regarding the chemical and physical properties of the phospholipids that were required for coagulant activity. The majority of the information was obtained by studying the clot-promoting activity of different kinds of phospholipid mixtures in coagulation assays. More recently, a better understanding of phospholipid involvement in coagulation factor activation was obtained by studying the binding and activation of purified coagulation factors at chemically and physically well-defined artificial membranes.

In the early investigations the chemical nature of procoagulant phospholipids was still a matter of debate. Both phosphatidylethanolamine[63-65] and phosphatidylserine[66,67] have been proposed to be the phospholipid catalytically active in blood coagulation. Other groups recognized that procoagulant membranes have to contain negatively charged phospholipids and observed that membranes prepared from mixtures of different phospholipids (i.e., phosphatidylserine with phosphatidylcholine or phosphatidylethanolamine) exhibited the highest procoagulant activity.[68-71]

It is now generally accepted that procoagulant membranes indeed must contain negatively charged phospholipids. Procoagulant activity can be obtained with membranes containing phosphatidylserine,[66-77] phosphatidic acid,[72,75-78] phosphatidylglycerol,[74,77] phosphatidylinositol,[78,79] or phosphatidylethanolamine at pH 8 to 9.[64] In 1961, Bangham[80] showed that there is an optimal net negative charge at which the membrane expresses maximal coagulant activity. His observation was later confirmed by Papahadjopoulos et al.[81] and Daemen et al.[72] for mixtures of phosphatidylserine with phosphatidylethanolamine or phosphatidylcholine. More recently, the same conclusions were reached on the basis of kinetic studies of coagulation factor activation in model systems. Pusey and Nelsestuen[82] and van Rijn et al.[77] have shown that the complete prothrombinase complex (Factor Xa, phospholipid, calcium ions, and Factor Va) is maximally active at low mole percentages of phosphatidylserine,[77,82] while in the absence of Factor Va the membranes must contain more phosphatidylserine in order to express optimal prothrombin-converting activity.[77] It is not known whether there are any special requirements with respect to the neutral phospholipids, since as yet there has not been a systematic study of the effect of such phospholipids on the procoagulant activity of membranes.

The activity of procoagulant membranes in coagulation factor activation strongly increases when the membranes are going through a phase transition from the gel state into the liquid-crystalline state. Sterzing and Barton[83] have shown that hydrogenation of a mixture of egg yolk phosphatidylcholine and beef brain phosphatidylserine results in a decrease of the procoagulant activity. Since the hydrogenation of the phospholipids used in the experiments caused a shift in the phase transition temperature from -14 to 72°C, they proposed that the phase transition of lipids effected the procoagulant activity. Tans et al.[84] have subsequently shown that there is indeed a direct correlation between the physical state of the membrane and the clot-promoting activity. Mixtures of dimyristoylphosphatidylserine and dipalmitoylphosphatidylcholine were considerably more active in the liquid-crystalline state than in the gel state. Recently, Higgins et al.[85] have shown that the membrane fluidity does not actually affect the catalytic activity of the prothrombinase complex (i.e., the steady-state rate of the conversion of prothrombin into thrombin), but influences the time required for the assembly of the prothrombinase complex at the procoagulant surface. They suggested that the diminished procoagulant activity of membranes in the gel state is caused by the fact that the prothrombinase complex is more slowly assembled at the surface of such membranes.

The majority of the information regarding the phospholipid requirements of blood coagulation has been obtained from coagulation tests or from assays in which the activity of the prothrombinase complex is determined (vide supra). The phospholipid requirements of the intrinsic Factor X activating complex have been very poorly studied. Most investigations on this complex have been carried out with ill-defined phospholipid mixtures such as brain cephalin and inosithin in assay systems (coagulation tests) that were also dependent upon the participation of the prothrombinase complex. Therefore, these studies do not provide explicit information about the phospholipids required for optimal activity of the intrinsic Factor X activator. The high degree of similarity between the prothrombinase and the intrinsic Factor X-activating complex suggests, however, that many of the observations on the phospholipid requirement of prothrombin activation presumably also apply to intrinsic Factor X activation.

More detailed studies are available on the role of phospholipids in extrinsic Factor X activation. This is likely caused by the fact that the protein cofactor of this complex (tissue factor) is a highly hydrophobic protein that is present in a wide variety of tissue membranes. Crude tissue factor preparations, also called (tissue) thromboplastin, consist of one or more protein components associated with phospholipid. Tissue factor apoprotein is insoluble in water and can only be isolated from tissue material by the use of detergents.[13-15] Purified tissue factor is only active in Factor VIIa-catalyzed Factor X activation when it is reconstituted with phospholipids. In the early days information about the phospholipid requirement of extrinsic Factor X activation was obtained by studying the phospholipid composition of different tissue thromboplastin preparations. It should be emphasized, however, that not all the phospholipids present in such preparations are necessarily involved in the activity of tissue factor. The phospholipid compositions of bovine brain and lung thromboplastin are

Table 1
PHOSPHOLIPID COMPOSITION OF DIFFERENT THROMBOPLASTINS[86]

	Bovine brain (%)[a]	Bovine lung (%)[a]
Phosphatidylethanolamine	15.1	14.8
Phosphatidylcholine	30.3	41.4
Phosphatidylserine	3.0	1.5
Phosphatidylinositol	3.0	1.0
Lysophosphatidylcholine	12.2	2.5
Sphingomyeline	36.3	38.3

[a] Values given are weight percent of the total amount of phospholipid present in the thromboplastin preparation.

presented in Table 1. It is clear that thromboplastin contains a wide variety of phospholipids, and that both negatively charged and neutral phospholipids are present. Although the fraction of negatively charged phospholipids is low, it may still be sufficient to support Factor VIIa-catalyzed Factor X activation. In that respect it should be noted that the prothrombinase complex functions optimally at membranes with a low phosphatidylserine content, provided that the protein cofactor Factor Va is present.[77,82]

More information about the phospholipid requirement of tissue factor was obtained by reconstitution of partially purified (delipidated) tissue factor apoprotein with different phospholipids or phospholipid mixtures.[74,86-90] Although thromboplastin activity could be restored with phosphatidylethanolamine or with phosphatidylcholine,[86,87] it was shown by Wijngaards et al.[74] that optimal activity required phospholipid mixtures that contained 30 to 50% negatively charged phospholipids such as phosphatidylglycerol or phosphatidylserine. It is possible that the activity observed with neutral phospholipid preparations is due to the presence of free fatty acids or a small amount of negatively charged phospholipids still present in the partially purified tissue factor preparations. Recently, highly purified tissue factor preparations were obtained from bovine and human sources, which contained less than 1 mol of phospholipid per mole of tissue factor.[13-15] These preparations exerted maximal activity at phospholipid to protein ratios (w/w) greater than 500. In these studies the phospholipid mixtures contained about 15% phosphatidylserine. It has been shown, however, that both binding of Factors VII and VIIa to the tissue factor-phospholipid complex[91] and Factor X activation by the tissue factor-phospholipid-Factor VIIa complex can occur at membranes which have no net negative charge.[15,92] Binding and Factor X-converting activity are, however, promoted by the presence of negatively charged phospholipids.[91,92]

V. BINDING OF COAGULATION FACTORS TO PHOSPHOLIPID SURFACES

In 1964, Papahadjopoulos and Hanahan[93] suggested that the formation of the prothrombinase complex involves four different components (Factor X_a, Factor V_a, phospholipid, and calcium ions) that interact in a stoichiometric manner and form a lipoprotein complex with maximal activity on prothrombin. Jobin and Esnouf[78] interpreted the stimulatory effect of phospholipids on the rate of prothrombin activation as being due to binding and proper localization of the interacting proteins at the phospholipid surface. Their conclusion was supported by experiments of Hemker et al.[94] who proposed that binding of the proteins to the phospholipid surface results in increased local coagulation factor concentrations, which will facilitate the interactions and reactions between the proteins that participate in prothrombin activation. With respect to the intrinsic Factor X-activating complex[95-98] it has also been suggested that the proteins (Factors X, IXa, and VIIIa) must bind to the phospholipid surface in order to obtain maximal rates of Factor X activation.

Of course, it has been realized that studies on the binding interactions of the coagulation factors with phospholipid membranes will provide essential information with respect to the mechanism of action of procoagulant membranes in coagulation factor activation. Indeed, there are many reports in literature on studies of coagulaiton factor binding to phospholipids. The majority of the binding experiments has been carried out with the proteins of the prothrombinase complex. The initial studies had a qualitative character, since the methods employed to detect binding, i.e., cochromatography of proteins and lipids during gelfiltration[75,76,99-101] or cosedimentation of protein with phospholipid upon centrifugation[76,78,101,102] gave only information as to whether a certain phospholipid preparation did or did not bind the protein. In such studies it was shown that Factor Xa[78,93,101] Factor Va,[75,78,93,101,102] the Factor Xa-Va complex,[75,93,101] and prothrombin[76,78,99,100] bind to phospholipid. Calcium ions are required for the binding of prothrombin, Factor Xa, and the Factor Xa-Va complex, while Factor Va associates with membranes in the absence of calcium.[75,78,93,101] The binding of prothrombin or Factor X is dependent on the presence of negatively charged phospholipids, such as phosphatidylglycerol,[100] phosphatidylserine,[75,76] phosphatidic acid,[75,76,78] or inosithine.[78]

Quantitative data (dissociation constants and binding sites) for the interaction of coagulation factors with well-defined phospholipid membranes were later produced by several laboratories. Since knowledge of such binding parameters is essential for the understanding of the kinetic and mechanistic effects of phospholipids in blood coagulation factor activation, we will discuss these binding studies in more detail below.

A. Binding of Vitamin K-Dependent Coagulation Factors to Phospholipid Membranes

All vitamin K-dependent proteins that participate in blood coagulation (prothrombin, protein C, protein S, and Factors VII, IX, and X) contain so-called γ-carboxyglutamic acid residues that play an important role in the binding of these proteins to phospholipid membranes. Since the vitamin K-dependent coagulant factors only bind in a calcium-dependent manner to membranes that contain negatively charged phospholipids, it is thought that binding occurs through calcium bridges between the γ-carboxyglutamic acid residues of the proteins and the polar head groups of the phospholipid molecules in the membrane surface.

A large number of techniques have been used to determine the binding parameters for the interaction of vitamin K-dependent coagulation factors with various membrane preparations. Bound and free ligands were quantitated by 90° light scattering,[103-107] centrifugation techniques,[91,108,109] gel filtration,[110] ellipsometry,[111,112] enzymatic techniques,[113] surface radioactivity measurements of phospholipid monolayers with bound radiolabeled proteins,[114-116] surface pressure changes of phospholipid monolayers,[116] or fluorescence polarization measurements.[117] There was not only a difference in the techniques used to determine binding parameters, but also different kinds of phospholipid preparations were used in these studies. The binding of vitamin K-dependent proteins to phospholipids was determined with micellar structures,[75] small unilamellar vesicles,[103-107,109,110,113,117] large volume unilamellar vesicles,[108] and planar phospholipid monolayers[111,112,114-116] or multilayers.[111] The binding parameters appear to be a function of pH, ionic strength, calcium concentration, type, and mole fraction of acidic phospholipid in the membrane and also seem to depend on the physical properties of the phospholipid preparation (micelles, monolayers, or vesicles). We will not attempt to give an exhaustive review of all binding parameters reported in literature, but instead present an overview of the effects of membrane structure and membrane composition on the binding parameters of vitamin K-dependent coagulation factors.

Nelsestuen et al.[105] compared the dissociation constants for protein-membrane complexes of various vitamin K-dependent coagulation factors with phospholipid vesicles composed of

Table 2
DISSOCIATION CONSTANTS FOR THE COMPLEXES BETWEEN PHOSPHOLIPIDS AND VITAMIN K-DEPENDENT PROTEINS[105]

Protein	$K_d(M)$
Factor X	0.25×10^{-6}
Prothrombin	0.6×10^{-6}
Factor IX	2×10^{-6}
Factor VII	15×10^{-6}
Protein C	17×10^{-6}

Note: The dissociation constants were determined at 2 m*M* $CaCl_2$ for phospholipid vesicles containing 20 mol% phosphatidylserine and 80 mol% phosphatidylcholine.

20 mol% phosphatidylserine and 80 mol% phosphatidylcholine (Table 2). The affinity of the coagulation factors for these membranes decreases in the order Factor X-prothrombin-protein S-Factor IX-Factor VII-protein C. Activation of the coagulation factors has a negligable effect on the membrane-binding affinity.[105] The affinity differences between Factor X, prothrombin, Factor IX, and Factor VII can also be inferred from other binding studies,[91,113,118] or from the effect of phospholipid vesicles on the kinetic parameters of prothrombin activation[77,119] and intrinsic[120,121] and extrinsic Factor X activation.[122]

1. The Effect of Type and Mole Fraction of Acidic Phospholipids

The type of acidic phospholipid that constitutes the procoagulant membrane is important for the actual values of the binding parameters of vitamin K-dependent coagulation factors. Phosphatidylserine- and phosphatidic acid-containing membranes have approximately the same affinity for coagulation factors,[103] while phosphatidylglycerol[103,113] is less effective in promoting protein-membrane interaction. The binding parameters are also strongly dependent on the mole fraction of acidic phospholipid in the membranes. Membranes which lack acidic phospholipids have no or a very low affinity for vitamin K-dependent coagulation factors. Introduction of acidic phospholipids and increase of the mole fraction causes a gradual decrease of the dissociation constant (increased binding affinity) for prothrombin,[103] as well as Factor X[103,113] (Figure 6). This phenomenon is observed for phosphatidylserine, phosphatidic acid, as well as phosphatidylglycerol. Also, the number of protein binding sites at the surface gradually increases when the amount of negatively charged phospholipid is increased. Between 0 and 25 mol% negatively charged phospholipid there is an almost linear increase in the number of binding sites. At higher mole percentages of acidic phospholipid there is no further increase in the binding capacity of the membrane surface. With some phospholipid preparations there is even a decrease in the number of binding sites at high mole fractions of negatively charged phospholipid (see Figure 6). This loss of binding sites is likely caused by calcium-induced aggregation of phospholipid vesicles.[113] Aggregation does not occur with phospholipid monolayers, hence, with these kinds of phospholipid surfaces it is possible to study binding of coagulation factors at high mole percentages of acidic phospholipid. Mayer et al.[116] reported that the binding parameters (K_d and number

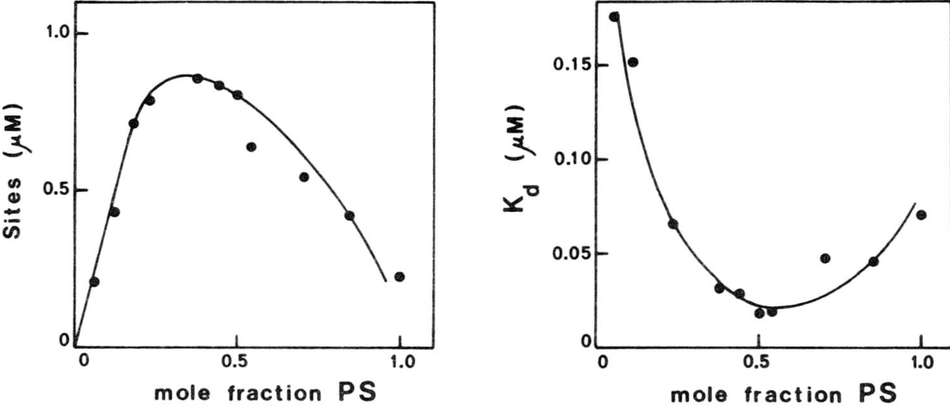

FIGURE 6. The effect of the phosphatidylserine content of vesicles on the binding parameters of Factor X.[113] The number of binding sites (μ*M*/100 μ*M* phospholipid) is plotted in the left graph and the dissociation constant (Kd) of the Factor X-phospholipid complex is plotted in the right graph.

of binding sites) of monolayers containing mole percentages of phosphatidylserine between 0 and 40% were very similar to those of single bilayer vesicles with the same composition. The binding parameters for phospholipid monolayers did not further change when the mole percentage of phosphatidylserine was increased to 80%. However, both Lecompte et al.[114] and Kop et al.[112] observed high affinity binding sites for prothrombin (K_d $8 \times 10^{-9} - 6 \times 10^{-10}$ *M*) at monolayers containing 80 and 100 mol% phosphatidylserine. These monolayers also display a second class of binding sites with much lower affinity ($K_d = 10^{-7}$ *M*) for prothrombin.[112] The binding capacity of phospholipid monolayers for vitamin K-dependent proteins (prothrombin and prothrombin fragment 1) reaches a maximum at about 20 mol% phosphatidylserine.[114,116] Mayer et al.[116] reported that between 0 and 20% phosphatidylserine the binding capacity was proportional with the phosphatidylserine content with a stoichiometry of about eight phosphatidylserine residues per bound protein molecule. This value is in agreement with earlier reported stoichiometries for small unilamellar vesicles.[103] For such membranes it can be calculated that 8 to 10 phosphatidylserine residues (two negative charges/molecule) or 19 phosphatidylglycerol residues (one negative charge/molecule) are required for the binding of one molecule of prothrombin or prothrombin fragment 1,[103,110,116] while 16 phosphatidylserines are required for the binding of Factor X.[113] Since the number of γ-carboxyglutamic acid residues is 10 in prothrombin and prothrombin fragment 1[41,42] and 12 to 14 in Factor X,[11,23,24] this indicates that at the phospholipid surface two negative charges are involved in the calcium-mediated interaction with the two carboxyl groups of γ-carboxyglutamic acid.

For membranes that contain high mole fractions of acidic phospholipid, there is no further increase of the number of binding sites. This saturation is not due to the fact that the membrane surface is fully occupied with protein molecules, since it can be calculated for small single bilayer vesicles[110,113,123] as well as for phospholipid monolayers[112,114,116] that the theoretical number of protein molecules which could be fit on the surface is two to three times higher than that practically observed. This indicates that some theoretical binding sites are sterically excluded.

2. *Molecular Models for Protein-Membrane Association*

The precise molecular interactions responsible for the binding of vitamin K-dependent coagulation factors to negatively charged phospholipids are still a matter of debate. Lecompte and Miller[115] have proposed that prothrombin and prothrombin fragment 1 penetrate into the

Table 3
DISSOCIATION CONSTANTS OF FACTOR Va-PHOSPHOLIPID COMPLEXES

Membrane composition (PS/PC; M/M)[a]	K_d (*M*)	n^b (mol/mol)	Ref.
0/100	No binding	No binding	—
5/95	4.2×10^{-7}	152	125
10/90	2.5×10^{-7}	115	125
15/85	7.1×10^{-8}	80	125
20/80	5.4×10^{-7}	62	107
	4.2×10^{-8}	71	125
	2.7×10^{-11}	250	124
25/75	1.7×10^{-7}	57	126
30/70	2.0×10^{-8}	75	125
	9.0×10^{-8}	120	107

[a] PS = phosphatidylserine, PC = phosphatidylcholine.
[b] n = lipid-to-protein ratio at saturation (mol/mol).

lipid layer, while the group of Nelsestuen argues that binding is not accompanied with protein insertion into the lipid neither with small unilamellar vesicles[123] nor with phospholipid monolayers.[116] Conflicting views also exist as to the nature of the calcium-dependent interaction between the γ-carboxyglutamic acid residues and the polar head groups of the phospholipid molecules in the membrane surface. Dombrose et al.[110] proposed that electrostatic interactions significantly contribute to protein-membrane association, since the binding of prothrombin fragment 1 to phospholipid vesicles containing phosphatidylglycerol is highly ionic strength dependent. A 40- to 100-fold decrease of the association constant was observed when the ionic strength was raised from 0.016 to 0.81 *M*. However, Resnick and Nelsestuen[106] showed that the binding of prothrombin to single bilayer membranes composed of 20% phosphatidylserine and 80% phosphatidylcholine was relatively insensitive to changes of pH and ionic strength. They proposed that the prothrombin-membrane binding can be explained with a chelation model in which calcium forms ionic bridges with the two carboxyl groups of γ-carboxyglutamic acid in the protein and two negative charges of the phospholipid molecule(s) in the membrane.

B. Binding of Protein Cofactors to Phospholipid Membranes

The protein cofactors of the prothrombin- and Factor X-activating complexes also bind with high affinity to phospholipid membranes. In contrast to the vitamin K-dependent coagulation factors, the cofactors do not possess γ-carboxyglutamic acid residues, hence, different interactions will be responsible for protein-membrane association. With respect to membrane binding properties, the most extensively studied protein cofactor is Factor Va. The binding of Factors V and Va to membranes is dependent on the presence of acidic phospholipids.[107,124,125] With phosphatidylserine as negatively charged phospholipid, the binding affinity as well as the number of protein binding sites for Factor Va increased when the amount of phosphatidylserine in the membrane bilayer was increased.[107,124,125]

In Table 3 we have summarized literature values reported for the binding parameters of Factor Va for phospholipid membranes that contain phosphatidylserine. In some of these studies the binding parameters for Factor Va were compared with those of Factor V. Pusey et al.[124] observed that the membrane binding properties of Factor V were similar to those of Factor Va. The group of Mann[107,126] reported, however, that Factor V binds with a four- to six-fold higher affinity than Factor Va to phospholipids and the small unilamellar vesicles employed in their studies did bind about four times more Factor Va than factor V per vesicle.

There are also large discrepancies with respect to the actual value of the K_d of the Factor Va-membrane complex that is observed in different laboratories. At similar experimental conditions Pusey et al.[124] observed a 10^4-fold tighter binding than the group of Mann and a 10^3-fold tighter binding than van de Waart et al.[125] Pusey et al.[124] noted that in their experiments not all unbound Factor Va could equilibrate with bound Factor Va and corrected the dissociation constant for the fraction of protein that did not participate in membrane-protein interaction. They concluded that the binding affinity of Factor Va for phospholipids reported by Bloom et al.[107] and Higgins and Mann[126] is underestimated, since these authors assumed that all unbound protein was in equilibrium with the membrane binding sites and, hence, used the total unbound concentration to calculate dissociation constants. It is questionable, however, whether the argumentation of Pusey et al.[124] is correct, since the experiments of van de Waart et al.[125] yield binding parameters that are similar to those reported by the group of Mann[107,126] and which were calculated from the concentrations of functionally active Factor Va. In the approach of van de Waart et al.,[125] the bound and unbound Factor Va concentrations were obtained after separating phospholipid-bound protein from soluble protein by centrifugation and determination of functionally active Factor Va in both the supernatant and pellet.

Although negatively charged phospholipids are required for the formation of the Factor Va-membrane complex, there is no calcium requirement for this interaction. It should be emphasized, however, that the light and heavy chains of Factor Va remain associated through calcium ions[50,52] and that calcium is required to stabilize membrane-bound Factor Va. Van de Waart et al.[125] even noted that high calcium concentrations inhibited the binding of Factor Va to phospholipid by competing with Factor Va for membrane binding sites.

Pusey et al.[124] and van de Waart et al.[125] observed large effects of ionic strength, pH, and charge density in the membrane on the dissociation constant of the Factor Va-phospholipid complex. Based on these findings, they suggested that Factor Va-phospholipid interaction is primarily the result of ionic (electrostatic) forces. The group of Mann[107] reported, however, that variation of the ionic strength hardly affects the dissociation constant of the Factor Va-phospholipid complex and concluded that the binding is not electrostatic in nature.

Isolated Factor Va consists of two polypeptide chains with M_r 95,000 (Factor Va heavy chain) and M_r 75,000 (Factor Va light chain) which are noncovalently associated in the presence of calcium ions.[50,52] In the presence of EDTA these polypeptides can be separated, and it is possible to study the interaction of the individual heavy and light chains with phospholipid. The heavy chain of Factor Va does not bind to phospholipid,[125,126] while the light chain, which is positively charged at physiological pH, has a high affinity for negatively charged membrane surfaces.[125-127] The binding parameters for the light chain-membrane interaction are similar to those of Factor Va-membrane interaction. This indicates that the light chain of Factor Va contains the peptide domain that is responsible for the binding of Factor Va to membrane surfaces.

Few quantitative data are available on the binding of Factor VIIIa to phospholipid membranes. Most studies deal with qualitative aspects of the binding of more or less purified Factor VIII-von Willebrand complex to phospholipid vesicles. Andersson and Brown[128] and Lajmanovich et al.[129] reported that incubation of the Factor VIII-von Willebrand complex with phospholipid vesicles that were composed of phosphatidylserine mixed with phosphatidylcholine or phosphatidylethanolamine results in the dissociation of the coagulation activity (Factor VIIIc) from the von Willebrand factor activity (Factor VIII R:WF) and binding of the Factor VIIIc moiety to the phospholipid surface. Factor VIIIc appears to have a high affinity for the phospholipid membranes, with a dissociation constant in the nanomolar range.[128] The binding of Factor VIII to phospholipid vesicles is not affected by increasing the ionic strength up to values of 1.0. Dissociation of Factor VIII from the phospholipid

Table 5
THE EFFECT OF PHOSPHOLIPID CONCENTRATION ON THE K_m FOR PROTHROMBIN[119]

Phospholipid conc (μM)	K_m (μM)
4	0.052
8	0.090
16	0.14
40	0.23
80	0.46
240	1.08

Note: Prothrombin was activated in the absence of Factor Va at pH 7.5, 37°C, in the presence of optimal $CaCl_2$ concentrations and phospholipid vesicles containing 50 mol phosphatidylserine and 50 mol% phosphatidylcholine.

minute per mole Factor Xa). Calcium ions hardly affect the K_m and the V_{max}, but phospholipids plus calcium and Factor Va have dramatic effects on the kinetic parameters. Phospholipid vesicles composed of 50% phosphatidylserine and 50% phosphatidylcholine (w/w) drastically decrease the K_m for prothrombin, and Factor Va causes a more than 2000-fold increase of the V_{max}. These effects of phospholipid and Factor Va on the kinetic parameters give an explanation for the physiologic requirement for these cofactors. Since the plasma prothrombin concentration is about 2 μ*M*, it is obvious that phospholipids are required to lower the K_m for prothrombin from a value far above to values considerably below the plasma prothrombin concentration. This assures that under physiological conditions saturation of Factor Xa with the substrate prothrombin is achieved so that Factor Xa can act at maximal catalytic activity. Factor Va subsequently enhances the catalytic capacity of Factor Xa to a level at which thrombin is formed at a rate sufficiently high to account for rapid and efficient thrombus formation.

The value of the K_m for prothrombin determined in the presence of phospholipids appears to be dependent on the amount of phospholipid present in the prothrombin activation mixture. At increasing phospholipid concentrations, increased values for the K_m for prothrombin[119] are observed (Table 5). This effect of phospholipid occurs in the presence as well as in the absence of Factor Va. An important additional effect with both mechanistic and physiologic implications has been observed when phospholipids with different binding affinities for coagulation factors were employed as procoagulant surface in prothrombin activation.[77,82] The binding affinity of phospholipid membranes for coagulation factors can be changed either by variation of mole percentage of negatively charged phospholipid in the membrane or by using different kinds of acidic phospholipids.[103] In Table 6 we have summarized the effects of various kinds of phospholipid vesicles on the kinetic parameters of prothrombin activation in the absence and presence of Factor Va. Changes of the binding parameters of prothrombin and Factor Xa for the phospholipid membranes are reflected in the kinetic

Table 6
KINETIC PARAMETERS OF PROTHROMBIN ACTIVATION FOR MEMBRANES CONTAINING VARIOUS AMOUNTS OF DIFFERENT NEGATIVELY CHARGED PHOSPHOLIPIDS[77]

Membrane phospholipid composition[a] (M/M)	K_m (μ*M*)	V_{max} (IIa/min/Xa)
Without Factor Va		
PS/PC (25/75)	0.11	2.56
PA/PC (25/75)	0.10	2.78
PG/PC (25/75)	1.81	0.17
PS/PC (5/95)	1.63	0.32
With Factor Va		
PS/PC (25/75)	0.14	4050
PA/PC (25/75)	0.11	4184
PG/PC (25/75)	0.04	3345
PS/PC (5/85)	0.057	4330

Note: The kinetic parameters were determined in the absence or presence of 5 n*M* Factor Va at 37°C, pH 7.9, 5 m*M* $CaCl_2$, and 50 μ*M* phospholipid.

[a] PS = phosphatidylserine, PA = phosphatidic acid, PG = phosphatidylglycerol, and PC = phosphatidylcholine.

parameters of prothrombin activation determined in the absence of Factor Va. Membranes with a high affinity for these proteins (vesicles containing a high mole percentage of phosphatidylserine or phosphatidic acid) have the most favorable kinetic parameters (low K_m and high V_{max}), while on membranes with a low affinity for coagulation factors (vesicles containing phosphatidylglycerol or a low mole percentage of phosphatidylserine) prothrombin is activated with a high K_m and a low V_{max}. In the presence of Factor Va there is, however, no correlation between the kinetic parameters of prothrombin activation and the binding affinities of prothrombin and Factor Xa for the membranes that constitute the prothrombinase complex.[77,82] When Factor Va is part of the prothrombinase complex, the V_{max} of prothrombin activation is not affected by the kind and mole percentage of negatively charged phospholipid in the membrane (Table 6). The K_m values determined on membranes with a high affinity for prothrombin are similar to those observed in the absence of Factor Va. However, on low affinity membranes Factor Va causes a drastic decrease of the K_m for prothrombin. Lipid membranes with low phosphatidylserine content or with phosphatidylglycerol, which are reported to have a very low affinity for prothrombin, even have the most favorable K_m for prothrombin. This effect of Factor Va is presumably of physiological significance, since activated blood platelets, which supposedly provide the procoagulant surface for in vivo prothrombin activation, expose a rather low amount of acidic phospholipid.[146]

The observation that membranes with a low affinity for prothrombin have a favorable K_m, provided that Factor Va is present, has important implications for the molecular mechanism by which phospholipids enhance prothrombin activation or, more generally, for the mechanism by which they promote the activation of vitamin K-dependent coagulation factors. These aspects will be discussed in the paragraph on the models for the mechanism of action of phospholipids in coagulation factor activation.

B. Kinetic Parameters of Extrinsic Factor X Activation

The actual effect of phospholipids (plus calcium) on the kinetic parameters of extrinsic

Table 7
KINETIC PARAMETERS OF FACTOR VIIa-CATALYZED ACTIVATION OF FACTOR X

	K_m (μM)	k_{cat} (sec^{-1})
Without tissue factor[a]	4.87	3.95×10^{-4}
With tissue factor		
Bovine brain thromboplastin[a]	0.45	1.15
Tissue factor + PC[b]	0.791	6.2
Tissue factor + PS/PC[b]	0.063	5.8

[a] In these experiments 10 m*M* benzamidine was present. In the absence of tissue factor rabbit brain cephalin was used as phospholipid source. Bovine brain thromboplastin was used as a source of phospholipid and tissue factor apoprotein.[122]

[b] In these experiments 2 μM dansyl-glu-gly-arg-chloromethylketone was present to prevent feedback reactions of Factor Xa. Tissue factor apoprotein was reconstituted with either phosphatidylcholine (PC) or with a mixture of phosphatidylserine (PS) and phosphatidylcholine (30/70; w/w). The K_m value given for PS/PC is based on the concentration of soluble Factor X available for interaction with the Factor VIIa-tissue factor-phospholipid complex.[92]

Factor X activation is not known, since there are as yet no reports of kinetic studies on the activation of Factor X by Factor VIIa in the absence of phospholipids. Silverberg et al.[122] have determined the kinetic parameters of Factor VIIa-catalyzed Factor X activation in the presence of phospholipid or phospholipid-containing tissue factor (Table 7). With rabbit brain cephalin as phospholipid source, they determined a K_m for Factor X of 4.87 μM and a k_{cat} of 3.9×10^{-4} sec^{-1}. In the presence of thromboplastin (crude phospholipid plus tissue factor) the K_m dropped to 0.34 μM and the k_{cat} increased to 32 sec^{-1}. Thus, tissue factor caused a 10-fold decrease of the K_m for Factor X and a 3000-fold increase of the k_{cat} of Factor X activation. It should be emphasized, however, that these kinetic assays were carried out in the presence of 10 m*M* benzamidine to prevent feedback reactions of Factor Xa on Factor X. Hence, it is possible that the K_m is overestimated and that the V_{max} may have been underestimated.[122]

In a recent paper Forman and Nemerson[92] reported the kinetic parameters for a Factor VIIa-tissue factor system containing phospholipid vesicles of pure phosphatidylcholine (Table 7). Although these vesicles did not bind Factor X, they observed a rather low K_m for Factor X (0.791 μM) and a high k_{cat} of Factor X activation (6.2 sec^{-1}). This indicates that the presence of negatively charged phospholipids is not a prerequisite for a membrane to be active in extrinsic Factor X activation.

C. Kinetic Parameters of Intrinsic Factor X Activation

The most extensive kinetic study of intrinsic Factor X activation has been carried out by van Dieijen et al.[120] Using bovine coagulation factors, they have determined the kinetic parameters of Factor IXa-catalyzed Factor X activation in the absence and presence of calcium ions, phospholipids, and Factor VIIIa (Table 8). In the absence of accessory components the K_m for Factor X is 299 μM and the V_{max} of Factor Xa formation is 0.022 mol Xa formed per minute per mole Factor IXa. Calcium ions have little effect on the kinetic parameters, but phospholipids plus calcium cause a dramatic decrease of the K_m for Factor X without having much effect on the V_{max} of the reaction. As in prothrombin activation, the K_m is

Table 8
KINETIC PARAMETERS OF FACTOR X ACTIVATION BY FACTOR IXa[120]

Activator	K_m (μ*M*)	V_{max} (Xa/min/IXa)
IXa	299	0.0022
IXa, Ca^{2+}	181	0.0105
IXa, Ca^{2+}, PL	0.058	0.00247
IXa, Ca^{2+}, VIIIa, PL	0.063	500

Note: Factor X activation was determined at pH 7.9 at 37°C with or without 7.5 m*M* $CaCl_2$, 11 clotting units Factor VIII/mℓ and 10 μM phospholipid (PL) vesicles (phosphatidylserine/phosphatidylcholine, 25/75; mol/mol).

dependent on the amount of phospholipid present and increases at increasing phospholipid concentrations. The complete intrinsic Factor X-activating complex (i.e., Factor IXa, Factor VIIIa, Ca^{2+} ions, and phospholipid) has a low K_m for Factor X and a very high V_{max} of 500 mol of Factor Xa formed per minute per mole of Factor IXa. The 200,000-fold increase of the V_{max} was attributed to the presence of the protein cofactor VIIIa.[120]

Kinetic studies with human blood coagulation factors also yielded unfavorable kinetic parameters (high K_m and low V_{max}) for Factor X activation by Factor IXa alone,[140] low Km values in the presence of negatively charged phospholipids,[134,140,143] and high V_{max} values when Factor VIIIa is part of the intrinsic Factor X-activation complex.[140,142,143] The magnitude of the Factor VIIIa-dependent increase of the catalytic efficiency of Factor IXa reported in these studies is, however, much less than observed by van Dieijen et al.[120,121] This is likely caused by the fact that in the latter case the kinetic parameters were determined at a saturating amount of Factor VIIIa, while suboptimal Factor VIIIa concentrations were used in the studies with human coagulation factors.[140,142,143] It should be further emphasized that, in contrast to van Dieijen et al.[120] who did not observe an effect of Factor VIIIa on the K_m for Factor X, the reports on human Factor X activation showed that Factor VIIIa caused a six- to tenfold decrease of the K_m for Factor X.[134,143] The latter effect might relate mechanistically to the Factor Va-dependent decrease of the K_m for prothrombin observed for procoagulant membranes that have a low affinity for coagulation factors.

VII. MODELS FOR THE MECHANISM OF ACTION OF PHOSPHOLIPIDS IN COAGULATION FACTOR ACTIVATION

It is now generally accepted that phospholipids function in the activation of vitamin K-dependent coagulation factors by providing a surface onto which the participating coagulation factors bind. In 1967 Jobin and Esnouf[78] and Hemker et al.[94] had already proposed that the stimulatory effect of phospholipids on prothrombin activation was the result of binding and proper localization of the proteins at the phospholipid surface, a condition which would facilitate the interactions and reactions between the proteins involved in prothrombin activation. More recent kinetic studies, the results of which were discussed in the previous paragraph, support the notion that the enzymatic unit of the complete prothrombin and Factor X activator consists of a three-component complex (Factor Xa-Factor Va-phospholipid, Factor VIIa-tissue factor-phospholipid, or Factor IXa-Factor VIIIa-phospholipid) that acts on their respective substrates prothrombin and Factor X. It is, however, still a matter of debate which molecular interactions between the coagulation factor-activating complexes and the substrates are essential for the expression of prothrombin- and Factor X-converting activity. Three models have been proposed to explain the stimulatory effect of phospholipids on prothrombin and Factor X activation. These models, which are depicted in Figure 7, can be characterized as follows.

Model 1 is the so-called "bound substrate model", in which it is hypothesized that the phospholipid-bound enzyme-cofactor complex acts on phospholipid-bound substrate.[119,147] In this model the overall substrate density at the phospholipid surface determines the rate of substrate activation. After binding of the substrate to phospholipid, the substrate concentration in a shell surrounding the phospholipid surface will greatly exceed its concentration in free solution. This will facilitate the interaction of substrate with phospholipid-bound enzyme and result in an increased rate of coagulation factor activation.

Model 2 is the so-called "free substrate model", in which the enzymatic unit acts on soluble substrate.[148] The affinity of the enzymatic unit for soluble substrate is determined by the additional free energies of substrate binding to the individual components of the activating complex, i.e., enzyme, protein cofactor, and the phospholipid molecules in the direct environment of the enzyme. The presence of phospholipids in the enzymatic unit is responsible for the increased affinity of the complete complex for its substrate, which explains the acceleration of substrate activation by phospholipid.

Model 3 is the so-called "conformation model" in which the phospholipid-bound enzymatic unit has a conformational state (denoted by an asterisk) that is different from the enzyme molecules in free solution. This conformational change of the enzyme, which is induced by binding to phospholipid, causes an increased affinity for soluble substrate molecules.[92,149]

The conformational model differs from the free substrate model with respect to the kind of interactions that are required for the binding of the substrate to the enzymatic unit. In the free substrate model the interaction of substrate with phospholipid is a prerequisite for the formation of the enzyme-substrate complex, while in the conformational model this interaction is absent and, hence, does not contribute to the binding of the substrate to the enzymatic unit.

The ultimate model for phospholipid involvement in the activation of vitamin K-dependent coagulation factors must explain:

1. The observation that phospholipids cause a 100- to 1000-fold decrease of the K_m for the substrates of the prothrombin-[119] and Factor X-activating complex.[120]
2. That the K_m observed in the presence of phospholipid has an apparent character. (The K_m is low at low phospholipid concentrations and increases again when the amount of phospholipid present in the reaction mixture is increased.[119,120])
3. That the kinetic parameters of the prothrombinase complex do not relate to the binding affinities of prothrombin and Factor Xa for the phospholipid component when Factor Va is present[77,82] (see Table 6) (phospholipid vesicles with a weak affinity for prothrombin have considerably lower K_m values in the presence of Factor Va than in its absence).
4. The observation of Forman and Nemerson[92] that extrinsic Factor X activation exhibits a low K_m for Factor X (0.79 μM) for a tissue factor-Factor VIIa system containing neutral phospholipids that do not bind Factor X.

Observations 1 and 2 actually led to the definition of the bound-substrate model in which the K_m (half-maximal saturation of surface-bound enzyme) is determined by the local concentration of surface-bound substrate. The fact that upon binding of the substrate to phospholipid its concentration at the surface will be higher than that in free solution explains why the K_m is decreased in the presence of phospholipid. Raising the phospholipid concen-

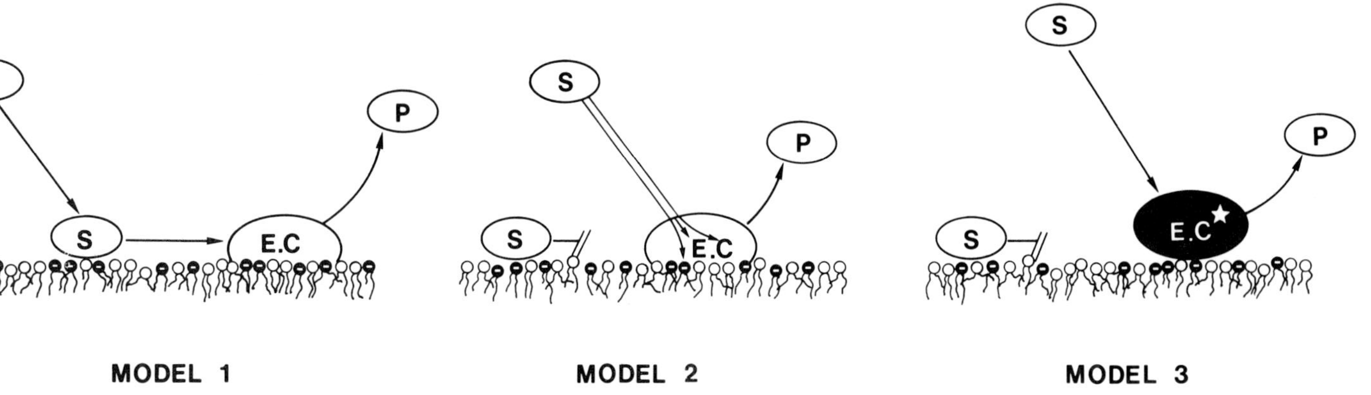

FIGURE 7. Models of the mode of action of phospholipids in the activation of vitamin K-dependent coagulation factors. Model 1 is the bound-substrate model, model 2 is the free-substrate model, and model 3 the conformational model. E = enzyme, C = protein cofactor, S = substrate, and P = product. ✪ denotes conformational change in enzymatic unit and ♀ are negatively charged phospholipid molecules present in the procoagulant surface.

trations results, however, in a decrease of the surface concentration of substrate, hence, more substrate has to be added to maintain the surface concentration required for half saturation of the surface-bound enzyme. Since the experimentally observed K_m (K_m^{app}) is expressed in terms of the total amount of substrate added, the K_m will increase at increasing phospholipid concentration.

The phospholipid-dependent decrease of the K_m can, however, also be explained in the free substrate and in the conformation model, since in both models the enzymatic unit is defined to have an increased affinity for its substrate. Also, the observation that the K_m increases again at high phospholipid concentrations can be fitted into these models, since excess phospholipid will bind substrate outside the enzymatic domain. This will lower the free substrate concentration available for interaction with the enzymatic unit and hence increase the observed K_m

The observation that the K_m for prothrombin of the complete prothrombinase complex (Xa, Va, Ca^{2+}, and phospholipid) does not relate to the binding parameters of prothrombin for the phospholipid component and is not a function of the surface density of prothrombin (observation 3) cannot be readily explained in model 1, but can be rationalized both in the free substrate model and in the conformational model. In these models the interaction of substrate with the phospholipid moiety is less important (free substrate model) or even absent (conformation model). Finally, the fact that extrinsic Factor X activation readily occurs on membranes composed of neutral phospholipids (observation 4) indicates that interaction of substrate with negatively charged phospholipids is not an absolute requirement for the formation of the enzyme-substrate complex. Such a phenomenon can only be explained in the conformational model. Application of this model does, however, raise questions about the purpose and function of the γ-carboxyglutamic acid residues in Factor X. Forman and Nemerson[92] speculate that the γ-carboxyglutamic acid domain may function in a Ca^{2+}-induced conformational change of Factor X (see Reference 150) which may render the cleavage site on Factor X more accessible to Factor VIIa.

Finally, we would like to emphasize that care should be taken in trying to define one unique model for the mechanism of action of phospholipid in three phospholipid-dependent coagulation factor-activating complexes. It is possible that different models for phospholipid involvement apply to the different complexes or even to the same complex dependent on the presence or absence of the protein cofactor. As examples of this, we like to mention that: (1) the prothrombin- and intrinsic Factor X-activating complexes have an absolute requirement for the presence of negatively charged phospholipids, while the extrinsic Factor X activator can apparently also function with neutral phospholipids, and that (2) prothrombin activation by Factor Xa-Ca^{2+}-phospholipid can be adequately explained with the bound-substrate model,[77] while the introduction of Factor Va in this complex results in kinetic observations that require the free substrate model for mechanistic evaluation.[77,82,148] We feel, however, that the experimental observations on a particular complex and the discussions on the hypothetical models will contribute to our knowledge of the other complexes and, hence, will finally result in a precise description of the chemical events which occur during the activation of vitamin K-dependent coagulation factors in the presence of protein cofactors and procoagulant phospholipids.

REFERENCES

1. **Suttie, J. W. and Jackson, C. M.,** Prothrombin structure, activation and biosynthesis, *Physiol. Rev.*, 57, 1, 1977.
2. **Davie, E. W., Fujikawa, K., and Kisiel, W.,** The role of serineproteases in the blood coagulation cascade, *Adv. Enzymol.*, 48, 277, 1979.
3. **Jackson, C. M. and Nemerson, Y.,** Blood coagulation, *Annu. Rev. Biochem.*, 49, 765, 1980.
4. **Cullis, P. R. and de Kruijff, B.,** Lipid polymorphism and the functional roles of lipids in biological membranes, *Biochim. Biophys. Acta*, 559, 399, 1979.
5. **Tilcock, C. P. S.,** Lipid polymorphism, *Chem. Phys. Lipids*, 40, 109, 1986.
6. **Cullis, P. R., Hope, M. J., and Tilcock, C. P. S.,** Lipid polymorphism and the roles of lipids in membranes, *Chem. Phys. Lipids*, 40, 127, 1986.
7. **Drakenberg, T., Fernlund, P., Roepstorff, P., and Stenflo, H.,** Hydroxyaspartic acid in vitamin K-dependent protein C, *Proc. Natl. Acad. Sci. U.S.A.*, 80, 1802, 1983.
8. **McMullen, B. A., Fujikawa, K., and Kisiel, W.,** The occurrence of β-hydroxyaspartic acid in the vitamin K-dependent blood coagulation zymogens, *Biochem. Biophys. Res. Commun.*, 115, 8, 1983.
9. **Church, W. R., Jernigan, R. L., Tode, J., Hewick, R., Knopf, J., Knutson, G. J., Nesheim, M. E., Mann, K. G., and Fass, D. N.,** Coagulation Factors V and VIII and ceruloplasmin constitute a family of structurally related proteins, *Proc. Natl. Acad. Sci. U.S.A.*, 81, 6934, 1984.
10. **Radcliffe, R. and Nemerson, Y.,** The activation and control of Factor VII by activated Factor X and thrombin, *J. Biol. Chem.*, 250, 388, 1975.
11. **DiScipio, R. G. and Davie, E. W.,** Characterization of protein S, a γ-carboxyglutamic acid containing protein from bovine and human plasma, *Biochemistry*, 18, 899, 1979.
12. **Radcliffe, R. and Nemerson, Y.,** The mechanism of activation of bovine Factor VII, *J. Biol. Chem.*, 251, 4797, 1976.
13. **Bach, R., Nemerson, Y., and Koningsberg, W.,** Purification and characterization of bovine tissue factor, *J. Biol. Chem.*, 256, 8324, 1981.
14. **Broze, G. J., Leykam, J. E., Schwarz, B. O., and Miletich, J. P.,** Purification of human brain tissue factor, *J. Biol. Chem.*, 260, 10917, 1985.
15. **Guha, A., Bach, R., Koningsberg, W., and Nemerson, Y.,** Affinity purification of human tissue factor: interaction of Factor VII and tissue factor in detergent micelles, *Proc. Natl. Acad. Sci, U.S.A.*, 83, 299, 1986.
16. **Jackson, C. M.,** Characterization of two glycoprotein variants of bovine Factor X and demonstration that the Factor X zymogen contains two polypeptide chains, *Biochemistry*, 11, 4873, 1972.
17. **Di Scipio, R. G., Hermodson, M. A., Yates, S. G., and Davie, E. W.,** A comparison of human prothrombin, Factor IX (Christmas Factor), Factor X (Stuart Factor), and protein S, *Biochemistry*, 16, 698, 1977.
18. **Di Scipio, R. G., Hermodson, M. A., and Davie, E. W.,** Activation of human Factor X (Stuart factor) by a protease from Russel's viper venom, *Biochemistry*, 16, 5253, 1977.
19. **Titani, K., Fujikawa, K., Enfield, D. L., Ericsson, L. H., Walsh, K. A., and Neurath, H.,** Bovine Factor X_1 (Stuart factor): amino acid sequence of the heavy chain, *Proc. Natl. Acad. Sci. U.S.A.*, 72, 3082, 1973.
20. **Enfield, D. L., Ericsson, L. H., Walsh, K. A., Neurath, H., and Titani, K.,** Bovine Factor X_1 (Stuart factor): primary structure of the light chain, *Proc. Natl. Acad. Sci. U.S.A.*, 72, 16, 1975.
21. **Leytus, S. P., Chung, D. W., Kisiel, W., Kurachi, K., and Davie, E. W.,** Characterization of a cDNA coding for human Factor X, *Proc. Natl. Acad. Sci. U.S.A.*, 81, 3699, 1984.
22. **Fung, M. R., Hay, C. W., and Mac Gillivray, R. T. A.,** Characterization of an almost full-length cDNA coding for human blood coagulation Factor X, *Proc. Natl. Acad. Sci. U.S.A.*, 82, 3591, 1985.
23. **Bucher, D., Nebelin, E., Thomson, J., and Stenflo, J.,** Identification of γ-carboxyglutamic acid residues in bovine Factor IX and X and in a new vitamin K-dependent protein, *FEBS Lett.*, 68, 293, 1976.
24. **Howard, J. B. and Nelsestuen, G. L.,** Isolation and characterization of vitamin K-dependent region of bovine blood clotting factor X, *Proc. Natl. Acad. Sci. U.S.A.*, 72, 1281, 1975.
25. **Leveson, J. E. and Esnouf, M. P.,** The inhibition of activated Factor X with diisopropylfluorophosphate, *Br. J. Haematol.*, 17, 173, 1969.
26. **Radcliffe, R. D. and Barton, P. G.,** The purification and properties of activated Factor X, *J. Biol. Chem.*, 247, 7735, 1972.
27. **Fujikawa, K., Legaz, M. E., Kato, H., and Davie, E. W.,** The mechanism of activation of bovine Factor IX (Christmas factor) by bovine Factor XIa (activated plasma thromboplastin antecedent), *Biochemistry*, 13, 4508, 1974.
28. **Osterud, B., Bouma, B. N., and Griffin, J. H.,** Human blood coagulation Factor IX. Purification, properties and mechanism of activation by activated Factor XI, *J. Biol. Chem.*, 253, 5946, 1978.

29. **Katayama, K., Ericsson, L. H., Enfield, D. L., Walsh, K. A., Neurath, H., Davie, E. W., and Titani, K.,** Comparison of amino acid sequence of bovine coagulation Factor IX (Christmas factor) with that of other vitamin K-dependent plasma proteins, *Proc. Natl. Acad. Sci. U.S.A.,* 76, 4990, 1979.
30. **Kurachi, K. and Davie, E. W.,** Isolation and characterization of a cDNA coding for human Factor IX, *Proc. Natl. Acad. Sci. U.S.A.,* 79, 6461, 1982.
31. **Choo, K. H., Gould, K. G., Rees, D. J. G., and Brownlee, G. G.,** Molecular cloning of the gene for human anti-haemophilic Factor IX, *Nature (London),* 299, 178, 1982.
32. **Tuddenham, E. G. D., Trabold, N. C., Collins, J. A., and Hoyer, L. W.,** The properties of Factor VIII coagulant activity prepared by immunoadsorbent chromatography, *J. Lab. Clin. Med.,* 93, 40, 1979.
33. **Vehar, G. A., Keyt, B., Eaton, D., Rodriguez, H., O'Brein, D. P., Rotblat, F., Opperman, H., Keck, R., Wood, W. I., Harkins, R. N., Tuddenham, E. G. D., Lawn, R. M., and Capon, D.,** Structure of human Factor VIII, *Nature (London),* 312, 337, 1984.
34. **Toole, J. J., Knopf, J. L., Wozney, J. M., Sultzman, L. A., Buecker, J. L., Pittman, D. D., Kaufman, R. J., Brown, E., Shoemaker, C., Orr, E. C., Amphlett, G. W., Foster, W. B., Coe, M. L., Knutson, G. J., Fass, D. N., and Hewick, R. M.,** Molecular cloning of a cDNA encoding human antihaemophilic factor, *Nature (London),* 312, 342, 1984.
35. **Wood, W. I., Capon, D. J., Simonson, C. C., Eaton, D. L., Gitschier, J., Keyt, B., Seeburg, P. H., Smith, D. H., Hollingshead, P., Wion, K. L., Delwart, E., Tuddenham, E. G. D., Vehar, G. A., and Lawn, R. M.,** Expression of active human Factor VIII from recombinant DNA clones, *Nature (London),* 312, 330, 1984.
36. **Rotblat, F., O'Brien, D. P., O'Brien, F. J., Goodall, A. H., and Tuddenham, E. G. D.,** Purification of human Factor VIII:C and its characterization by Western blotting using monoclonal antibodies, *Biochemistry,* 24, 4294, 1985.
37. **Fulcher, C. A., Roberts, J. R., Holland, L. Z., and Zimmerman, T. S.,** Human Factor VIII procoagulant protein. Monoclonal antibodies define precursor-product relationships and functional epitopes, *J. Clin. Invest.,* 76, 117, 1985.
38. **Eaton, D., Rodriguez, H., and Vehar, G. A.,** Proteolytic processing of human Factor VIII. Correlation of specific cleavages by thrombin, Factor Xa, and activated protein C with activation and inactivation of Factor VIII coagulant activity, *Biochemistry,* 25, 505, 1986.
39. **Fass, D. N., Knutson, G. J., and Katzmann, J. A.,** Monoclonal antibodies to porcine Factor VIII coagulant and their use in the isolation of active coagulant protein, *Blood,* 59, 594, 1982.
40. **Magnusson, S., Petersen, T. E., Sottrup-Jensen, L., and Claeys, H.,** Complete primary structure of prothrombin, in *Proteases and Biological Control,* Reich, E., Rifkin, D. B., and Shaw, W., Eds., Cold Spring Harbor Laboratory, Cold Spring Harbor, N.Y., 1975, 123.
41. **Magnusson, S., Sottrup-Jenssen, L., and Petersen, T. E.,** Primary structure of the vitamin K-dependent part of prothrombin, *FEBS Lett.,* 44, 189, 1975.
42. **Walz, D. A., Hewett-Emmett, H. D., and Seegers, W. H.,** Amino acid sequence of human prothrombin fragments 1 and 2, *Proc. Natl. Acad. Sci. U.S.A.,* 74, 1969, 1977.
43. **Esmon, C. T. and Jackson, C. M.,** The conversion of prothrombin into thrombin, IV. The function of the fragment 2 region during activation in the presence of Factor V, *J. Biol. Chem.,* 249, 7791, 1974.
44. **Butkowski, R. J., Elion, J., Downing, M. R., and Mann, K. G.,** Primary structure of human prethrombin 2 and γ-thrombin, *J. Biol. Chem.,* 252, 4942, 1977.
45. **Esmon, C. T., Owen, W. G., and Jackson, C. M.,** The conversion of prothrombin into thrombin. III. The Factor Xa-catalyzed activation of prothrombin, *J. Biol. Chem.,* 249, 7782, 1974.
46. **Rosing, J., Tans, G., Govers-Riemslag, J. W. P., Zwaal, R. F. A., and Hemker, H. C.,** The role of phospholipids and Factor Va in the prothrombinase complex, *J. Biol. Chem.,* 255, 274, 1980.
47. **Rosing, J., Zwaal, R. F. A., and Tans, G.,** Formation of meizothrombin as intermediate in Factor Xa-catalyzed prothrombin activation, *J. Biol. Chem.,* 261, 4224, 1986.
48. **Krishnaswamy, S., Mann, K. G., and Nesheim, M. E.,** The prothrombinase-catalyzed activation of prothrombin proceeds through the imtermediate meizothrombin in an ordered sequential reaction, *J. Biol. Chem.,* 261, 8977, 1986.
49. **Nesheim, M. E. and Mann, K. G.,** Thrombin-catalyzed activation of single chain bovine Factor V, *J. Biol. Chem.,* 254, 1326, 1979.
50. **Esmon, C. T.,** The subunit structure of thrombin-activated Factor V, *J. Biol. Chem.,* 254, 964, 1979.
51. **Suzuki, K., Dahlbäck, B., and Stenflo, J.,** Thrombin-catalyzed activation of human coagulation Factor V, *J. Biol. Chem.,* 257, 6556, 1982.
52. **Hibbard, L. S. and Mann, K. G.,** The calcium binding properties of bovine Factor V, *J. Biol. Chem.,* 255, 638, 1980.
53. **Huang, C.,** Studies on phosphatidylcholine vesicles: formation and physical characteristics, *Biochemistry,* 8, 344, 1969.
54. **Batzri, S. and Korn, E. D.,** Single bilayer liposomes prepared without sonication, *Biochim. Biophys. Acta,* 298, 1015, 1973.

55. **Deamer, D. and Bangham, A. D.,** Large volume liposomes by an ether vaporization method, *Biochim. Biophys. Acta,* 443, 629, 1976.
56. **Brunner, J., Skrabal, P., and Hauser, H.,** Single bilayer vesicles prepared without sonication; physicochemical properties, *Biochim. Biophys. Acta,* 455, 322, 1976.
57. **Birell, G. B. and Griffith, O. H.,** Cytochrome c induced lateral phase separation in a diphosphatidylglycerol steroid-spin-label model membrane, *Biochemistry,* 15, 2925, 1976.
58. **Boggs, J. M., Wood, D. D., Moscarello, M. A., and Papahadjopoulos, D.,** Lipid phase separation induced by a hydrophobic protein in phosphatidylserine-phosphatidylcholine vesicles, *Biochemistry,* 16, 2325, 1977.
59. **Onishi, S. and Ito, T.,** Calcium-induced phase separations in phosphatidylserine-phosphatidylcholine mixtures, *Biochemistry,* 13, 881, 1974.
60. **Ito, T. and Onishi, S.,** Ca^{2+}-induced lateral phase separations in phosphatidic acid-phosphatidylcholine membranes, *Biochim. Biophys. Acta,* 352, 29, 1974.
61. **Papahadjopoulos, D., Poste, G., Schaeffer, D. E., and Vail, W. J.,** Membrane fusion and molecular segregation in phospholipid vesicles, *Biochim. Biophys. Acta,* 352, 10, 1974.
62. **Jacobson, H. and Papahadjopoulos, D.,** Phase transitions and phase separations in phospholipid membranes induced by changes in temperature, pH and concentration of bivalent cations, *Biochemistry,* 14, 152, 1975.
63. **Rouser, G., White, S. G., and Schloredt, D.,** Phospholipid structure and thromboplastic activity. I. The phosphatide fraction active in recalcified normal human plasma, *Biochim. Biophys. Acta,* 28, 71, 1958.
64. **Wallach, D. F. H., Maurice, P. A., Steele, B. B., and Surfenor, D. M.,** Studies on the relationship between the colloidal state and clot-promoting activity of pure phosphatidylethanolamines, *J. Biol. Chem.,* 234, 2829, 1959.
65. **Turner, D. L., Holburn, R. R., De Sipin, M., Silver, M. J., and Tocantins, L. M.,** Thromboplastic activity of phosphatidylethanolamine from natural and synthetic sources, *J. Lipid Res.,* 4, 52, 1963.
66. **Troup, S. B. and Reed, C. F.,** Platelet thromboplastic factor. Its chemical nature, in vitro activity and the identification of similar thromboplastic substances in red blood cells, *J. Clin. Invest.,* 37, 937, 1958.
67. **Marcus, A. J.,** The role of lipids in blood coagulation, *Adv. Lipid Res.,* 4, 1, 1966.
68. **Rapport, M. M.,** Activation of phospholipid thromboplastin by lecithin, *Nature,* 178, 591, 1956.
69. **Troup, S. B., Reed, C. F., Marinetti, G. V., and Swisler, S. N.,** Thromboplastic factors in platelets and red blood cells: observations on their chemical nature and function in in vitro coagulation, *J. Clin. Invest.,* 39, 342, 1960.
70. **Hecht, E. and Slotta, K. H.,** The chemical nature of the lipid activator in blood coagulation, *Am. J. Clin. Pathol.,* 37, 126, 1962.
71. **Grisdale, P. J. and Okany, A.,** Phospholipids. II. A correlation of chemical structure with thromboplastic activity, *Can. J. Biochem.,* 43, 1465, 1965.
72. **Daemen, F. J. M., van Arkel, C., Hart, H. C., van der Drift, C., and van Deenen, L. L. M.,** Activity of synthetic phospholipids in blood coagulation. *Thromb. Diath. Haemorrh.,* 13, 194, 1965.
73. **Walsh, P. N.,** Different requirements for intrinsic factor-Xa forming activity and platelet factor 3 activity and their relationship to platelet aggregation and secretion, *Br. J. Haemtol.,* 40, 311, 1978.
74. **Wijngaards, G., van Deenen, L. L. M., and Hemker, H. C.,** Reconstitution and lipid requirements of porcine tissue thromboplastin, *Biochim. Biophys. Acta,* 488, 161, 1977.
75. **Subbaiah, P. V., Bajwa, S. S., Smith, C. M., and Hanahan, D. J.,** Interactions of the components of the prothrombinase complex, *Biochim. Biophys. Acta,* 444, 131, 1976.
76. **Bull, R. K., Jevons, S., and Barton, P. G.,** Complexes of prothrombin with calcium ions and phospholipids, *J. Biol. Chem.,* 247, 2747, 1972.
77. **van Rijn, J. L. M. L., Govers-Riemslag, J. W. P., Zwaal, R. F. A., and Rosing, J.,** Kinetic studies of prothrombin activation: effect of Factor Va and phospholipids on the formation of the enzyme-substrate complex, *Biochemistry,* 23, 4557, 1984.
78. **Jobin, F. and Esnouf, M. P.,** Studies on the formation of the prothrombin-converting complex, *Biochem. J.,* 102, 666, 1967.
79. **Varadi, K. and Hemker, H. C.,** Kinetics of the formation of the Factor X activating enzyme of the blood coagulation system, *Thromb. Res.,* 8, 303, 1976.
80. **Bangham, A. D.,** A correlation between surface charge and coagulant action of phospholipids, *Nature,* 192, 1197, 1961.
81. **Papahadjopoulos, D. P., Hougie, C., and Hanahan, D. J.,** Influence of surface charge of phospholipids on their clot promoting activity, *Proc. Soc. Exp. Biol. Med.,* 111, 412, 1962.
82. **Pusey, M. L. and Nelsestuen, S. L.,** The physical significance of K_m in the prothrombinase reaction, *Biochem. Biophys. Res. Commun.,* 114, 526, 1983.
83. **Sterzing, P. R. and Barton, P. G.,** The influence of cholesterol on the activity of phospholipids in blood coagulation: requirement for a liquid-crystalline lipid phase, *Chem. Phys. Lipids,* 10, 137, 1973.

84. **Tans, G., van Zutphen, H., Comfurius, P., Hemker, H. C., and Zwaal, R. F. A.,** Lipid phase transitions and procoagulant activity, *Eur. J. Biochem.*, 95, 449, 1979.
85. **Higgins, D. L., Callahan, P. J., Prendergast, F. G., Nesheim, M. E., and Mann, K. G.,** Lipid mobility in the assembly and expression of the activity of the prothrombinase complex, *J. Biol. Chem.*, 260, 3604, 1985.
86. **Liu, D. T. H. and McCoy, L. E.,** Phospholipid requirements of tissue thromboplastin in blood coagulation, *Thromb. Res.*, 7, 213, 1975.
87. **Nemerson, Y. and Pitlick, F. A.,** Purification and characterisation of the protein component of tissue factor, *Biochemistry,* 9, 5105, 1970.
88. **Bjorklid, E. and Storm, E.,** Purification and some properties of the protein component of tissue thromboplastin from human brain, *Biochem. J.*, 165, 89, 1977.
89. **Gonmori, H. and Takeda, Y.,** Properties of human tissue thromboplastins from brain, lung arteries and placenta, *Thromb. Haemoastis,* 36, 99, 1976.
90. **Howell, R. M. and Rezvan, H.,** Circular dichroic, infrared and other studies on the protein component of pig brain thromboplastin, *Biochem. J.*, 189, 209, 1980.
91. **Bach, R., Gentry, R., and Nemerson, Y.,** Factor VII binding to tissue factor in reconstituted phospholipid vesicles: induction of cooperativity by phosphatidylserine, *Biochemistry,* 25, 4007, 1986.
92. **Forman, S. D. and Nemerson, Y.,** Membrane-dependent coagulation reaction is independent of the concentration of phospholipid-bound substrate: fluid phase Factor X regulates the extrinsic system, *Proc. Natl. Acad. Sci. U.S.A.*, 83, 4675, 1986.
93. **Papahadjopoulos, D. and Hanahan, D. J.,** Observations on the interaction of phospholipids and certain clotting factors in prothrombin activator formation, *Biochim. Biophys. Acta,* 90, 436, 1964.
94. **Hemker, H. C., Esnouf, M. P., Hemker, P. W., Swart, A. C., and MacFarlane, R. G.,** Formation of prothrombin converting activity, *Nature,* 215, 248, 1967.
95. **Lundblad, R. L. and Davie, E. W.,** The activation of Stuart factor (Factor X) by activated antihemophilic factor (activated Factor VIII), *Biochemistry,* 4, 113, 1965.
96. **McFarlane, R. G., Biggs, R., Ash, B. J., and Denson, K. W. E.,** The interaction of Factors VIII and IX, *Br. J. Haematol.*, 10, 530, 1964.
97. **Hemker, H. C. and Kahn, M. J. P.,** Reaction sequence of blood coagulation, *Nature,* 215, 1201, 1967.
98. **Barton, P. G.,** Sequence theories of blood coagulation re-evaluated with reference to lipid-protein interactions, *Nature,* 215, 1508, 1967.
99. **Barton, P. G. and Hanahan, D. J.,** Some lipid-protein interactions involved in prothrombin activation, *Biochim. Biophys. Acta,* 187, 319, 1969.
100. **Jackson, C. M., Owen, W. G., Gitel, S. N., and Esmon, C. T.,** The chemical role of lipids in prothrombin conversion, *Thromb. Diath. Haemorrh.*, 57(Suppl.), 273, 1974.
101. **Cole, E. R., Koppel, J. L., and Olwin, J. H.,** Phospholipid-protein interactions in the formation of the prothrombin activator, *Thromb. Diath. Haemorrh.*, 14, 431, 1965.
102. **Kandall, C. L., Shohet, S. B., Akinbami, T. K., and Colman, R. W.,** Determinants of the formation and activity of Factor V-phospholipid complexes. II. Molecular properties of the complexes, *Thromb. Diath. Haemorrh.*, 34, 271, 1975.
103. **Nelsestuen, G. L. and Broderius, M.,** Interaction of prothrombin and blood-clotting Factor X with membranes of varying composition, *Biochemistry,* 16, 4172, 1977.
104. **Nelsestuen, G. L. and Lim, T. K.,** Equilibria involved in prothrombin- and blood-clotting Factor X-membrane binding, *Biochemistry,* 16, 4177, 1977.
105. **Nelsestuen, G. L., Kisiel, W., and di Scipio, R. G.,** Interaction of vitamin K dependent proteins with membranes, *Biochemistry,* 17, 2134, 1978.
106. **Resnick, R. M. and Nelsestuen, G. L.,** Prothrombin-membrane interaction. Effects of ionic strength, pH and temperature, *Biochemistry,* 19, 3028, 1980.
107. **Bloom, J. W., Nesheim, M. E., and Mann, K. G.,** Phospholipid-binding properties of bovine Factor V and Factor Va, *Biochemistry,* 18, 4419, 1979.
108. **van der Waart, P., Hemker, H. C., and Lindhout, T.,** Interaction of prothrombin with Factor Va-phospholipid complexes, *Biochemistry,* 23, 2838, 1984.
109. **Mertens, K., Cupers, R., van Wijngaarden, A., and Bertina, R. M.,** Binding of human blood-coagulation factors IXa and X to phospholipid membranes, *Biochem. J.*, 223, 599, 1984.
110. **Dombrose, F. A., Gitel, S. N., Zawalich, K., and Jackson, C. M.,** The association of bovine prothrombin fragment 1 with phospholipid, *J. Biol. Chem.*, 254, 5027, 1984.
111. **Cuypers, P. A., Corsel, J. W., Janssen, M. P., Kop, J. M. M., Hermens, W. Th., and Hemker, H. C.,** The adsorption of prothrombin to phosphatidylserine multilayers quantitated by ellipsometry, *J. Biol. Chem.*, 258, 2426, 1983.
112. **Kop, J. M. M., Cuypers, P. A., Lindhout, T., Hemker, H. C., and Hermens, W. Th.,** The adsorption of prothrombin to phospholipid monolayers quantitated by ellipsometry, *J. Biol. Chem.*, 259, 13993, 1984.

113. **van Dieijen, G., Tans, G., van Rijn, J., Zwaal, R. F. A., and Rosing, J.,** Simple and rapid method to determine the binding of blood coagulation Factor X to phospholipid vesicles, *Biochemistry,* 20, 7096, 1981.
114. **Lecompte, M. F., Miller, I. R., Elion, J., and Benarous, R.,** Interaction of prothrombin and its fragments with monolayers containing phosphatidylserine. I. Binding of prothrombin and its fragment 1 to phosphatidylserine-containing monolayers, *Biochemistry,* 19, 3434, 1980.
115. **Lecompte, M. F. and Miller, I. R.,** Interaction of prothrombin and its fragments with monolayers containing phosphatidylserine. II. Electrochemical determination of lipid layer perturbation by interacting prothrombin and its fragments, *Biochemistry,* 19, 3439, 1980.
116. **Mayer, L. D., Nelsestuen, G. L., and Brockman, H. L.,** Prothrombin association with phospholipid monolayers, *Biochemistry,* 22, 316, 1983.
117. **Nesheim, M. E., Kettner, C., Shaw, E., and Mann, K. G.,** Cofactor dependence of Factor Xa incorporation into the prothrombinase complex, *J. Biol. Chem.,* 256, 6537, 1981.
118. **Beals, J. M. and Castellino, F. J.,** The interaction of bovine Factor IX, its activation intermediate Factor IX and its activation products Factor IXaα and Factor IXaβ with acidic phospholipid vesicles of various compositions, *Biochem. J.,* 236, 861, 1986.
119. **Rosing, J., Tans, G., Govers-Riemslag, J. W. P., Zwaal, R. F. A., and Hemker, H. C.,** The role of phospholipids and Factor Va in the prothrombinase complex, *J. Biol. Chem.,* 255, 274, 1980.
120. **van Dieijen, G., Tans, G., Rosing, J., and Hemker, H. C.,** The role of phospholipid and Factor VIIIa in the activation of bovine Factor X, *J. Biol. Chem.,* 256, 3433, 1981.
121. **van Dieijen, G., van Rijn, J. L. M. L., Govers-Riemslag, J. W. P., Hemker, H. C., and Rosing, J.,** Assembly of the intrinsic Factor X activating complex — interactions between Factor IXa, Factor VIIIa and phospholipid, *Thromb. Haemostasis,* 52, 396, 1985.
122. **Silverberg, S. A., Nemerson, Y., and Zur, M.,** Kinetics of the activation of blood coagulation Factor X by components of the extrinsic pathway, *J. Biol. Chem.,* 252, 8481, 1977.
123. **Lim, T. K., Bloomfield, V. A., and Nelsestuen, G. L.,** Structure of prothrombin- and blood-clooting Factor X-membrane complexes, *Biochemistry,* 16, 4177, 1977.
124. **Pusey, M. L., Mayer, L. D., Jason Wei, G., Bloomfield, A., and Nelsestuen, G. L.,** Kinetic and hydrodynamic analysis of blood clotting Factor V-membrane binding, *Biochemistry,* 21, 5262, 1982.
125. **van de Waart, P., Bruls, H., Hemker, H. C., and Lindhout, T.,** Interaction of bovine blood clotting Factor Va and its subunits with phospholipid vesicles, *Biochemistry,* 22, 2427, 1983.
126. **Higgins, D. L. and Mann, K. G.,** The interaction of bovine Factor V and Factor V-derived peptides with phospholipid vesicles, *J. Biol. Chem.,* 258, 6503, 1983.
127. **Pusey, M. L. and Nelsestuen, G. L.,** Membrane binding properties of blood coagulation Factor V and derived peptides, *Biochemistry,* 23, 6202, 1984.
128. **Andersson, L.-O. and Brown, J. E.,** Interaction of Factor VIII-von Willebrand factor with phospholipid vesicles, *Biochem. J.,* 200, 161, 1981.
129. **Lajmanovich, A., Hudrey-Clergeon, G., Freyssinet, J. M., and Margueri, G.,** Human Factor VIII procoagulant activity and phospholipid interaction, *Biochim. Biophys. Acta,* 678, 132, 1981.
130. **Andersson, L.-O., Phuc Thuy, L., and Brown, J. E.,** Affinity chromatography of coagulation Factors II, VIII, IX, and X on matrix-bound phospholipid vesicles, *Thromb. Res.,* 23, 481, 1981.
131. **Nesheim, M. E., Eid, S., and Mann, K. G.,** Assembly of the prothrombinase complex in the absence of prothrombin, *J. Biol. Chem.,* 256, 9874, 1981.
132. **Nesheim, M., Taswell, J. B., and Mann, K. G.,** The contribution of bovine Factor V and Factor Va to the activity of prothrombinase, *J. Biol. Chem.,* 254, 10952, 1979.
133. **Lindhout, T., Govers, Riemslag, J. W. P., van de Waart, P., Hemker, H. C., and Rosing, J.,** Factor Va-Factor Xa interaction. Effects of phospholipid vesicles of varying composition, *Biochemistry,* 21, 5494, 1982.
134. **Griffith, M. J., Reisner, H. M., Lundblad, R. L., and Roberts, H. R.,** Measurement of human Factor IXa activity in an isolated Factor X activation system, *Thromb. Res.,* 27, 289, 1982.
135. **Svendsen, L., Blomback, B., Blomback, M., and Olsen, P.,** Synthetic chromogenic substrates for determination of tryspin, thrombin, and thrombin-like enzymes, *Thromb. Res.,* 1, 267, 1972.
136. **Aurell, L., Friberger, P., Karlsson, G., and Claeson, G.,** A new sensitive and highly specific chromogenic peptide substrate for Factor Xa, *Thromb. Res.,* 11, 595, 1977.
137. **Lottenberg, R., Christensen, U., Jackson, C. M., and Coleman, P. L.,** Assay of coagulation proteases using peptide chromogenic and fluorogenic substrates, *Methods Enzymol.,* 80, 341, 1982.
138. **Nesheim, M. E., Prendergast, F. G., and Mann, K. G.,** Interactions of a fluorescent active-site directed inhibitor of thrombin: dansylarginine-*N*-(3-ethyl-1,5-pentanediyl)amide, *Biochemistry,* 18, 996, 1979.
139. **Zur, M. and Nemerson, Y.,** Radiometric assays for blood coagulation factors, *Methods Enzymol.,* 80, 237, 1982.
140. **Mertens, K. and Bertina, R. M.,** The contribution of Ca^{2+} and phospholipids to the activation of human

blood coagulation Factor X by activated Factor IX, *Biochem. J.*, 223, 607, 1984.

141. **Morrision, S. A.,** Kinetics of activation of human prothrombin. Use of a fluorescein-labeled derivative to obtain kinetic constants as a function of Factor V concentration and activation state, *Biochemistry,* 22, 4053, 1983.
142. **Mertens, K., van Wijngaarden, A., and Bertina, R. M.,** The role of Factor VIII in the activation of human blood coagulation Factor X by activated Factor IX, *Thromb. Hameostasis,* 54, 654, 1985.
143. **Hultin, M. B.,** Role of human Factor VIII in Factor X activation, *J. Clin. Invest.*, 69, 950, 1982.
144. **Link, R. P. and Castellino, F. J.,** Kinetic comparison of bovine blood coagulation Factors IXaα and IXaβ toward bovine Factor X, *Biochemistry,* 22, 4033, 1983.
145. **Kosow, D. P. and Orthner, C. L.,** Kinetics of the activation of human prothrombin by human coagulation Factor Xa, *J. Biol. Chem.*, 254, 9448, 1979.
146. **Bevers, E. M., Comfurius, P., van Rijn, J. L. M. L., Hemker, H. C., and Zwaal, R. F. A.,** Generation of prothrombin-converting activity and the exposure of phosphatidylserine at the outer surface of platelets, *Eur. J. Biochem.*, 122, 429, 1982.
147. **Nesheim, M. E., Tracy, R. P., and Mann, K. G.,** "Clotspeed", a mathematical simulation of the functional properties of prothrombinase, *J. Biol. Chem.*, 259, 1447, 1984.
148. **Nelsestuen, G. L.,** Interactions of vitamin K-dependent proteins with calcium ions and phospholipid membranes, *Fed. Proc. Fed. Am. Soc. Exp. Biol.*, 37, 2621, 1978.
149. **van Rijn, J. L. M. L., Zwaal, R. F. A., Hemker, H. C., and Rosing, H.,** Role of accessory components in the activation of vitamin K-dependent coagulation factors, *Haemostasis,* 16, 216, 1986.
150. **Nelsestuen, G. L., Broderius, M., and Martin, G.,** Role of γ-carboxyglutamic acid. Cation specificity of prothrombin and Factor X-phospholipid binding, *J. Biol. Chem.*, 251, 6886, 1976.

Chapter 8

ROLE OF PLATELETS IN FACTOR X AND PROTHROMBIN ACTIVATION

Edouard M. Bevers and Robert F. A. Zwaal

TABLE OF CONTENTS

I. INTRODUCTION

Normal hemostasis requires a mutual interaction between platelets and coagulation factors present in plasma. Bleeding caused upon vessel wall injury is efficiently ceased by a plug of aggregated platelets which is formed rapidly when platelets contact subendothelial structures. The simultaneously initiated coagulation process leads to the formation of insoluble fibrin strands, reinforcing the primary hemostatic plug to a stable thrombus. Platelets are intimately involved in several steps of the coagulation pathway. Moreover, thrombin formed in the final stage of coagulation is considered to be the most potent platet activator. The interplay between platelets and coagulation factors, therefore, plays an essential role in the hemostatic process.

Platelets contain several proteins involved in the coagulation process either as activators or as inhibitors. These proteins are located predominantly in the storage granules and can be released upon platelet activation. Although the level of these proteins is rather low compared to their plasma concentration, one should bear in mind that these proteins are released from a platelet aggregate. Since this will lead to a much higher local concentration of these proteins, their relative importance in coagulation could become significant. Platelet storage proteins, including those involved in coagulation, have been reviewed elsewhere and will — apart from factor V — not be discussed in this chapter.

Binding of coagulation proteins to cell surfaces forms an important mechanism in the regulation of the coagulation process. Binding may lead to modification of the activity of enzymes or proenzymes or may facilitate a proper aposition of enzyme and substrate. In particular, platelets are suitable for binding of coagulation factors probably because the ability to aggregate provides an additional means to rapidly increase the total surface area at those sites where coagulation is required.

The platelet surface has procoagulant properties, but also regulates certain anticoagulant reactions in hemostasis. Inactivation of serine proteases in coagulation by plasma protease inhibitors such as antithrombin III (ATIII) can be regulated through binding of these proteases to the platelet surface.[1] For instance, binding of factor Xa to phospholipids present in the platelet surface protects this protein from inactivation by ATIII.[2,3] On the other hand, the increased activity of platelet-bound activated protein C which activates factors Va and VIIIa might provide an important negative feedback mechanism in the coagulation cascade.[4,5] Moreover, it was shown recently that platelets also contain protein S, which upon release acts as an accessory component to activated protein C.[6] One of the earliest observations of the stimulating effects of platelets in the coagulation process was the shortening of the clotting time of plasma initiated by Russell's viper venom, which activates factors X and V.[7] This probably most powerful procoagulant activity of platelets, previously termed platelet factor 3 (PF3), reflects the contribution of platelets in the activation of prothrombin to thrombin by a complex of factors Xa and Va. Similarly, platelets also stimulate the intrinsic factor X activation by a complex of factors IXa and VIIIa. Since both reactions occur in sequence, the presence of platelets causes a large amplification of the overall process in which thrombin is formed. Both procoagulant activities of platelets are normally unavailable in the circulating intact platelet, but become unmasked when platelets are activated by specific stimuli. This chapter will focus on these two procoagulant activities of platelets and describes the conditions for expression, as well as the nature, of these activities.

II. PHOSPHOLIPIDS AS A CATALYTIC SURFACE FOR FACTOR X AND PROTHROMBIN ACTIVATION

As early as 1954, Bell and Alton[8] reported that the platelet component in the thromboplastin generation test can be replaced by phospholipids. Later it was found that not a certain phospholipid class was responsible for the clot-promoting activity in vitro, but that negatively charged phospholipids such as phosphatidylserine, phosphatidylinositol, phosphatidylglycerol, or phosphatidic acid in a mixture with neutral phospholipids like phosphatidylcholine or phosphatidylethanolamine form an essential part of a procoagulant phospholipid surface.[9-11] More insight into the function of phospholipids on prothrombin and intrinsic factor X activation was obtained from kinetic studies by Rosing et al.[12] and van Dieijen et al.[13] (see Chapter 3).

In summary, phospholipids decrease the K_M for prothrombin and factor X to values below the physiological concentrations in the plasma. The effect can best be explained by the increased local concentration of coagulation factors resulting from the binding to the phospholipid surface. This binding is accomplished through a Ca^{2+}-mediated interaction between the negatively charged γ-carboxyglutamic acid residues of the vitamin K-dependent coagulation factors (IX, X, and prothrombin) and the polar headgroups of the negatively charged phospholipids.[14] As to the role of the accessory components, factors Va and VIIIa, it was found that the major effect was on the k_{cat} of both reactions, which were dramatically increased. With respect to factor Va, the increased turnover number of prothrombin activation can be explained by at least two different effects: an increase in one of the forward rate constants of the reaction[12] and an increased affinity of factor Xa for phospholipids in the presence of factor Va.[15]

III. PLATELET PROTHROMBIN- AND FACTOR X-CONVERTING ACTIVITY

A. Assay System

Prothrombin-converting activity of platelets can be measured in a one-stage prothrombinase assay, using delipidated plasma and Russell's viper venom to activate factors X and V. Although the assay as such can be made dependent on the presence of procoagulant phospholipids, release and activation of factor V from the platelet granules might significantly contribute to a reduction in the clotting time.[16] Moreover, the rectangular hyperbolic relationship between the clotting time and the concentration of procoagulant phospholipid hampers a clear interpretation of the results. In particular, minor cell lysis which is inevitable in platelet handling may give rise to serious misinterpretation of the data. Furthermore, factor X activation has to be measured in a two-stage clotting assay, introducing additional pitfalls. Better results are, therefore, obtained from a spectrophotometric method using specific chromogenic substrates to measure factor Xa and thrombin.[17,18] In this assay, washed platelets are incubated with highly purified coagulation factors in the presence of Ca^{2+} ions. The incubation conditions are chosen to meet kinetic requirements; rates of thrombin or factor Xa formation are linear in time and proportional to the amount of (platelet)-phospholipids. This implicates that exogenous factor Va is added in the prothrombinase assay to rule out any contribution of endogenous platelet factor V. Samples from the incubation mixture are transferred to a cuvette containing a buffer with EDTA to stop the reaction. Factor Xa and thrombin are determined spectrophotometrically, using specific chromogenic substrates. The amount of factor Xa or thrombin formed is calculated using calibration curves made with known amounts of active site-titrated factor Xa or thrombin.

B. Activity of Nonstimulated Platelets

A direct relationship between the rate of prothrombin activation and the amount of Factor Xa bound to platelets was first demonstrated by Miletich and co-workers.[19] Binding of ^{125}I-labeled factor Xa to platelets was shown to be specific, reversible, and saturable and was enhanced in the presence of factor Va, which could be provided either by the platelets through activation with thrombin or added exogenously.[20] Binding of factor Xa and concomitant thrombin formation were inhibited by antifactor V Fab fragments, as well as by an acquired antibody to factor V.[21,22] Impaired factor Xa binding to platelets from patients with congenital factor V deficiency could be restored by addition of the supernatant of thrombin-stimulated normal platelets. Tracy et al.[22] showed that factors Xa and Va bind to platelets in a stoichiometric 1:1 complex. Nesheim and co-workers[15] demonstrated that factor Va promotes the binding of factor Xa to phospholipid, with an apparent dissociation constant of the same order of magnitude as observed for the binding of factor Xa to platelet-bound factor Va. Moreover, similar specific activities for factor Xa were found when plasma factor Va plus phospholipids were substituted by activated platelets.

Approximately 200 to 300 high-affinity binding sites for factor Xa are present at human platelets (Kd 30 to 70 p*M*).[24] From equilibrium studies, the number of factor Va binding sites was estimated at 2000 to 3000. This difference in the number of binding sites led to the suggestion that some other platelet component is limiting the binding of factor Xa. However, it cannot be excluded that a limiting concentration of either factor Xa or Va or both was used in this study. In contrast, 800 to 900 high-affinity sites for factor Va (Kd 400 p*M*) and a similar number of factor Xa binding sites (Kd 600 p*M*) were found for bovine platelets, indicating that all high-affinity bound factor Va participates in factor Xa binding.[22,25]

In an indirect manner, the number of functional factor Xa-Va binding sites could be calculated from the rate of thrombin formation in the presence of platelets, using conditions approaching saturating concentrations of factors Xa, Va, and prothrombin.[18] Assuming the same turnover number for prothrombinase as found in the presence of phospholipids, Rosing et al. calculated a number of 2550 sites for prothrombinase complexes present at the outer surface of nonstimulated human platelets. This number is in agreement with the number of factor Va binding sites obtained from equilibrium binding studies.[24] Similar to the calculation of the number of functional factor Xa-Va binding sites, Rosing et al. found about 920 binding sites for the factor X-activating complex composed of factors IXa and VIIIa.[18] Data from direct binding studies with these coagulation factors are not available at present. The difference in binding sites for factor X activation and prothrombin activation does not necessarily mean that we are dealing with two sites of different nature at the platelet surface, but may reflect differences in optimal phospholipid requirement for both complexes. Moreover, it was found that the prothrombinase activity at the platelet surface can be inhibited by factors VIIIa and IXa, while the factor X activation is inhibited by factors Va and Xa.[18] This mutual competition strongly suggests the involvement of similar binding sites at the platelet outer surface involved in factor X and prothrombin activation.

Finally, it should be emphasized that the number of binding sites for both complexes could be an overestimation due to a minor amount of lysed cells present in all platelet preparations. On the other hand, partial "activation" of the platelets as might occur either during circulation in vivo or upon isolation may also increase the number of binding sites.

C. The Nature of the Binding Sites for Factor X- and Prothrombin-Activating Complexes

High-affinity binding of factor Xa to platelets requires the presence of factor Va.[15,24] For this reason, factor Va was defined as the receptor for factor Xa at the platelet surface, although this does not conform to the classical concept of a membrane receptor. However, factor Va is not exclusively responsible for the high-affinity binding of factor Xa. Des-(1-44)-factor Xa is a modified form of factor Xa which lacks the N-terminal 44 amino acid residues containing the γ-carboxyglutamic acid residues.[24,26,27] The enzymatic activity of this modified protein towards prothrombin, as well as the affinity to factor Va in solution, is virtually unchanged compared to native factor Xa. Nevertheless, it was demonstrated that des-(1-44)-factor Xa has a 100-fold lower affinity than factor Xa for platelet-associated factor

Table 1
EFFECT OF PLATELETS IN PROTHROMBIN AND INTRINSIC FACTOR X ACTIVATION

Platelet activator	Prothrombin activation (nM IIa · min^{-1})	Factor X activation (nM Xa · min^{-1})
None	34	2
ADP (10 μ*M*)	36	2
Thrombin (2 n*M*)	40	3
Collagen (10 μg/mℓ)	98	18
Collagen + thrombin	351	47
A23187 (1 μ*M*)	843	94

Va. Moreover, Skogen and co-workers[28] found that the rate of thrombin formation by des-(1-44)-factor Xa is 300-fold less than that measured with factor Xa in a system of phospholipids and factor Va. In 1983, Dahlbäck and co-workers[29] isolated a particular lupus antibody specific for negatively charged phospholipids and showed that this antibody completely blocks prothrombinase activity in the presence of platelets as well as phospholipids. These observations indicate the importance of negatively charged phospholipids for the activation of prothrombin at the platelet surface. This notion was supported by the finding that both the prothrombinase activity and factor X-activating activity of nonactivated platelets are destroyed by the action of phospholipases.[18,30] The abolishment of both procoagulant activities cannot be observed with phospholipases that do attack membrane phospholipids, but are unable to degrade phosphatidylserine. In addition, proteolytic treatment of unstimulated platlets did not affect the ability to stimulate the two coagulation reactions. Further evidence for phospholipid as the major determinant of the binding sites for the prothrombin- and factor X-activating complexes came from a patient with a moderately severe bleeding disorder.

In conclusion, the data indicate that the binding sites for both complexes of factors Xa-Va and factors IXa-VIIIa are not essentially different from each other and predominantly consist of negatively charged phospholipids at the outer surface of the platelet. Although the major negatively charged phospholipid-phosphatidylserine is confined mainly to the inner leaflet of the platelet membrane, the presence of minor amounts of this lipid in the outer surface cannot be excluded.[17,31-33]

D. Activity of Stimulated Platelets

Table 1 shows the factor X- and prothrombin-converting activities of human platelets after stimulation by a variety of agonists. Prothrombin-converting activity is measured in the presence of excess exogenous factor Va to rule out any contribution of endogenous factor V(Va) which can be released from the alpha-granules by some of the different stimulators. Consistent with the binding data of Kane et al.[20] and Miletich et al.,[21] no significant rise in prothrombinase- or factor X-converting activity is seen upon stimulation with thrombin. This suggests that activation with thrombin, which causes the platelets to release granule contents and to aggregate, hardly results in the formation of additional binding sites for prothrombin- or factor X-activating complexes. Other platelet agonists such as ADP, epinephrine, arachidonic acid, platelet activating factor (PAF), or serotonin are also without effect on the two procoagulant activities. However, rates of thrombin and factor X activation are substantially increased in the presence of platelets stimulated by collagen. This effect of collagen on platelets can be amplified by the simultaneous action of thrombin, producing a 10-fold rate enhancement of prothrombin activation and a 20-fold increase in rate of factor Xa formation. Similar increase in prothrombin-converting activity of platelets simultaneously activated by collagen and thrombin has been reported by Blajchman and co-workers[34] and Ellis and co-workers.[1] Tracy et al. could not find an effect of collagen plus thrombin on the platelet prothrombin-converting activity, possibly due to significant differences in experimental conditions which did not allow optimal platelet activation.[35]

Although vessel wall injury *in situ* inevitably leads to action of collagen and thrombin on circulating platelets, it still remains unclear why two of the most potent stimuli are required simultaneously to evoke optimal procoagulant activity. The increased levels of prothrombin- or factor X-converting activity observed with collagen plus thrombin-stimulated platelets cannot be found with increased concentrations of either one of these stimuli separately. This might suggest that thrombin potentiates the effect of collagen or vice versa, in such a way that a final result is obtained which differs from the effect of each trigger separately. The active center of thrombin is required to enhance the effect of collagen on the procoagulant activity of platelets, because DIP-thrombin (thrombin blocked by diisopropylfluorophosphate) is unable to replace thrombin in combined action with collagen.[36] Thrombin can be substituted by γ-thrombin, trypsin, and to a lesser extent by α-clostripain, but not by chymotrypsin and thermolysin, suggesting the requirement of a specific proteolytic event in conjunction with the action of collagen. Whether or not this indicates the necessity of a rapid and specific hydrolysis of glycoprotein V remains to be established.[37,38] The most potent platelet stimulator with respect to the capacity of platelets to promote factor X and prothrombin activation is Ca^{2+}-ionophore A23187. This nonphysiological platelet activator evokes 60 to 70% of the maximal procoagulant activity that is observed with completely lysed platelets, presumably representing a situation where the maximal amount of procoagulant phospholipids is exposed to the coagulation factors.

The increased prothrombin- and factor X-converting activities obtained after various platelet treatments are almost completely abolished upon subsequent treatment with phospholipase A_2 from *Najanaja*.[18] This indicates that the additionally exposed sites for prothrombin- and factor X-activating complexes are also determined predominantly by phospholipids. Furthermore, it should be noted that the binding sites can be considered to be associated with the cell surface, since the procoagulant activity cosediments with the platelets at 7000 $\times$ *g* for 5 min. Since both procoagulant activities were measured under saturating conditions approaching maximal velocities of factor X and prothrombin conversion, the increase in enzymatic activity upon stimulation is proportional to the increase in functional binding sites at the platelet surface. Assuming that productive enzyme-substrate complexes are formed only at the platelet surface and have the same catalytic efficiency as observed in the presence of phospholipid vesicles, the number of functional binding sites can be calculated directly from the observed rates of thrombin or factor Xa formation. Thus, the highest state of activation by physiological stimuli, i.e., collagen plus thrombin, would represent some 26, 120 binding sites for the complex of factors Xa and Va and about 19,000 sites for the complex of factors IXa and VIIIa. The relatively small difference in the number of sites presumably reflects differences in optimal phospholipid requirement for factor Xa-Va and factor IXa-VIIIa complexes.

IV. RELATION BETWEEN CHANGES IN SURFACE PHOSPHOLIPID COMPOSITION AND PROCOAGULANT ACTIVITY OF PLATELETS

From the foregoing, it will be clear that platelet phospholipids play an essential role in the assembly of the factor X- and prothrombin-activating complexes at the membrane surface. The large difference in procoagulant activity between resting platelets and stimulated platelets suggests that stimulation is accompanied by alterations in the structural organization of the plasma membrane phospholipids. This was indeed demonstrated using phospholipases as a tool to establish the distribution of the various phospholipid classes in both leaflets of the platelet plasma membrane before and after stimulation.[17,31] It appeared that an increased

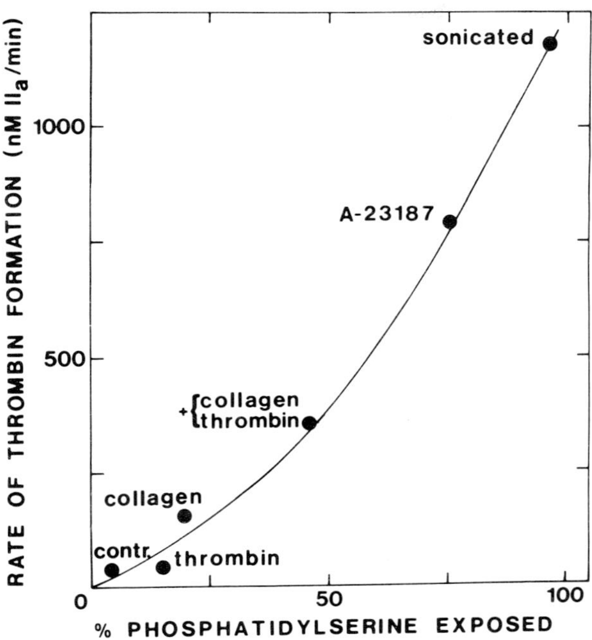

FIGURE 1. Relationship between prothrombin-converting activity and phosphatidylserine exposure at the surface of human platelets. Different activation procedures are indicated in the figure.

procoagulant activity was accompanied by a progressive loss of the asymmetric distribution of phospholipids in the platelet membrane. (A detailed discussion of these observations is given in the next chapter.) With respect to the platelet procoagulant activity, it is important to consider the distribution of the negatively charged phospholipids in the plasma membrane, in particular phosphatidylserine (phosphatidylinositol plays a minor role as procoagulant lipid in platelets).

Figure 1 shows the relationship between the prothrombinase activity and the amount of phosphatidylserine that is exposed at the platelet surface under varying conditions. The almost exclusive localization of phosphatidylserine in the inner monolayer of the plasma membrane of nonstimulated platelets is reflected by the large difference in prothrombinase activity between intact cells and lysed platelets. Various platelet treatments result in increasing amounts of phosphatidylserine exposed at the outer surface and a corresponding increase in prothrombinase activity. A similar correlation is observed between phosphatidylserine exposure and factor X-converting activity. The nonlinearity of the relationship might be caused by the modulating effect of other phospholipids on both procoagulant activities. For instance, sphingomyelin, which is less exposed at the outer surface upon stimulation of platelets with collagen plus thrombin (or diamide, or A23187), has an inhibitory effect on the conversion of prothrombin and factor X (unpublished observation). A modulating effect of phosphatidylethanolamine on both procoagulant activities has also been found. Therefore, a precise relation between the alterations in phospholipid composition of the outer leaflet of the platelet membrane and the procoagulant activity is extremely complicated.

At this point it is important to note that the platelet release reaction is accompanied by an increase in phospholipid content and possibly also a change in phospholipid composition of the plasma membrane due to fusion with the granule membranes. However, no significant increase in phosphatidylserine exposure or corresponding prothrombinase (or factor X-converting) activity is observed upon stimulation with thrombin, although the extent of granule release is similar to that found with the combined action of collagen and thrombin. Moreover, treatment of platelets with diamide completely blocks the release reaction, but evokes the same prothrombinase activity as observed with collagen plus thrombin.[31]

V. INHIBITION OF PLATELET PROCOAGULANT ACTIVITY

Expression of procoagulant activity by collagen plus thrombin is inhibited after pretreatment of the platelet suspension with prostacyclin or dibutyryl-cAMP.[39] In contrast, aspirin treatment in vitro appeared to be ineffective, which excludes the involvement of thromboxane A_2 in the development of procoagulant activity.

Stimulation of platelets by collagen plus thrombin or by ionophore A23187 in the presence of EDTA significantly inhibits the exposure of a procoagulant surface.[40] This suggests that either extracellular Ca^{2+} is required or that intracellular Ca^{2+}, which is directly or indirectly necessary for the changes in the plasma membrane, is drained from the cytoplasma by the extracellular bulk of EDTA. Using A23187 in a Ca^{2+}-buffered system, platelet procoagulant activity was measured as a function of the extracellular Ca^{2+} concentration. Under the assumption that the ionophore equilibrates the intra- and extracellular Ca^{2+} concentrations of the platelets, the minimal intracellular Ca^{2+} concentration required to evoke platelet procoagulant activity was estimated to be 10 to 15 μM.[41] Another indication for the importance of intracellular Ca^{2+} comes from the observation that platelets loaded with the intracellular Ca^{2+} indicator (and chelator) Quin-2 exhibit a diminished procoagulant activity upon stimulation with collagen plus thrombin.[41]

Inhibition of exposure of procoagulant activity by specific interference with the platelet-collagen interaction was found with a synthetic octapeptide derived from collagen.[42] Half-maximal exposure of platelet prothrombin converting activity, evoked either by collagen alone or by combined action of collagen plus thrombin, requires octapeptide concentrations of 0.5 and 0.9 m*M*, respectively, suggesting a modifying effect of thrombin on the platelet collagen interaction. Octapeptide is unable to prevent the generation of procoagulant activity by A23187.

Platelet prothrombin-converting activity and, by extension, also platelet factor X-converting activity can be inhibited also by β_2-glycoprotein I (apoprotein H) from human plasma.[43] A preferential interaction of this protein with negatively charged phospholipids has been demonstrated and is likely to be responsible for its inhibiting effect on platelets. β_2-glycoprotein I does not prevent the expression of procoagulant activity induced by collagen plus thrombin or by A23187, but causes a time-dependent inhibition once the procoagulant surface has been generated. This led to the assumption that β_2-glycoprotein I plays a regulatory role in hemostasis by acting in a feedback-like manner, gradually inhibiting the prothrombinase activity of activated platelets in order to prevent a persisting activity over longer periods of time.

VI. PLATELET PROCOAGULANT ACTIVITY IN HEREDITARY PLATELET DISORDERS

Further understanding in the role of various platelet structures or functions involved in the development of a procoagulant surface was obtained from studies on patients with hereditary disorders of platelet function.[44] The gray platelet syndrome is a bleeding disorder characterized by the absence of α-granules as visualized by electron microscopy and by a deficiency of specific α-granule proteins, including factor V.[45-47] Procoagulant activity of these platelets measured at saturating concentrations of coagulation factors did not differ significantly from normal platelets, either in the resting state or activated by collagen plus thrombin. Similarly, no significant differences in procoagulant activity were found between normal platelets and storage pool-deficient platelets which lack most of their dense bodies (Hermansky-Pudlak syndrome). These observations led to the conclusion that neither release of α-granules nor release of dense bodies forms a prerequisite for the expression of a procoagulant platelet surface. This finding is consistent with the notion outlined earlier that the negatively charged phosphatidylserine is not brought to the outer surface during the fusion between granule and plasma membrane as a result of the release reaction.[31]

Platelets from patients with Glanzmann's Thrombasthenia are almost completely devoid of glycoproteins IIb and III.[48-50] The complex between these two glycoproteins is generally considered to be the receptor for fibrinogen.[51-53] The absence of this membrane glycoprotein complex is the primary cause of the impaired platelet aggregation and defective clot retraction responsible for the observed prolongation of the bleeding time.[37] Although thrombasthenic platelets also failed to aggregate upon stimulation with collagen plus thrombin, normal development of procoagulant activity was found. Also, in the nonactivated state the procoagulant activity of thrombasthenic platelets did not differ from that of normals. This allowed the conclusion that aggregation is not required, and glycoproteins IIb and III are not involved in the expression of platelet procoagulant activity.[44]

Increased procoagulant activities were found for platelets from patients with Bernard-Soulier syndrome.[44] This was particularly manifested in the procoagulant activity of nonstimulated platelets, which appeared to be approximately tenfold higher than found for normal platelets measured at the same platelet concentration.[54,55] Bernard-Soulier platelets are predominantly characterized by the large size and the absence of membrane glycoproteins Ib, V, and IX.[56-59] Although glycoprotein Ib is considered to be the high-affinity binding site for thrombin and glycoprotein V, the surface substrate that is cleaved by thrombin,[37] the procoagulant activity can still be increased upon treatment with thrombin, though to a somewhat smaller extent than in normal platelets. Maximal procoagulant activity after stimulation by collagen plus thrombin is only twofold larger than for normal platelets. This probably reflects the increased size (and, hence, increased surface area) of the Bernard-Soulier platelets. The difference in size, however, is not sufficient to explain the increased activity of the nonstimulated Bernard-Soulier platelets. More likely, the increased basal procoagulant activity of these platelets is related to an increased exposure of phosphatidylserine and phosphatidylethanolamine together with a diminished exposure of sphingomyelin at the outer surface of the plasma membrane.[60] It is tempting to speculate that glycoproteins Ib, V, or IX or a combinaiton of these proteins is involved somehow in the maintenance of the phospholipid asymmetry of the plasma membrane. However, an altered phospholipid orientation in Bernard-Soulier platelets might reflect also a partially activated state of the platelets induced during circulation, caused by a possible increased susceptibility towards activators. This might be caused by the increased platelet size. In this respect, it is of interest to mention that a positive relationship between platelet procoagulant activity and platelet size has been observed in a number of patients with diabetes mellitus.[61]

In 1985 Nieuwenhuis and co-workers[62] described a patient with a hemorrhagic disorder and excessively prolonged bleeding time. Coagulation studies were normal and von Willebrands disease was excluded, but the patient's platelets were totally unresponsive to collagen. This defect appeared to be associated with a marked reduction in the glycoprotein Ia content of the platelets. Normal physiological responses were seen with several other platelet agonists. Procoagulant activity of the nonstimulated platelets from this patient was normal. However, stimulation by collagen plus thrombin resulted only in a minor increase in procoagulant activity, which was comparable to the increased activity observed upon stimulation with thrombin alone. In contrast, stimulation of these platelets with A23187 evoked a normal increase in procoagulant activity, indicating that the mechanism of expression of a procoagulant platelet surface is not impaired.

An isolated deficiency of platelet procoagulant activity was found in a patient with a moderately severe bleeding disorder, known as Scott Syndrome, which was first described by Weiss et al. in 1979.[63] The only abnormalities found were an impaired prothrombin consumption test, a decreased platelet factor 3 availability, and, as demonstrated by Miletich and co-workers,[64] a decreased number of factor Xa-Va binding sites at the patient's platelets.[64] No abnormalities were found in platelet factor V content nor in phospholipid content or composition of the platelets. Initially, it was proposed that these platelets lack a specific receptor protein for factor Va which mediates the high affinity binding of factor Xa to platelets. However, Rosing et al.[65] demonstrated that the number of functional binding sites for both the factor Xa-Va complex and the factor IXa-VIIIa complex were significantly decreased. Platelet activation by thrombin plus collagen revealed a lower exposure rate and lower final level of prothrombin- and factor X-converting activity in the patient's platelets. Moreover, it was demonstrated that the patient's platelets showed a diminished exposure of phosphatidylserine at the outer surface upon activation with collagen plus thrombin. This strongly suggests that the combined impairment of prothrombin- and factor X-converting activity in this patient is due to a defect in the mechanism by which phosphatidylserine becomes exposed at the surface of stimulated platelets (see also Chapter 7).

VII. CONCLUDING REMARKS

Two sequential reactions in blood coagulation — activation of factor X and activation of prothrombin — are enhanced significantly in the presence of a negatively charged phospholipid surface. A similar enhancement of prothrombin and factor X conversion is observed when phospholipids are substituted by a suspension of lysed platelets, since the negatively charged phospholipid phosphatidylserine is almost exclusively located at the cytoplasmic side of the plasma membrane, being exposed upon lysis. This asymmetric distribution of phosphatidylserine also explains the low rates of factor X and prothrombin-conversion observed for intact platelets. Stimulation by collagen plus thrombin, Ca ionophore, or treatment with diamide increases both procoagulant activities of platelets. The increased activities are not a consequence of increased platelet lysis, but are the result of an increased exposure of phosphatidylserine at the outer surface of the stimulated platelets. As will be discussed in the following chapter, exposure of phosphatidylserine is presumably due to an increased transbilayer movement of phospholipids, which tends to randomize the different phospholipid classes over both leaflets of the plasma membrane. A model explaining the appearance of platelet prothrombin converting activity upon stimulation by collagen plus thrombin is schematically depicted in Figure 2. The release reaction as such does not evoke a significant increase in procoagulant activity as seen, for instance, upon stimulation with thrombin. However, in a system without exogenous factor Va, thrombin-induced release and subsequent activation of endogenous factor V from the α-granules will significantly contribute to an increase in prothrombin-converting activity.

Expression of a procoagulant surface requires Ca^{2+}, as will be discussed in the following chapter. Prostacyclin or dibutyryl-cAMP can prevent the generation of a procoagulant surface which reflects interference with the stimulus-response coupling mechanism. Direct interference with the agonist-receptor interaction is observed with a synthetic octapeptide derived from collagen, which inhibits expression of procoagulant activity induced by collagen plus thrombin, but is without effect when Ca ionophore is used as a stimulus. Once a procoagulant platelet surface has been developed, β_2-glycoprotein I can act as an inhibitor by binding to the platelet surface.

Studies with pathological platelets have shown that neither release of α-granules or dense bodies nor aggregation is essential to provoke procoagulant activity. The increased phosphatidylserine exposure in resting Bernard-Soulier platelets and the diminshed exposure of this lipid upon stimulation of Scott syndrome platelets are in good agreement with the

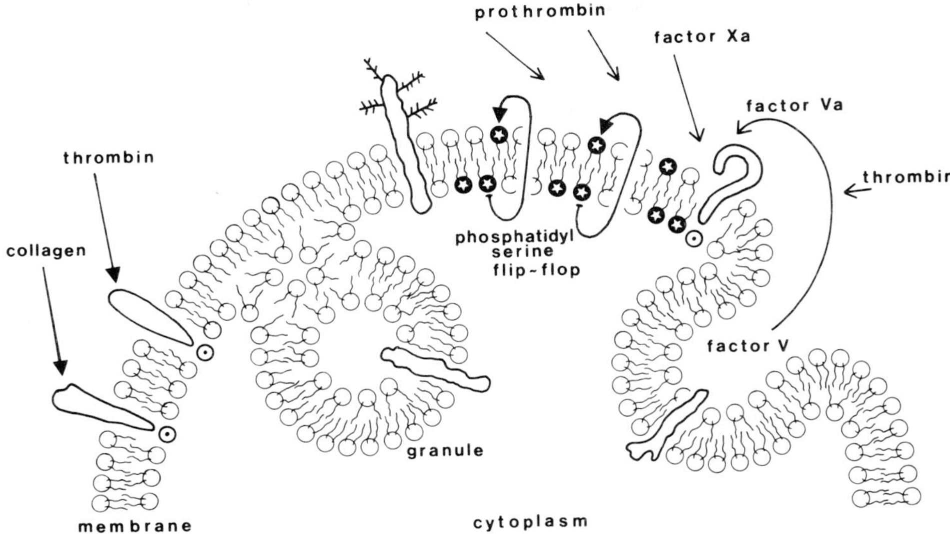

FIGURE 2. Appearance of platelet prothrombin-converting activity. Simultaneous action of collagen and thrombin initiates the platelets to release the granule contents. Among the components liberated from the α-granules is factor V, which is immediately converted to factor Va by the action of thrombin. Factor Va enhances the binding of factor Xa to the platelet surface. In addition, an increased transbilayer movement of phospholipids, induced by the simultaneous action of collagen and thrombin, tends to randomize the different phospholipid classes over both leaflets of the plasma membrane. This results in an increased exposure of phosphatidylserine, thus creating a negatively charged phospholipid surface, which enables an increased number of prothrombinase complexes to be formed at the platelet surface.

observed alterations in procoagulant activities of these abnormal platelets. A detailed description of the alterations in the platelet membrane during stimulation and a discussion of the possible mechanisms involved are presented in the following chapter.

REFERENCES

1. **Ellis, V., Scully, M. F., and Kakkar, V. V.,** Inhibition of prothrombinase complex by plasmaproteinase inhibitors, *Biochemistry,* 23, 5882, 1984.
2. **Marciniak, E.,** Factor Xa activation by antithrombin III. Evidence for biological stabilization of factor Xa by factor V-phospholipid complex, *Br. J. Haematol.,* 24, 391, 1973.
3. **Walker, F. J. and Esmon, C. T.,** The effects of phospholipid and factor Va on the inhibition of factor Xa by antithrombin III, *Biochem. Biophys. Res. Commun.,* 90, 641, 1979.
4. **Stenflo, J.,** Structure and function of protein C, *Sem. Thromb. Haemostasis,* 10, 109, 1984.
5. **Harris, K. W. and Esmon, C. T.,** Protein S is required for bovine platelets to support activated protein C binding and activity, *J. Biol. Chem.,* 260, 2007, 1985.
6. **Schwarz, H. P., Heeb, M. J., Wencel-Drake, J. D., and Griffin, J. H.,** Identification and quantitation of protein S in human platelets, *Blood,* 66, 1452, 1985.
7. **Zwaal, R. F. A.,** Membrane and lipid involvement in coagulation, *Biochim. Biophys. Acta,* 515, 163, 1978.
8. **Bell, W. N. and Alton, H. G.,** A brain extract as a substitute for platelet suspensions in the thromboplastin generation test, *Nature,* 174, 880, 1954.
9. **Bangham, A. D.,** A correlation between surface charge and coagulant action of phospholipids, *Nature,* 192, 1197, 1961.
10. **Papahadjopoulos, D. P., Hougie, C., and Hanahan, D. J.,** Influence of surface charge of phospholipids on their clot promoting activity, *Proc. Soc. Exp. Biol. Med.,* 111, 412, 1962.

11. **Daemen, F. J. M., van Arkel, C., Hart, H. C., van der Drift, C., and van Deenen, L. L. M.,** Activity of synthetic phospholipids in blood coagulation, *Thromb. Diath. Haemorrh.*, 13, 194, 1965.
12. **Rosing, J., Tans, G., Govers-Riemslag, J. W. P., Zwaal, R. F. A., and Hemker, H. C.,** The role of phospholipids and factor Va in the prothrombinase complex, *J. Biol. Chem.*, 255, 274, 1980.
13. **van Dieijen, G., Tans, G., Rosing, J., and Hemker, H. C.,** The role of phospholipid and factor VIIIa in the activation of bovine factor X, *J. Biol. Chem.*, 256, 3433, 1981.
14. **Suttie, J. W. and Jackson, C. M.,** Prothrombin structure, activation and biosynthesis, *Physiol. Rev.*, 57, 1, 1977.
15. **Nesheim, M. E., Taswell, J. B., and Mann, K. G.,** The contribution of bovine factor V and factor Va to the activity of prothrombinase assay, *Haemostasis,* 12, 268, 1982.
16. **Bevers, E. M., Comfurius, P., Hemker, H. C., and Zwaal, R. F. A.,** On the clot-promoting activity of human platelets in a one-stage prothrombinase assay, *Haemostasis,* 12, 268, 1982.
17. **Bevers, E. M., Comfurius, P., van Rijn, J. L. M. L., Hemker, H. C., and Zwaal, R. F. A.,** Generation of prothrombin-converting activity and the exposure of phosphatidylserine at the outer surface of platelets, *Eur. J. Biochem.*, 122, 429, 1982.
18. **Rosing, J., van Rijn, J. L. M. L., Bevers, E. M., van Dieijen, G., Comfurius, P., and Zwaal, R. F. A.,** The role of activated human platelets in prothrombin and factor X activation, *Blood,* 65, 319, 1985.
19. **Miletich, J. P., Jackson, C. M., and Majerus, P. W.,** Interaction of coagulation factor Xa with human platelets, *Proc. Natl. Acad. Sci. U.S.A.*, 74, 4033, 1977.
20. **Kane, W. H., Lindhout, M. J., Jackson, C. M., and Majerus, P. W.,** Factor Va-dependent binding of factor Xa to human platelets, *J. Biol. Chem.*, 255, 1170, 1980.
21. **Miletich, J. P., Jackson, C. M., and Majerus, P. W.,** Properties of the Xa binding site on human platelets, *J. Biol. Chem.*, 253, 6908, 1978.
22. **Tracy, P. B., Nesheim, M. E., and Mann, K. G.,** Coordinate binding of factor Va and factor Xa to the unstimulated platelet, *J. Biol. Chem.*, 256, 743, 1981.
23. **Miletich, J. P., Majerus, D. W., and Majerus, P. W.,** Patients with congenital factor V deficiency have decreased factor Xa binding sites on their platelets, *J. Clin. Invest.*, 62, 824, 1978.
24. **Kane, W. H. and Majerus, P. W.,** The interaction of human coagulation factor Va with platelets, *J. Biol. Chem.*, 257, 3963, 1982.
25. **Tracy, P. B., Peterson, J. M., Nesheim, M. E., McDuffie, F. C., and Mann, K. G.,** Interaction of coagulation factor V and factor Va with platelets, *J. Biol. Chem.*, 254, 10345, 1979.
26. **Morita, T., Kane, W. H., Majerus, P. W., and Jackson, C. H.,** Enzymatic properties of a derivative or activated factor X from which the γ carboxyglutamic acid domains has been removed, in *The Regulation of Coagulation,* Mann, K. G. and Taylor, F. B., Eds., Elsevier/North-Holland, New York, 1980, 187.
27. **Morita, T. and Jackson, C. M.,** Preparation and properties of derivatives of bovine factor X and factor Xa from which the γ-carboxyglutamic acid containing domain has been removed, *J. Biol. Chem.*, 261, 4015, 1986.
28. **Skogen, W. F., Esmon, C. T., and Cox, A. C.,** Comparison of coagulation factor Xa and *des*(1-44)factor Xa in assembly of prothrombinase, *J. Biol. Chem.*, 259, 2306, 1984.
29. **Dahlbäck, B., Nilsson, I. M., and Frohm, B.,** Inhibition of platelet prothrombinase activity by a lupus anticoagulant, *Blood,* 62, 218, 1983.
30. **Bevers, E. M., Comfurius, P., and Zwaal, R. F. A.,** The nature of the binding site for prothrombinase at the platelet surface as revealed by lipolytic enzymes, *Eur. J. Biochem.*, 122, 81, 1982.
31. **Bevers, E. M., Comfurius, P., and Zwaal, R. F. A.,** Changes in membrane phospholipid distribution during platelet activation, *Biochim. Biophys. Acta,* 736, 57, 1983.
32. **Perret, B., Chap, H., and Douste-Blazy, L.,** Asymmetric distribution of arachidonic acid in the plasma membrane of human platelets, *Biochim. Biophys. Acta,* 556, 434, 1979.
33. **Chap, H., Zwaal, R. F. A., and van Deenen, L. L. M.,** Action of highly purified phospholipases on blood platelets, *Biochim. Biophys. Acta,* 467, 146, 1977.
34. **Blajchman, M. A., Ozge-Anwar, A. H., Senyi, A., and Klein, M.,** Evidence for independent pathway for the induction of platelet prothrombin-coverting activity by thrombin and collagen, *Thromb. Res.*, 35, 719, 1984.
35. **Tracy, P. B., Eide, L. L., and Mann, K. G.,** Human prothrombinase complex assembly and function on isolated peripheral blood cell populations, *J. Biol. Chem.*, 260, 2119, 1985.
36. **Zwaal, R. F. A., Bevers, E. M., and Comfurius, P.,** Platelets and coagulation, in *New Comprehensive Biochemistry,* Vol. 13, Zwaal, R. F. A. and Hemker, H. C., Eds., Elsevier/North Holland, New York, 1986, 141.
37. **Berndt, M. C. and Phillips, D. R.,** Platelet membrane proteins: composition and receptor function, in *Platelets in Biology and Pathology,* Gordon, J. L., Ed., Elsevier/North Holland, New York, 1981, 44.
38. **Berndt, M. C. and Phillips, D. R.,** Interaction of thrombin with platelets: purification of the thrombin substrate, *Ann. N.Y. Acad. Sci.*, 370, 87, 1981.

39. **Zwaal, R. F. A., Comfurius, P., Hemker, H. C., and Bevers, E. M.,** The inhibition of platelet prothrombinase activity by prostacyclin, *Haemostasis,* 14, 320, 1984.
40. **Comfurius, P., Bevers, E. M., and Zwaal, R. F. A.,** The involvement of cytoskeleton in trans-bilayer movement of phospholipids in human blood platelets, *Biochim. Biophys. Acta,* 815, 143, 1985.
41. **Verhallen, P. F. J., Beavers, E. M., Comfurius, P., and Zwaal, R. F. A.,** Correlation between calpain-mediated cytoskeletal degradation and expression of platelet procoagulant activity, *Biochim. Biophys. Acta,* 903, 206, 1987.
42. **Bevers, E. M., Karniguian, A., Legrand, Y. J., and Zwaal, R. F. A.,** Collagen derived octapeptide inhibits platelet procoagulant activity induced by the combined action of collagen and thrombin, *Thromb. Res.,* 37, 365, 1985.
43. **Nimpf, J., Bevers, E. M., Bomans, P. H. H., Till, U., Wurm, H., Kostner, G. M., and Zwaal, R. F. A.,** Prothrombinase activity of human platelets is inhibited by β_2-glycoprotein-I, *Biochim. Biophys. Acta,* in press.
44. **Bevers, E. M., Comfurius, P., Nieuwenhuis, H. K., Levy-Toledano, S., Enouf, J., Belluci, S., Caen, J. P., and Zwaal, R. F. A.,** Platelet prothrombin converting activity in hereditary disorders of platelet function, *Br. J. Haematol.,* 63, 335, 1986.
45. **Raccuglia, G.,** Gray platelet syndrome. A variety of qualitative platelet disorders, *Am. J. Med.,* 51, 818, 1971.
46. **Gerrard, J. M., Phillips, D. R., Rao, G. H. R., Plow, E. F., Walz, D. A., Ross, R., Harker, L. A., and White, J. G.,** Biochemical studies of two patients with the gray platelet syndrome, *J. Clin. Invest.,* 66, 102, 1982.
47. **Baruch, D., Lindhout, M. J., Dupuy, E., and Caen, J. P.,** Thrombin-Induced Platelet Factor Va Formation in Patients with a Gray Platelet Syndrome, Ph.D. thesis, University of Limburg, Maastricht, 1985.
48. **Nurden, A. T. and Caen, J. P.,** Role of surface glycoproteins in human platelet function, *Thromb. Haemostasis,* 35, 139, 1976.
49. **Nurden, A. T. and Caen, J. P.,** The different glycoprotein abnormalities in thromboasthenic and Bernard-Soulier platelets, *Sem. Hematol.,* 16, 234, 1979.
50. **Phillips, D. R. and Poh Agin, P.,** Platelet membrane defects in Glanzmann's thrombasthenia, *J. Clin. Invest.,* 64, 1392, 1979.
51. **Bennett, J. S. and Vilaire, G.,** Exposure of platelet fibrinogen receptors by ADP and epinephrine, *J. Clin. Invest.,* 64, 1392, 1979.
52. **Nachman, R. L. and Leung, L. L. K.,** Complex formation of platelet membrane glycoprotein IIb and IIIa with fibrinogen, *J. Clin. Invest.,* 69, 263, 1982.
53. **Marguerie, G. A., Thomas-Maison, N., Ginsberg, M. H., and Plow, E. F.,** The platelet-fibrinogen interaction, *Eur. J. Biochem.,* 139, 5, 1984.
54. **Evensen, S. A., Solum, N. O., Grøttum, K. A., and Hovig, T.,** Familial bleeding disorder with a moderate thrombocytopenia and giant blood platelets, *Scand. J. Haematol.,* 13, 203, 1974.
55. **McGill, M., Jamieson, G. A., Drouin, J., Cho, M. S., and Rock, G. A.,** Morphometric analysis of platelets in Bernard-Soulier syndrome: size and configurations in patients and carriers, *Thromb. Haemostasis,* 52, 37, 1984.
56. **Tobelem, G., Levy-Toledano, S., Bredoux, R., Michel, H., Nurden, A. T., and Caen, J. P.,** New approach to determination of specific functions of platelet membrane sites, *Nature,* 263, 427, 1976.
57. **Degos, L., Tobelem, G., Lethielleux, P., Levy-Toledano, S., Caen, J. P., and Colombain, J.,** Molecular defects in platelets with Bernard-Soulier syndrome, *Blood,* 50, 899, 1977.
58. **Clemetson, K. J., McGregor, J. L., James, E., Dechavanne, H., and Lüscher, E.,** Characterization of the platelet membrane glycoprotein abnormalities in Bernard-Soulier syndrome and comparison with normal by surface-labeling techniques and high-resolution two-dimensional gel electrophoresis, *J. Clin. Invest.,* 70, 403, 1982.
59. **Berndt, M. C., Gregory, C., Chang, B. H., Zola, H., and Castaldi, P. A.,** Additional glycoprotein defects in Bernard-Soulier syndrome: confirmation of genetic basis by parental analysis, *Blood,* 62, 800, 1983.
60. **Perret, B., Levy-Toledano, S., Plantavid, M., Bredoux, R., Chap, H., Tobelem, G., Douste-Blazy, L., and Caen, J. P.,** Abnormal phospholipid organization in Bernard-Soulier platelets, *Thromb. Res.,* 31, 529, 1983.
61. **Rao, A. K., Goldberg, R. E., and Walsh, P. N.,** Platelet coagulant activities in diabetes mellitus, *J. Lab. Clin. Med.,* 103, 82, 1984.
62. **Nieuwenhuis, H. K., Akkerman, J. W. N., Houdijk, W. P. M., and Sixma, J. J.,** Human blood platelets showing no response to collagen fail to express surface glycoprotein Ia, *Nature,* 318, 470, 1985.
63. **Weiss, H. J., Vicic, W. J., Lages, B. A., and Rogers, J.,** Isolated deficiency of platelet procoagulant activity, *Am. J. Med.,* 67, 206, 1979.

64. **Miletich, J. P., Kane, W. H., Hofmann, S. L., Stanford, N., and Majerus, P. W.,** Deficiency of factor Xa-factor Va binding sites on the platelets of a patient with a bleeding disorder, *Blood,* 54, 1015, 1979.
65. **Rosing, J., Bevers, E. M., Comfurius, P., Hemker, H. C., van Dieijen, G., Weiss, H. J., and Zwaal, R. F. A.,** Impaired factor X and prothrombin activation associated with decreased phospholipid exposure in platelets from a patient with a bleeding disorder, *Blood,* 65, 1557, 1985.

Chapter 9

MEMBRANE PHENOMENA AND COAGULANT PROPERTIES OF PLATELETS

Robert F. A. Zwaal and Edouard M. Bevers

TABLE OF CONTENTS

I. INTRODUCTION

The platelet plasma membrane has gained increasing interest in the last decade as a model membrane for probing the more general aspects of membrane structure and function. Gradually, the popularity rating for studying the platelet membrane approaches that of the red cell membrane. In some respects, the platelet plasma membrane may be a more rewarding object to study because it surrounds a highly reactive cell, which better reflects the behavior and metabolic activities of other cells in the body than does the erythrocyte with its rather one-sided functional specialization. Also, the study of the platelet membrane has provided important insights in disease-related membrane defects[1,2] that may have a profound impact on our understanding of abnormal behavior of other cells.

Although many biological activities have been assigned to the platelet, the main function is to participate in the arrest of bleeding upon vessel wall injury.[3] Platelets circulate in the blood for 8 to 11 days as smooth discoid cells. The potential reactivity becomes apparent upon vessel wall injury (compare also Chapter 3). When endothelial cells are damaged or removed, platelets rapidly adhere to the exposed subendothelial fibrils and collagen, become sticky, and aggregate with each other to form a primary hemostatic plug. This platelet plug prevents blood loss from the vessel, as occurs during normal hemostasis, or obstructs the blood circulation within the vessel, as occurs in thrombosis and in the reaction of platelets to a severe atherosclerotic lesion. The platelet aggregate is stabilized by fibrin, which is formed as the end product of the coagulation cascade (see Chapter 1). Some of the reactions in the coagulation cascade are dramatically accelerated by activated platelets (see Chapter 8) and, in fact, depend on the exposition of anionic phospholipids which provide a catalytic surface for interacting coagulation factors (see Chapter 7). An important aspect of this is that thrombin formed in the coagulation process not only converts fibrinogen into fibrin, but also activates a variety of other processes not the least of which is platelet activation itself.

Obviously, the platelet plasma membrane plays a pivotal role in virtually all phenomena associated with platelet activation. The membrane contains receptors for external stimuli,[4] transduces the signal into the cell, and plays a part in the execution of the platelet response. Part of this response consists of a cellular shape change, including pseudopod formation, and a secretory event involving fusion of intracellular membranes with the plasma membrane.[5] Moreover, the platelet membrane undergoes a number of different alterations in molecular architecture, enabling it to interact with a variety of different plasma proteins, such as von Willebrand factor, fibrinogen, and the coagulation factors involved in the activation of factor X and prothrombin.[6] The concerted action of these processes is an essential prerequisite for normal hemostasis to occur, witnessed from the fact that a variety of hemostatic disorders originate from defects in structural composition or functional behavior of the platelet plasma membrane. A selected number of membrane phenomena that are of crucial importance for the hemostatic activities of blood platelets will be discussed in this chapter.

II. STRUCTURAL ASPECTS OF THE PLATELET MEMBRANE

The plasma membrane of blood platelets has many features in common to plasma membranes from other cells in that its molecular organization is an example of the fluid mosaic membrane structure described by Singer and Nicolson.[7] From a structural point of view, it displays a rather unusual aspect because it not only surrounds the cell, but also invaginates to the cell interior to form a sponge-like system of channels that burrow their way to the cytoplasm.[8] This so-called open canalicular system strongly increases the surface area of the cell in contact with the aqueous environment and serves as a channel in which secretion

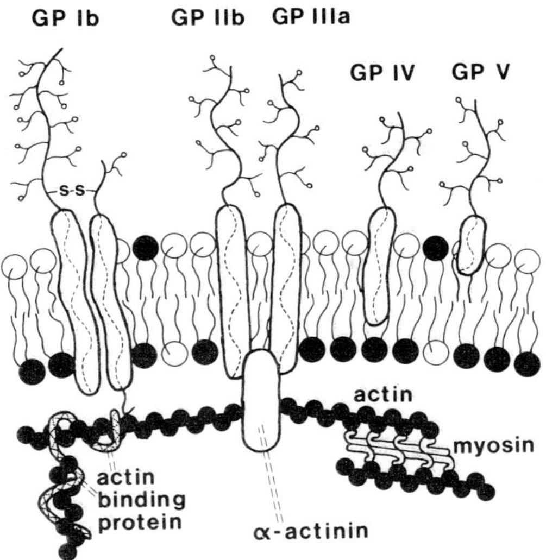

FIGURE 1. Structural aspects of the human platelet plasma membrane. GP = glycoprotein.

granules release their contents upon platelet activation. Under the electron microscope the platelet membrane displays the characteristic trilaminar image of some 70 Å in diameter, reflecting the lipid bilayer structure.[8] Specific carbohydrate staining techniques applied to electron microscopic preparations reveal an electron-dense glycocalyx extending outward as much as 25 nm beyond the unit bilayer, representing the carbohydrate-rich domains of more than 30 membrane glycoproteins exposed at the cell surface.[4] A schematic representation of the essential features of the platelet plasma membrane is shown in Figure 1. The major membrane glycoproteins are Ib, IIb, IIIa, and IV. The functional roles including that of glycoprotein V are beginning to be understood. Glycoproteins Ib, IIb, and IIIa have been shown to span the unit bilayer from one side to the other, allowing them to interact with cytoskeletal proteins at the inner aspect of the membrane.[9,10] These interactions involve an attachment of glycoprotein Ib with actin-binding protein (filamin) and a presumed binding of the glycoprotein IIb-IIIa complex with α-actinin. The cytoskeletal proteins undergo structural alterations during platelet activation.[11] These alterations involve polymerization of actin into filaments that associate with myosin, being regulated by the level of phosphorylation of the myosin light chains. Actin polymerization is regulated by a number of proteins such as profilin and gelsolin, while α-actinin also serves as the membrane attachment site for actin filaments. Moreover, branching of actin filaments into a network is brought about by actin-binding protein. A number of cytoskeletal proteins are also subject to partial proteolytic breakdown by an endogenous calcium-dependent protease during platelet activation.[12,13] This process influences the direct interactions between cytoskeletal proteins and the lipid bilayer.[14] As in most biological membranes, the lipid bilayer forms the core of the membrane to which peripheral membrane proteins (such as cytoskeletal proteins) are attached via polar interactions, and which is interrupted to allow hydrophobic interactions with integral membrane proteins (e.g., the hydrophobic domains of glycoproteins). The lipid bilayer contains 70% phospholipids by weight, the remainder being composed of cholesterol and minor amounts of glycolipids. Five major phospholipid classes have been identified in human platelets:[15,16] phosphatidylcholine (38%), phosphatidylethanolamine (27%), sphingomyelin (19%), phosphatidylserine (10%), and phosphatidylinositol (5%). The lipid composition of the plasma membrane resembles that of the intracellular membranes, although it contains more sphingomyelin, phosphatidylserine, and cholesterol. As in erythrocytes,[17] the phospholipids are asymmetrically distributed over the bilayer.[6,16,18-20] The outer leaflet of the plasma membrane contains most of the sphingomyelin, whereas phosphatidylserine and phosphatidylinositol are mainly confined to the inner monolayer of the membrane. Phosphatidylcholine is almost equally distributed between both halves of the bilayer, while phosphatidylethanolamine is more abundant at the inside.

III. GLYCOPROTEINS AND HEMOSTATIC FUNCTIONS

Some of the platelet membrane glycoproteins have been recognized as binding sites for plasma proteins. These interactions are necessary for platelet adhesion to subendothelial microfibrils as well as for platelets to interact with each other to form an aggregate. Both processes are essential for normal hemostatic plug formation to occur. In particular, glycoprotein Ib has been shown to be intimately involved in platelet adhesion, whereas glycoproteins IIb and IIIa are essential for platelet aggregation.

Glycoprotein Ib is a sialoglycoprotein composed of two glycopolypeptides connected by at least one disulfide bond.[21,22] The larger subunit, or α chain, has an apparent molecular weight of 145 kdaltons on SDS-polyacrylamide gel electrophoresis under reduced conditions, whereas the smaller β chain has a molecular weight of 22 kdaltons. Glycoprotein Ib has been implicated as the major receptor for von Willebrand Factor. This is a protein synthesized by endothelial cells[23] that circulates as a series of high molecular weight multimeric structures[24] and is the necessary component for platelet adhesion.[3] The evidence that glycoprotein Ib is the main functional binding site for von Willebrand Factor comes from a significant part from studies on platelets from patients with an inherited bleeding disorder known as Bernard-Soulier syndrome. These platelets are deficient in glycoprotein Ib[25] and fail to adhere to subendothelial structures.[26]

Defective platelet adhesion is also apparent in von Willebrand's disease, in which von Willebrand Factor is absent or defective.[27] Normally in plasma, von Willebrand Factor does not interact with glycoprotein Ib at the platelet surface. However, after interaction with subendothelial microfibrils, it undergoes a calcium-dependent conformational change after which it recognizes glycoprotein Ib,[28,29] thus leading to adhesion of platelets to subendothelium. When the α-chain of GPIb is cleaved from the platelet surface by a calcium-dependent protease, the binding site for von Willebrand Factor is lost, which indicates this site to be located on the α-chain.[22]

The function of the β chain is thought to exert some influence in maintaining the correct conformation of the α-chain. Moreover, immunoinhibitory probes using both polyclonal and monoclonal antisera against glycoprotein Ib also suggest that this glycoprotein is the receptor for von Willebrand Factor.[30,31] Other studies using antibodies as inhibitory probes also suggest the glycoprotein IIb-IIIa complex to be involved in binding von Willebrand Factor.[32] Binding of von Willebrand Factor to glycoprotein IIb-IIIa is apparent when platelets are stimulated with thrombin or ADP. Whether or not this plays a function in platelet adhesion to subendothelium is unclear, moreso as this glycoprotein complex plays a crucial role in platelet aggregation.

Glycoprotein IIb consists of two subunits linked by at least one disulphide bond.[22,23] The larger α-subunit has an apparent molecular weight of 130 kdaltons, while the small β-subunit has a molecular weight of 23 kdaltons. Glycoprotein IIIa is a single chain polypeptide, contains at least two intramolecular disulfide bridges, and has an apparent molecular weight of 114 kdaltons upon reduction.[21-22] Glycoproteins IIb and IIIa are present in platelet plasma membranes in an apparent 1:1 stoichiometry, and together account for 15 to 20% of the total membrane protein.[33] Complex formation between these two glycoproteins during platelet activation is required to form a binding site for fibrinogen,[34-36] a process essential for platelet aggregation to occur.[37,38] In platelets from patients with an inherited bleeding disorder known as Glanzmann's thrombasthenia, both glycoproteins are markedly diminished to absent.[1,25] These platelets do not aggregate in response to any stimulus in spite of normal release reaction[2] and fail to express increased binding of fibrinogen, as occurs with normal platelets in the presence of calcium and ADP. Monoclonal antibodies directed against glycoproteins IIb and IIIa prevent fibrinogen binding and aggregation of normal platelets.[39] In the unstimulated platelet, both glycoproteins are exposed but the binding properties for fibrinogen are not expressed.

Receptor induction following membrane stimulation is a prerequisite for fibrinogen binding and cell aggregation. The nature of this receptor formation process is not fully understood, but is thought to involve either complex formation between both glycoproteins or a conformational change of a preexisting glycoprotein complex resulting in the acquisition of a binding function. Also, treatment of platelets with chymotrypsin exposes fibrinogen binding sites, presumably because parts of the shielding N-terminal domains of both glycoproteins are clipped off.[40] There are approximately 40,000 fibrinogen binding sites per platelet and a similar number of glycoprotein IIb-IIIa complexes. The fibrinogen molecule exposes a major interaction site on the carboxy-terminal region of each γ chain.[36,41] Two sites per fibrinogen molecule thus enable two adjacent activated platelets to bridge, forming an adhesive intermediate in platelet aggregation.

Whereas glycoproteins Ib and IIb-IIIa are intimately involved in binding of the adhesive proteins von Willebrand Factor and fibrinogen, respectively, most of the other surface-exposed (glyco) proteins are thought to function as typical receptors for external agonists or antagonists, transmitting their signal to the cell interior, leading to initiation or inhibition of a cellular response. Recently, however, another membrane glycoprotein has been implicated in the adhesive properties of platelets to collagen. Platelets from a patient with an excessively long bleeding time were found to be nonresponsive to collagens type I and III and to exhibit an isolated deficiency in glycoprotein Ia.[42] This glycoprotein is known as a single chain molecule of 168 kdalton containing at least one intramolecular disulfide bond.[21] The observations with these glycoprotein Ia-deficient platelets suggest a role for this membrane protein as the principal binding site involved in adhesion of platelets to subendothelial collagen. It should be mentioned that, unlike platelet adhesion to microfibrils, von Willebrand Factor is not a necessary component for platelet adhesion to collagen.

IV. PHOSPHOLIPID ORGANIZATION AND THE FUNCTION IN HEMOSTASIS

Alterations in the molecular organization of the platelet plasma membrane are not restricted to membrane proteins, but involve the membrane lipids as well. Among the very early events in a stimulated membrane is the breakdown of phosphatidylinositols by a specific phospholipase C, which leads to the formation of two intracellular second messenger, diacylglycerol and inositol-triphosphate. Diacylglycerol stimulates a protein kinase which phosphorylates a 43-kdalton protein,[43] while inositol-triphosphate is involved in liberating calcium from the dense tubular system, thus raising the cytoplasmic calcium concentration.[44] Moreover, the metabolic events during the PI-cycle also result in the formation of free arachidonic acid, which can be converted to thromboxane A_2, a potent cofactor in platelet activation.[45]

The importance of anionic platelet phospholipids in the activation of two sequential reactions in the coagulation cascade, i.e., factor X and prothrombin activation (see Chapter 7), has evoked an interest in possible changes in exposure of phospholipids at the outer surface during platelet activation. As a matter of fact, the virtual absence of negatively charged phospholipids (in particular, phosphatidylserine) from the outer surface of platelets explains why intact unactivated cells have little procoagulant activity as compared to lysed cells.[6,19] The same phenomenon is also observed with other blood cells, including endothelial

Table 1
COMPOSITION OF PHOSPHOLIPID FRACTIONS HYDROLYZED BY PHOSPHOLIPASE A_2 AND SPHINGOMYELINASE TREATMENT OF ACTIVATED HUMAN PLATELETS

		Activated by				
	Unactivated	Thrombin	Collagen	Collagen + thrombin	Diamide	A23187
PS	2.4	4.9	6.0	11.2	13.4	12.6
PC	31.0	39.3	41.4	33.9	39.0	29.5
PE	9.5	15.5	17.0	36.0	25.8	35.8
SM	57.1	40.2	35.6	18.7	21.7	22.0
Hydrolyzed fraction as % of total phospholipid	21	32	34	44	39	65

Note: Values are expressed as percentage of the hydrolyzed fraction. PS, phosphatidylserine; PC, phosphatidylcholine; PE, phosphatidylethanolamine; and SM, sphingomyelin.

cells lining the blood vessel.[46] Alterations in the surface exposure of negatively charged phospholipids during platelet activation are to be expected, in view of the increased ability of stimulated platelets to catalyze prothrombin and factor X activation. Two inherent difficulties arise during the determination of the orientation of the membrane phospholipids in stimulated platelets. First, platelet activation usually leads to platelet aggregation, and the intimate platelet-platelet contact may, therefore, reduce the amount of outer surface being accessible for the probing agent. Second, the platelet release reaction involves a secretory event during which granular membranes fuse with the plasma membrane, thus increasing the amount of phospholipids in the surface membrane or even altering the overall phospholipid composition. Both phenomena impose certain limitations concerning the accuracy with which the amount and composition of phospholipids exposed at the outer surface can be detected. Therefore, the best one can say is that the lipids which react with a nonpermeable probing agent at the outer surface of stimulated, but intact, platelets are (at least temporarily) located at the outer surface, but the location of the lipids which do not react remains uncertain.

The first indication for an alteration in phospholipid orientation during platelet activation was obtained by comparing the reaction of the nonpermeable probe trinitrobenzene sulfonate (TNBS) on thrombin-activated and control platelets in the presence of EDTA to avoid platelet aggregation.[20,47,48] In platelets treated by thrombin, some 25% of the phosphatidylethanolamine could be labeled which is twice as much as observed with unactivated platelets. No labeling of phosphatidylserine could be detected, either in thrombin-treated or in control platelets. The main disadvantage of using chemical probes such as TNBS is that the reaction is generally slow (particularly with phosphatidylserine), incomplete, and limited to aminophospholipids.

A more extensive insight into alterations in phospholipid exposure during platelet activation has been obtained using highly purified phospholipases as tools to probe the phospholipid orientation in the plasma membrane. This technique has the advantage over chemical reagents in that a proper combination of phospholipases can, in principle, react with all phospholipid classes, and that reaction goes to completion. Although there are a number of pitfalls in using phospholipases in sidedness studies,[46,49] it appears possible to obtain detailed information on the orientation of phospholipids in the surface membrane of a variety of activated platelets.[50,51] Table 1 shows the maximum attainable amount, as well as the composition, of those phospholipids which are degraded by treatment of activated and control platelets with a mixture of sphingomyelinase and phospholipase A_2 in the absence of or prior to the onset of cell lysis.[51] The hydrolyzed fractions are interpreted to represent the phospholipids that are mainly present in the outer leaflet of the plasma membrane during the time period of the phospholipase treatment (20 to 30 min). With allegedly unactivated platelets, about 21% of the total platelet phospholipids can be hydrolyzed in the absence of cell lysis. This fraction is mainly composed of choline-phospholipids, i.e., sphingomyelin and phosphatidylcholine, whereas the exposure of aminophospholipids (particularly phosphatidylserine) is limited. Activation of platelets, either by collagen or by thrombin followed by treatment with phospholipases, leads to 32 to 35% of phospholipid hydrolysis. Compared to unactivated platelets, the surface-exposed fraction is somewhat less rich in sphingomyelin, while the glycerophospholipids are increased. It is, however, difficult to ascertain if the slight increase in phosphatidylserine exposure is significant in thrombin- or collagen-activated platelets in view of the relatively small quantities involved. Activation of platelets by a mixture of collagen plus thrombin produces a progressive change in the phospholipid pattern susceptible to exogenously added phospholipases The composition of the hydrolyzed phospholipid fraction shows a substantial increase in phosphatidylserine and phosphatidylethanolamine and a remarkable decrease in sphingomyelin. As a result, this composition tends to approach the overall phospholipid composition of the platelet membrane, suggesting a randomization of the phospholipids over both leaflets of the membrane. A similar progressive loss in phospholipid asymmetry is also observed with platelets treated with Ca ionophore A23187 or with diamide. The alterations in phospholipid composition of the outer membrane leaflet of platelets activated by thrombin or collagen alone can be attributed mainly to arise from the secretory event (release reaction), which involves fusion of granular membranes with the plasma membrane.[51] On the other hand, the progressive loss in phospholipid asymmetry in platelets activated by collagen plus thrombin, diamide, or ionophore presumably reflects an abrupt increase in transbilayer movement of phospholipids as a result of the activation procedure.

V. POSSIBLE MECHANISMS INVOLVED IN EXPOSURE OF PROCOAGULANT LIPID

Since phosphatidylserine is the major anionic, and thus procoagulant, phospholipid in platelet membranes, the increased exposure in the exterior half of the platelet plasma membrane during cell activation is strictly correlated to the procoagulant properties of activated platelets (see Chapter 8). The ability of platelets to alter their membrane phospholipid orientation upon platelet activation can be expected to require participation of other platelet (membrane) components. It is becoming increasingly evident that flip-flop of phospholipids, which is the process whereby lipids migrate from one monolayer of the membrane to the other, can occur at significant rates when irregularities in the bilayer structure occur. In artificial bilayer vesicles, transbilayer movement can be induced by creating different physical properties between outer and inner monolayer, by insertion of bilayer-spanning proteins, and by triggering the formation of nonbilayer arrangements in the lipid bilayer.[52,53] In addition, increased phospholipid flip-flop in red cell membranes has been shown to occur when organization of cytoskeletal proteins becomes disturbed (see Chapter 2).[54-57] Moreover, flip-flop of aminophospholipids from the external to the internal leaflet of red cell membranes has been demonstrated to be an ATP-dependent process,[58-60] although ATP-depletion does not necessarily lead to a loss of membrane lipid asymmetry.[60] Some evidence has been obtained that formation of nonbilayer structures as well as changes in cytoskeleton organization upon platelet activation might be involved in phospholipid flip-flop across the plasma membrane, leading to an increased exposure of phosphatidylserine providing the activated platelet with a procoagulant surface.

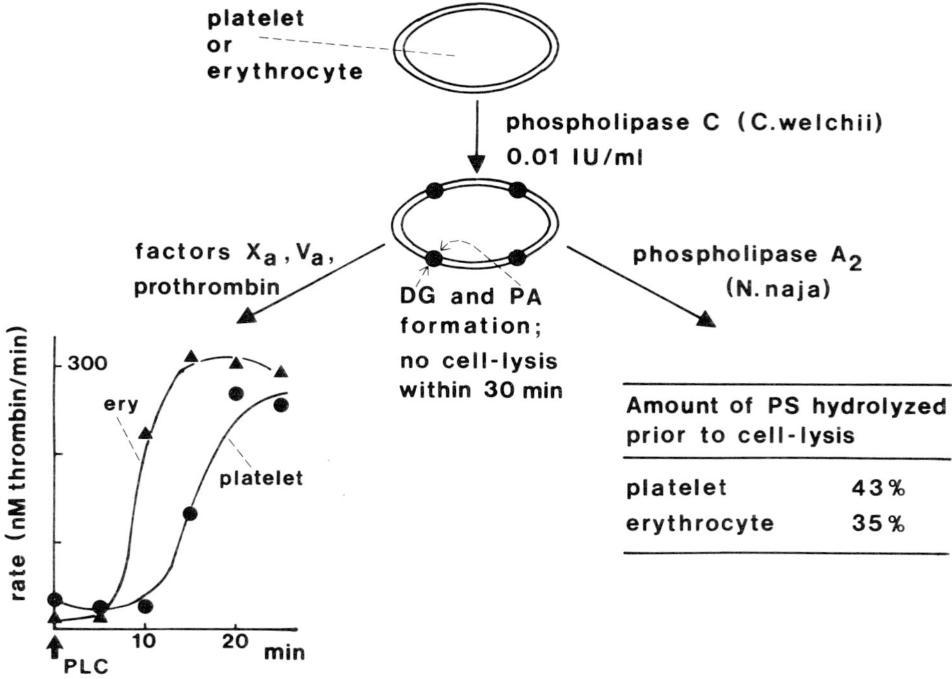

FIGURE 2. Prothrombinase activity of platelets and erythrocytes and exposure of phosphatidylserine during treatment with minor amounts of *C. welchii* phospholipase C. DG = diacylglycerol, PA = phospatidic acid, PS = phosphatidylserine, PLC = phospholipase C.

A. Formation of Nonbilayer Structures

Hydrated lipids can adopt a variety of phases in addition to the bilayer phase.[61] Moreover, certain lipids do not accommodate easily to the bilayer structure and tend to form nonbilayer arrangements within the bilayer itself.[53] These structures have been demonstrated using ^{31}P-NMR and freeze-fracture electron microscopy. They are composed of cylindrical hexagonal phases, as well as inverted lipid micelles known as lipidic particles. In particular, lipids which have a molecular shape in the form of a cone, with the polar head group at the smaller end of the cone, tend to adopt hexagonal structures with the polar head group inside. Examples of these are phosphatidic acid and diacylglycerol. It has been shown both for platelets[62] and red cells[63] that production of diacylglycerol in the membrane by the action of exogenously added phospholipase C from *Clostridium welchii* results in the formation of phosphatidic acid. This demonstrates a transbilayer movement of diacylglycerols, formed in the outer monolayer, to the inner leaflet of the membrane, where diacylglycerol kinase and ATP are available. Treatment of platelets with this phospholipase C also elicits release and aggregation and eventually leads to lysis of the cells.[64] However, using a particular combination of phospholipases, it could be shown that before the onset of lysis, substantial amounts of phosphatidylserine appear at the external surface.[65] This phenomenon is accompanied by a markedly enhanced ability of these platelets to promote thrombin formation by the prothrombinase complex (Figure 2). This behavior is not restricted to platelets, as red cells also acquire the property of stimulating prothrombinase activity during phospholipase C treatment. The amount of negatively charged phosphatidic acid produced during these incubations is 2 to 4% of total phospholipid, too low to account for the observed prothrombinase activity. The amount of phosphatidic acid is, however, of the same order as that formed in activated platelets during triggering of the phosphatidylinositol cycle.[66,67] In the initial steps of this cycle, (poly)phosphoinositides are converted to diacylglycerol by an endogenous phospholipase C, followed by a phosphorylation catalyzed by diacyl glycerol kinase to form phosphatidic acid.[68] It is conceivable that triggering of the phosphatidylinositol cycle may, under certain conditions, produce transient amounts of diacylglycerol and phosphatidic acid which exceed the threshold concentrations required to elicit nonbilayer arrangements in the membrane bilayer. These may produce microenvironmental perturbations of bilayer structure to form a locus for flip-flop of phospholipids, leading to increased exposure of phosphatidylserine in the outer membrane leaflet.

B. Involvement of Cytoskeletal Proteins

There is increasing evidence that in red cells cytoskeletal proteins play a role in the maintenance of membrane phospholipid asymmetry.[54-57] Therefore, loss of the asymmetric orientation can be suspected to be preceded by or accompanied with changes in the structural organization of cytoskeletal proteins. The first indication for involvement of cytoskeletal proteins in phospholipid asymmetry was obtained from treatment of red cells with SH-oxidizing agents like diamide or tetrathionate.[54] Inner layer phospholipids were shown to move to the outer leaflet upon oxidation of spectrin SH groups to disulfide bonds, which is paralleled by cross-linking of spectrin to form oligomers. Also, treatment of platelets with diamide results in extensive polymerization of cytoskeletal proteins, particularly filamin, myosin, and actin.[69] This process is also accompanied by increased exposure of aminophospholipids,[51] formerly present in the internal leaflet of the membrane. Apart from polymerization, hydrolysis of actin-binding protein (filamin) and talin (P235) has been shown to occur by an endogenous calcium-dependent protease upon activation of platelets with Ca ionophore A23187 in the presence of exogenous calcium chloride.[12-14,70,71]

Stimulation of endogenous calcium-dependent protease can also occur upon platelet stimulation with physiological activators. Depending upon the platelet stimulation procedure, different extents of degradation of cytoskeletal proteins filamin, talin, but also myosin are observed.[14] The highest extent of proteolysis was observed with Ca ionophore A23187 and decreased on going from A23187 > collagen plus thrombin > collagen > thrombin = ADP. The same order of potency is found for the ability of these activators to induce exposure of anionic phosphatidylserine in the outer leaflet of the platelet plasma membrane (compare Table 1), and to stimulate platelets to become procoagulant (see Chapter 8). Also, platelets from a patient with an isolated deficiency in prothrombin- and factor X-converting activity resulting from a reduced exposure of phosphosphatidylserine (see Chapter 8)[72] were found to have a diminished extent of degradation of cytoskeletal proteins upon platelet stimulation with collagen plus thrombin.[14]

Finally, the action of local anesthetics dibucaine and tetracaine towards platelets also leads to extensive degradation of cytoskeletal protein,[73] accompanied by a strongly increased ability of these platelets to stimulate prothrombinase activity.[74] This is also consistent with the view that cytoskeletal organization plays a regulatory role in transbilayer movement of phosphatidylserine in platelets. At least two different types of mechanisms may be involved (Figure 3). It is conceivable that degradation of cytoskeletal proteins will produce alterations in cytoskeletal organization, leading to a disturbance in presumed interactions with phosphatidylserine. Therefore, this lipid may acquire more freedom of motion so as to participate in transbilayer movement once microenvironmental perturbations of the bilayer structure occur. On the other hand, the action of calcium-dependent protease towards myosin splits the head from the tail portion.[75] As far as generation and maintenance of phospholipid asymmetry in platelets would also be ATP dependent, myosin may play a significant role being the major membrane associated ATPase activity.[76] Cleavage of membrane-bound myosin may either inactivate myosin-ATPase activity or detach this activity from the membrane proper, because the globular head portion containing ATPase is readily water soluble,

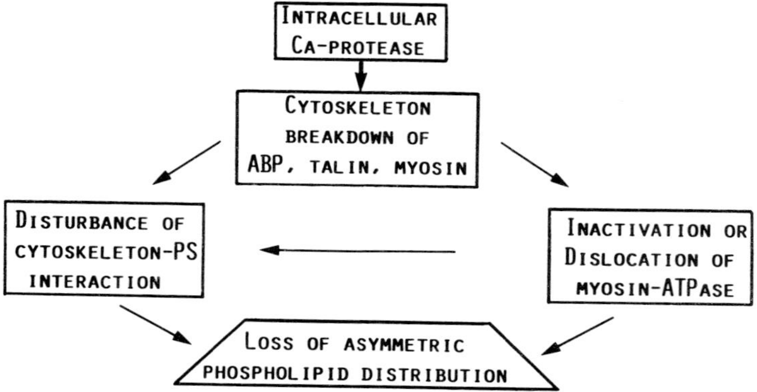

FIGURE 3. Possible mechanisms involved in phosphatidylserine exposure at the outer surface of activated platelets.

unlike the rod portion of the molecule. Observations with red cells suggest that movement of aminophospholipids towards the inner aspect of the membrane is ATP-dependent.[58-60] Therefore, dislocation or inactivation of myosin ATPase may deprive the membrane of energy, thus leading to a progressive loss of membrane phospholipid asymmetry.

REFERENCES

1. **Nurden, A. T. and Caen, J. P.,** Membrane glycoproteins and human platelet function, *Br. J. Haematol.*, 38, 155, 1978.
2. **Weiss, H. J.,** Congenital disorders of platelet function, *Semin. Hematol.*, 17, 228, 1980.
3. **Weiss, H. J.,** Physiology and abnormalities of platelet function, *N. Engl. J. Med.*, 293, 531, 1975.
4. **Berndt, M. C. and Phillips, D. R.,** Platelet membrane proteins: composition and receptor function, in *Platelets in Biology and Pathology 2*, Gordon, J. L., Ed., Elsevier/North-Holland, 1981, chap. 3.
5. **Skaer, R. J.,** Platelet degranulation, in *Platelets in Biology and Pathology 2*, Gordon, J. L., Ed., Elsevier/North-Holland, 1981, chap. 13.
6. **Zwaal, R. F. A.,** Membrane and lipid involvement in blood coagulation, *Biochim. Biophys. Acta*, 515, 63, 1978.
7. **Singer, S. J. and Nicolson, G. L.,** The fluid mosaic model of the structure of cell membranes, *Science*, 175, 720, 1972.
8. **White, J. G.,** Interaction of membrane systems in blood platelets, *Am. J. Pathol.*, 66, 295, 1972.
9. **Fox, J. E. B.,** Identification of ABP as the protein linking the membrane skeleton to glycoproteins on platelet plasma membranes, *J. Biol. Chem.*, 260, 11970, 1985.
10. **Fox, J. E. B.,** Linkage of a membrane skeleton to integral membrane glycoproteins in human platelets. Identification of one of the glycoproteins as glycoprotein Ib, *J. Clin. Invest.*, 76, 1673, 1985.
11. **Fox, J. E. B. and Phillips, D. R.,** Polymerization and organisation of actin filaments with platelets, *Semin. Hematol.*, 20, 243, 1983.
12. **White, G. C.,** Calcium-dependent proteins in platelets. Response of calcium-activated protease in normal and thrombasthenic platelets to aggregating agents, *Biochim. Biophys. Acta*, 631, 130, 1980.
13. **Fox, J. E. B., Goll, D. E., Reynolds, C. C., and Phillips, D. R.,** Identification of two proteins (ABP and P235) that are hydrolyzed by endogenous Ca^{2+}-dependent protease during platelet aggregation, *J. Biol. Chem.*, 260, 1060, 1985.
14. **Comfurius, P., Bevers, E. M., and Zwaal, R. F. A.,** The involvement of cytoskeleton in the regulation of transbilayer movement of phospholipids in human blood platelets, *Biochim. Biophys. Acta*, 815, 43, 1985.
15. **Marcus, A. J.,** The role of lipids in platelet function with particular reference to the arachidonic pathway, *J. Lipid Res.*, 19, 793, 1978.

16. **Perret, B., Chap, H. J., and Douste-Blazy, L.,** Asymmetric distribution of arachidonic acid in the plasma membrane of human platelets. A determination using purified phospholipases and a rapid method for membrane isolation, *Biochim. Biophys. Acta,* 556, 434, 1979.
17. **Zwaal, R. F. A., Roelofsen, B., Comfurius, P., and van Deenen, L. L. M.,** Organization of phospholipids in human red cell membranes, *Biochim. Biophys. Acta,* 406, 33, 1975.
18. **Chap, H. J., Zwaal, R. F. A., and van Deenen, L. L. M.,** Action of highly purified phosphlipases on blood platelets, *Biochim. Biophys. Acta,* 467, 146, 1977.
19. **Zwaal, R. F. A., Comfurius, P., and van Deenen, L. L. M.,** Membrane asymmetry and blood coagulation, *Nature,* 268, 358, 1977.
20. **Schick, P. K.,** The role of platelet membrane lipids in platelet hemostatic activities, *Semin. Hematol.,* 16, 221, 1979.
21. **Phillips, D. R. and Poh-Agin, P.,** Platelet plasma membrane glycoproteins: evidence for the presence of nonequivalent disulphide two-dimensional gel electrophoresis, *J. Biol. Chem.,* 252, 2121, 1977.
22. **Clemetson, K. J.,** Glycoproteins of the platelet plasma membrane, in *Platelet Membrane Glycoproteins,* George, J. N., Nurden, A. T., and Phillips, D. R., Eds., Plenum Press, New York, 1985, chap. 3.
23. **Jaffe, E. A., Hoyer, L. W., and Nachman, R. L.,** Synthesis of von Willebrand factor by cultured human endothelial cells, *Proc. Natl. Acad. Sci. U.S.A.,* 71, 1906, 1974.
24. **Counts, R. B., Poskell, S. L., and Elgeen, S. K.,** Disulfide bonds and the quarternary structure of Factor VIII/von Willebrand factor, *J. Clin. Invest.,* 62, 702, 1978.
25. **Nurden, A. T. and Caen, J. P.,** Further studies on the glycoprotein composition of normal human, Bernard-Soulier, and thrombasthenic platelets, *Thromb. Haemostasis,* 39, 200, 1977.
26. **Weiss, H. J., Tschopp, T. B., and Baumgartner, H. R.,** Decreased adhesion of giant (Bernard-Soulier) platelets to subendothelium, *Am. J. Med.,* 57, 920, 1974.
27. **Tschopp, T. B., Weiss, H. J., and Baumgartner, H. R.,** Decreased adhesion of platelets to subendothelium in von Willebrand's disease, *J. Lab. Clin. Med.,* 83, 296, 1974.
28. **Sakariassen, K. S., Bolhuis, P. A., and Sixma, J. J.,** Human blood platelet adhesion to artery subendothelium is mediated by factor VIII-von Willebrand factor bound to the subendothelium, *Nature,* 279, 636, 1979.
29. **Kao, K. J., Pizzo, S. V., and McKee, P. A.,** Demonstration and characterization of specific binding sites for factor VIII/von Willebrand factor on human platelets, *J. Clin. Invest.,* 63, 656, 1979.
30. **Nachman, R. L., Jaffe, E. A., and Wekster, B. W.,** Immunoinhibition of ristocetin induced platelet aggregation, *J. Clin. Invest.,* 59, 143, 1977.
31. **Ruan, C., Tobelem, G., McMichael, A. J., Drouet, L., Legrand, Y., Degos, L., Kieffer, N., Lee, H., and Caen, J. P.,** Monoclonal antibody to human platelet glycoprotein I, *Br. J. Haematol.,* 49, 511, 1981.
32. **Gralnick, H. and Coller, B.,** Platelets stimulated with thrombin and ADP bind von Willebrand factor to different sites than platelets stimulated with ristocetin, *Clin. Res.,* 31, 482, 1983.
33. **Jennings, L. K. and Phillips, D. R.,** Purification of glycoproteins IIb and III from human platelet plasma membranes and characterization of a calcium-dependent glycoprotein IIb-III complex, *J. Biol. Chem.,* 257, 10488, 1982.
34. **Bennett, J. S. and Vilaire, G.,** Exposure of platelet fibrinogen receptors by ADP and epinephrine, *J. Clin. Invest.,* 64, 1393, 1979.
35. **Marguerie, G. A., Plow, E. F., and Edgington, T. S.,** Human platelets possess an inducible and saturable receptor specific for fibrinogens, *J. Biol. Chem.,* 254, 5357, 1979.
36. **Marguerie, G. A., Ardaillon, N., Cherel, G., and Plow, E. F.,** The binding of fibrinogen to its platelet receptor, *J. Biol. Chem.,* 257, 11872, 1982.
37. **Peerschke, E. I. and Zucker, M. B.,** Fibrinogen receptor exposure and aggregation of human blood platelets produced by ADP and chilling, *Blood,* 57, 663, 1981.
38. **Lee, H., Nurden, A., Thomaidis, A., and Caen, J. P.,** Relationship between fibrinogen binding and the platelet glycoprotein deficiencies in Glanzmann's thrombasthenia type I and type II, *Br. J. Haematol.,* 48, 47, 1981.
39. **McEver, R. P., Bennett, E. M., and Martin, M. N.,** Identification of two structurally and functionally distinct sites on human platelet membrane glycoprotein IIb-IIIa using monoclonal antibodies, *J. Biol. Chem.,* 258, 5264, 1983.
40. **McGregor, J. L., Clezardin, P., James, E., McGregor, L., Dechavanne, M., and Clemetson, K. J.,** Identification and characterization of fragments of major glycoproteins from platelet membranes after chymotrypsin treatment, *Eur. J. Biochem.,* 148, 97, 1985.
41. **Hawiger, J., Timmons, S., Kloczewiak, M., Strong, D. D., and Doolittle, R. R.,** Gamma chains of human fibrinogen possess sites reactive with human platelet receptors, *Proc. Natl. Acad. Sci. U.S.A.,* 79, 2068, 1982.
42. **Nieuwenhuis, H. K., Akkerman, J. W., Houdijk, W. P. M., and Sixma, J. J.,** Human blood platelets showing no response to collagen fail to express surface glycoprotein Ia, *Nature,* 318, 470, 1985.

43. **Kawahara, Y., Takai, Y., Minakuchi, R., Sano, K., and Nishizuka, Y.**, Phospholipid turnover as a possible transmembrane signal for protein phosphorylation during human platelet activation by thrombin, *Biochem. Biophys. Res. Commun.*, 97, 309, 1980.
44. **Billah, M. M. and Lapetina, E. G.**, Rapid decrease of phosphatidylinositol 4,5-biphosphate in thrombin-stimulated platelets, *J. Biol. Chem.*, 257, 12705, 1982.
45. **Hamberg, M., Svensson, J., and Samuelson, B.**, Thromboxanes: a new group of biologically active compounds derived from prostaglandin endoperoxides, *Proc. Natl. Acad. Sci. U.S.A.*, 72, 2994, 1975.
46. **Zwaal, R. F. A. and Bevers, E. M.**, Platelet phospholipid asymmetry and its significance in hemostasis, *Sub. Cell. Biochem.*, 9, 299, 1983.
47. **Schick, P. K., Kurica, K. B., and Chacko, G. K.**, Location of phosphatidylethanolamine in the human platelet plasma membrane, *J. Clin. Invest.*, 57, 1221, 1976.
48. **Schick, P. K.**, The organization of aminophospholipids in human platelet membranes: selective changes induced by thrombin, *J. Lab. Clin. Med.*, 91, 802, 1978.
49. **Op den Kamp, J. A. F.**, Lipid asymmetry in membranes, *Ann. Rev. Biochem.*, 48, 47, 1979.
50. **Bevers, E. M., Comfurius, P., van Rijn, J. L. M. L., Hemker, H. C., and Zwaal, R. F. A.**, Generation of platelet prothrombin converting activity and the exposure of phosphatidylserine at the platelet outer surface, *Eur. J. Biochem.*, 122, 429, 1982.
51. **Bevers, E. M., Comfurius, P., and Zwaal, R. F. A.**, Changes in membrane phospholipid distribution during platelet activation, *Biochim. Biophys. Acta*, 736, 57, 1983.
52. **van Deenen, L. L. M.**, Topology and dynamics of phospholipids in membranes, *FEBS Lett.*, 123, 3, 1981.
53. **Cullis, P. R. and de Kruijff, B.**, Lipid polymorphism and the functional role of lipids in biological membranes, *Biochim. Biophys. Acta*, 559, 399, 1979.
54. **Haest, C. W. M., Plasa, G., Kamp, D., and Deuticke, B.**, Spectrin as a stabilizer of the phospholipid asymmetry in the human erythrocyte membrane, *Biochim. Biophys. Acta*, 509, 21, 1978.
55. **Dressler, V., Haest, C. W. M., Plasa, G., Deuticke, B., and Erusalimsky, J. D.**, Stabilizing factors of phospholipid asymmetry in the erythrocyte membrane, *Biochim. Biophys. Acta*, 775, 189, 1984.
56. **Williamson, P., Bateman, J., Kozarsky, K., Mattocks, K., Hermanowicz, N., Choe, H. R., and Schlegel, R. A.**, Involvement of spectrin in the maintenance of phase-state asymmetry in the erythrocyte membrane, *Cell*, 30, 725, 1982.
57. **Franck, P. F. H., Bevers, E. M., Lubin, B. H., Comfurius, P., Chiu, D. T.-Y., Op den Kamp, J. A. F., Zwaal, R. F. A., van Deenen, L. L. M., and Roelofsen, B.**, Uncoupling of the membrane skeleton from the lipid bilayer. The cause of accelerated phospholipid flip-flop leading to an enhanced procoagulant activity of sickled cells, *J. Clin. Invest.*, 75, 183, 1985.
58. **Seigneuret, M. and Devaux, P. F.**, ATP-dependent asymmetric distribution of spin-labeled phospholipids in the erythrocyte membrane: relation to shape changes, *Proc. Natl. Acad. Sci. U.S.A.*, 81, 3751, 1984.
59. **Daleke, D. L. and Huestis, W. H.**, Incorporation and translocation of aminophospholipids in human erythrocytes, *Biochemistry*, 24, 5406, 1985.
60. **Tilley, L., Cribier, S., Roelofsen, B., Op den Kamp, J. A. F., and van Deenen, L. L. M.**, ATP-dependent translocation of amino phospholipids across the human erythrocyte membrane, *FEBS Lett.*, 194, 21, 1986.
61. **Luzatti, V. and Husson, F.**, The structure of the liquid-crystalline phase of lipid-water systems, *J. Cell Biol.*, 12, 207, 1962.
62. **Mauco, G., Chap, H., Simon, M. F., and Douste-Blazy, L.**, Phosphatidic acid and lysophosphatidic acid production in phospholipase C and thrombin-treated platelets. Possible involvement of platelet lipase, *Biochimie*, 60, 653, 1978.
63. **Allan, D., Low, M. G., Finean, J. B., and Michell, R. H.**, Changes in lipid metabolism and cell morphology following attack by phospholipase C (C. perfringens) on red cells or lymphocytes, *Biochim. Biophys. Acta*, 413, 309, 1975.
64. **Chap, H. and Douste-Blazy, L.**, Phospholipase C induced release reaction in platelets, *Eur. J. Biochem.*, 48, 351, 1974.
65. **Comfurius, P., Bevers, E. M., and Zwaal, R. F. A.**, Stimulation of prothrombinase activity of platelets and erythrocytes by sublytic treatment with phospholipase C from *Clostridium welchii*, *Biochem. Biophys. Res. Commun.*, 117, 803, 1983.
66. **Lapetina, E. G. and Cuatrecasas, P.**, Stimulation of phosphatidic acid production in platelets precedes the formation of arachidonate and parallels in the release of serotonin, *Biochim. Biophys. Acta*, 573, 394, 1979.
67. **Bell, R. L. and Majerus, P. W.**, Thrombin-induced hydrolysis of PI in human platelets, *J. Biol. Chem.*, p. 255, 1970.
68. **Rittenhouse, S. E.**, Human platelets contain phospholipase C that hydrolyzes polyphosphoinositides, *Proc. Natl. Acad. Sci. U.S.A.*, 80, 5417, 1983.

69. **Davies, G. E. and Palek, J.,** Platelet protein organization: analysis by treatment with membrane-permeable cross-linking reagents, *Blood,* 59, 502, 1982.
70. **Truglia, J. A. and Stracher, A.,** Purification and characterization of a calcium-dependent sulfhydryl protease from human platelets, *Biochem. Biophys. Res. Commun.,* 100, 814, 1981.
71. **McGowan, E. B., Yeo, K. T., and Detwiler, T. C.,** The action of calcium-dependent protease on platelet surface glycoproteins, *Arch. Biochem. Biophys.,* 227, 287, 1983.
72. **Rosing, J., Bevers, E. M., Comfurius, P., Hemker, H. C., van Dieijen, G., Weiss, H. J., and Zwaal, R. F. A.,** Impaired factor X and prothrombin activation associated with decreased phospholipid exposure in platelets from a patient with a bleeding disorder, *Blood,* 65, 1557, 1985.
73. **Solum, N. O. and Olsen, T. M.,** Effects of diamide and dibucaline on platelet glycoprotein Ib, actin-binding protein and cytoskeleton, *Biochim. Biophys. Acta,* 817, 249, 1985.
74. **Verhallen, P. F. J., Comfurius, P., Bevers, E. M., and Zwaal, R. F. A.,** On the regulatory role of the cytoskeleton in the expression of platelet procoagulant activity, *Agents Action,* 20, 181, 1986.
75. **Adelstein, R. S., Pollard, T. D., and Kuehl, M. W.,** Isolation and characterization of myosin and two myosin fragments from human blood platelets, *Proc. Natl. Sci. U.S.A.,* 68, 2703, 1971.
76. **Peleg, I., Muhlrad, A., Eldor, A., Groschel-Stewart, U., and Kahane, I.,** Characterization of the ATPase activities of myosins isolated from the membrane and the cytoplasmic fractions of human platelets, *Arch. Biochem. Biophys.,* 234, 442, 1984.

INDEX

I

J

K

L

M

N

O

P

Q

R

S

T

U

V

X

Z